D1209908

Regulating Doctors' Fees

Regulating Doctors' Fees

Competition, Benefits, and Controls under Medicare

Edited by H. E. Frech III

The AEI Press

Publisher for the American Enterprise Institute
WASHINGTON, D.C.

1991

Distributed by arrangement with

University Press of America, Inc.
4720 Boston Way   3 Henrietta Street
Lanham, Md. 20706   London WC2E 8LU England

Library of Congress Cataloging-in-Publication Data

Frech, H. E.
 Regulating doctor's fees : competition, benefits, and controls
under medicare / edited by H. E. Frech.
   p.   cm. — (AEI Studies : 518)
 ISBN 0-8447-3742-9
 1. Medical fees—Government policy—United States.
 2. Medicare. 3. Physicians—Salaries, etc.—United States.
 I. Title.   II. Series.
 R728.5.F74   1991
 331.2'81362173'0973—dc20   91-10943
                                                          CIP

ISBN 0-8447-3742-9

1   3   5   7   9   10   8   6   4   2

AEI Studies 518

THE AEI PRESS
Publisher for the American Enterprise Institute
1150 Seventeenth Street, N.W., Washington, D.C. 20036

Printed in the United States of America

Contents

CONTENTS

CONTENTS

Contributors

H. E. FRECH III is a professor of economics at the University of California at Santa Barbara. He has been a visiting professor at the University of Chicago and at Harvard. His current research focuses on health economics, and he is writing a book entitled *Competition in Medical Care*. Mr. Frech received his Ph.D. in economics from the University of California at Los Angeles.

ROBIN ALLEN is an economist in the Antitrust Division, U.S. Department of Justice. Her research is in competition and incentives in the health care industry. In 1986–1987, she was Kramer Fellow in Law and Economics at the University of Chicago Law School.

JOSEPH R. ANTOS is director of the Office of Research and Demonstration of the Health Care Financing Administration, where he oversees the budget for the Medicare and Medicaid programs. Mr. Antos has worked on health, income maintenance, and labor policy issues at the Council of Economic Advisers, the Office of Management and Budget, the U.S. Department of Health and Human Services, and the U.S. Department of Labor. He received his Ph.D. in economics from the University of Rochester.

LEE BENHAM is a professor in the Economics Department at Washington University. He has also taught in the Graduate School of Business at the University of Chicago. Mr. Benham's research interest is medical economics, including the regulation of the professions. He received his Ph.D. in economics from Stanford University.

ROBERT A. BERENSON is in private practice in internal medicine and serves as a health policy consultant specializing in physician payment policy, relative value schedule and fee schedule development, managed care organizations, and the politics of health care. He has worked on the Domestic Policy Staff at the White House and at the

U.S. Department of Health, Education, and Welfare. He received his M.D. from Mount Sinai School of Medicine.

DAVID C. COLBY is a senior analyst at the Physician Payment Review Commission. He has written articles and conducted research on varied social programs and issues, including physician reimbursement, AIDS policies, health planning, and Medicare and Medicaid expenditures. Previously, Mr. Colby was coordinator of the Masters of Policy Sciences Program at the University of Maryland Graduate School, Baltimore. He received his Ph.D. from the University of Illinois.

JERRY CROMWELL is president of Health Economics Research, Inc. He received his Ph.D. in economics from Harvard University in 1974. He has published extensively on options for Medicare reimbursement of physicians and hospitals. He has also conducted several studies on the diffusion of medical technology, including the impact of Medicare's Prospective Payment System on technology diffusion.

DAVID DRANOVE is an associate professor of business economics in the Graduate School of Business at the University of Chicago. His research and teaching interests include medical economics, health services policy analysis, and financial management of health care organizations. Mr. Dranove received his Ph.D. in economics from Stanford University.

DANIEL L. DUNN is a research associate in the Department of Health Policy and Management, Harvard School of Public Health. Mr. Dunn's research focuses on the economics of doctor reimbursement schemes. His recent research concerns reimbursement based on diagnosis related groups and physician responses to the Resource-based Relative Value Study. Mr. Dunn received his Ph.D. in economics from the University of New Hampshire.

JOEL IRA FRANCK is chief of the Section of Neurosurgery at Central Maine Medical Center, St. Mary's Hospital in Lewiston, Maine. He serves as secretary and re-founder of the Maine Neurosurgical Society and as Maine delegate to the Joint Council of State Neurosurgical Societies. Mr. Franck has published extensively on the subjects of neurosurgery, neurophysiology, neuroanatomy, and economics. He received his M.D. from the Yale University School of Medicine.

PAUL B. GINSBURG is the executive director of the Physician Payment Review Commission. He has experience in a wide variety of health care financing issues, including physician payment, hospital payment, and health insurance. Mr. Ginsburg has served as a senior economist at the RAND Corporation and as deputy assistant director for Income Security and Health at the Congressional Budget Office. He earned a doctorate in economics at Harvard University.

GLENN M. HACKBARTH is vice president of the Harvard Community Health Plan. His past positions include service with the Health Care Financing Administration and the Office of the Assistant Secretary for Planning and Evaluation, both in the U.S. Department of Health and Human Services and with the Center for Health Policy Research at the American Enterprise Institute. Mr. Hackbarth received J.D. and M.A. degrees from Duke University's School of Law and Institute for Policy Studies and Public Affairs.

JACK HADLEY is codirector of the Center for Health Policy Studies in the Department of Community and Family Medicine at Georgetown University. He is engaged in full-time health services research covering a wide range of topics, including physician payment methods in Medicare and Medicaid, hospital care for the poor and uninsured, the impact of Medicare's Prospective Payment System on hospitals, and hospital cost variations. Mr. Hadley received his Ph.D. in economics from Yale University.

GLENN T. HAMMONS is deputy director of the Physician Payment Review Commission and is on leave from the Department of Pathology of the University of Iowa College of Medicine, where he is medical director of the Clinical Chemistry Laboratories for the University of Iowa Hospitals and Clinics. His recent work has focused on health policy, including an assessment of the expected impact of alternative physician payment methods on quality of care. He received his M.D. from Washington University.

CLARK C. HAVIGHURST is the William Neal Reynolds Professor of Law at Duke University, where he teaches courses in antitrust law, economic regulation, and health care law and policy. He has recently published a law school casebook entitled *Health Care Law and Policy: Readings, Notes and Questions* and in 1982 published *Deregulating the Health Care Industry*. Mr. Havighurst is an adjunct scholar at the American Enterprise Institute.

JESSE S. HIXSON is director of Public Policy Studies in the Center for Health Policy Research at the American Medical Association. Before joining the AMA, Mr. Hixson worked for the U.S. Department of Health and Human Services, where he worked in the Office of Research and Statistics (Social Security Administration), the Bureau of Health Manpower, and the National Institutes of Health. He received his Ph.D. in economics from Michigan State University.

JOHN HOLAHAN is director of the Health Policy Research Center of the Urban Institute. He received a Ph.D. in economics from Georgetown University. His work has focused on Medicare-Medicaid programs in general and on hospital, nursing home, and physician payment issues specifically. He is currently studying the effect of the prospective payment system on physician practice patterns and on the use of nursing home and home health services.

WILLIAM C. HSIAO is a professor of economics and health policy at the Harvard University School of Public Health, and he directed Harvard's Center for Health Financing and Regulations. Mr. Hsiao was named by the editorial board of McGraw-Hill Health Publications as the 1988 Person of the Year for Medicine and Health for his work in developing a resource-based relative value scale for physician payment. He served as an adviser to the Carter administration on the planning of national health insurance and has worked as a consultant for several congressional committees. Mr. Hsiao received his Ph.D. in economics from Harvard University.

DAVID A. JUBA is a senior analyst at the Physician Payment Review Commission. His work there has ranged from evaluating the effects of imposing a Medicare fee schedule to analyzing geographic variation in physicians' Medicare fees. He has conducted and published research in the areas of Medicare physician and hospital payment policy for the past ten years. Prior to joining the commission's staff, Mr. Juba was senior analyst at ABT Associates Inc., the Urban Institute, and Policy Analysis Incorporated.

WILLIAM D. MARDER is senior economist at ABT Associates Inc., where his research currently focuses on physician supply projections, the PPS/DRG system, and other investigations solicited by public and private agencies. Previously, he served as director of the Department of Manpower and Demographic Studies in the American Medical Association's Center for Health Policy Research. Mr. Marder received his Ph.D. in economics from the University of Chicago.

THOMAS G. MCGUIRE is a professor of economics at Boston University and also serves as a senior research associate at Brandeis University and a senior economist at the Health Data Institute. His major fields of interest include the economics of health and mental health, public finance, and market organization. Mr. McGuire received his Ph.D. from Yale University.

JANET B. MITCHELL is president of the Center for Health Economics Research and a member of the National Advisory Committee for the Robert Wood Johnson Health Care Finance Fellows. She also serves as a consultant for the Veterans Administration and the Health Care Financing Administration and has worked as an adviser to the Physician Reimbursement Study for the Congressional Budget Office. She received her Ph.D. from the Heller Graduate School, Brandeis University.

JOSEPH P. NEWHOUSE is the John D. and Catherine T. MacArthur Professor of Health Policy and Management at Harvard University and director of the Division of Health Policy Research and Education. He is a member of the faculty of the John F. Kennedy School of Government, the Harvard Medical School, and the Harvard School of Public Health. Mr. Newhouse is currently the codirector of the Rand/ UCLA/Harvard Center on Health Care Financing Policy, which is supported by the Health Care Financing Administration. He is the founding editor of the *Journal of Health Economics*.

ROGER G. NOLL is the director of the Public Policy Program at Stanford University, where he is also a Professor by Courtesy in the Department of Political Science and the Graduate School of Business. His research interests include applied microeconomics, social control of business, and political economics. Dr. Noll received his Ph.D. in economics from Harvard University.

MARK V. PAULY is a professor of health care systems and public management, the Wharton School, and a professor of economics, School of Arts and Sciences at the University of Pennsylvania. He is also executive director of the Leonard Davis Institute of Health Economics and Robert D. Eilers Professor of Health Care Management and Economics. He has served as a consultant to the Office of Management and Budget, the National Institutes of Health, the Veterans Administration, and the Organization for Economic Cooperation and Development in Paris, France. Mr. Pauly received his Ph.D. in economics from the University of Virginia.

CHARLES E. PHELPS is professor and chair, Department of Community and Preventive Medicine, and professor of political science and economics at the University of Rochester. He has served as a senior economist at the RAND Corporation. Dr. Phelps's current research interests include medical technology evaluation, and reduction of drunk driving. He received his Ph.D. in business economics from the University Chicago.

JAMES B. RAMSEY is a professor of economics at New York University, where he previously served as chairman of the Department of Economics. He has held teaching positions at Michigan State University and the University of Birmingham, England, and has worked as a consultant for Governor Carey of New York and for the American Medical Association. Mr. Ramsey received the U.S. Department of Health, Education, and Welfare's Human Resources Administration grant for his work on physician ambulatory care production behavior. He received his Ph.D. from the University of Wisconsin in Madison.

ROGER A. REYNOLDS is a principal economist at the American Medical Association, where he has served as the director of the Department of Medical Practice Economics. Mr. Reynolds has worked at De Paul University, the University of Chicago, and the Health Care Financing Administration. He received his Ph.D. in economics from the University of Chicago.

JAMES F. RODGERS is director of the Center for Health Policy Research of the American Medical Association. He is responsible for the association's socioeconomic research program and physician practice surveys. Mr. Rodgers received his Ph.D. in economics from the University of Iowa.

MARGO L. ROSENBACH is vice president of Health Economics Research, Inc. She received her Ph.D. in health policy from the Heller Graduate School, Brandeis University. She has performed numerous studies of physician reimbursement under Medicare, as well as studies of Medicare options for paying nurse anesthetists. She is currently project director of a study on the impact of hospital closures on access to care.

MARK A. SATTERTHWAITE is the Earl Dean Howard Professor of Managerial Economics at the Kellogg Graduate School of Management at Northwestern University. His research has concentrated on the effect of consumer information on the competitiveness of medical care markets. Mr. Satterthwaite received his Ph.D. in economics from the University of Wisconsin.

JODY L. SINDELAR is an associate professor in the Department of Epidemiology and Public Health at the Yale School of Medicine. She also holds joint appointments in Yale University's Institution for Social and Policy Studies and in the Yale School of Management. She received her Ph.D. in economics from Stanford University.

FRANK A. SLOAN is Centennial Professor and chairman, Department of Economics and Business Administration, and director of the Health Policy Center at the Vanderbilt Institute for Public Policy Studies, Vanderbilt University. He is currently conducting research on medical malpractice and has recently completed studies on the effects of Medicare's Prospective Payment System and its cost in capital to hospitals. Mr. Sloan received his Ph.D. in economics from Harvard University.

WILLIAM B. STASON is currently vice president of Health Economics Research, Inc. Previously, he was director of the Northeast Health Services Research and Development Field Program for the Veterans Administration, West Roxbury, Massachusetts. He received his M.D. degree from Harvard Medical School and his M.S. in epidemiology from Harvard Public School of Health. He has published extensively on physician reimbursement policy and on quality assessment/medical effectiveness.

FINIS WELCH is a professor of economics at the University of California at Los Angeles. He is also chairman of Unicon Research Corporation and president of Welch Associates. His previous academic positions include acting director of the Institute for Social Science Research at UCLA and director of the Labor and Population Studies Program at the Rand Corporation. In addition, Mr. Welch has served as chairman of the Advisory Committee on the Status of Women and Minorities of the U.S. Commission on Civil Rights. He received a Ph.D. in economics from the University of Chicago.

RICHARD J. WILLKE is a senior economist at the Center for Health Policy Research of the American Medical Association. His research concerns physician human capital and labor supply and earnings, particularly the accumulation of practice capital and physician-hospital relationships, as well as some analyses of patient behavior. Dr.

Willke received his Ph.D. in economics from Johns Hopkins University.

STEPHEN ZUCKERMAN is a senior research associate at the Health Policy Center of the Urban Institute. His work has explored state-level systems covering Medicaid and other payers as well as the nationally oriented Medicare Prospective Payment System. He has also studied variation in physician practice costs and service utilization, and hospital responses to government rate-setting programs. Mr. Zuckerman received his Ph.D. in economics from Columbia University.

PETER ZWEIFEL is a professor of economics at the University of Zurich and a member of the Federal Commission for Economic Stabilization. He is also a member of the board of editors for the *Journal of Health Economics*. Mr. Zweifel received his Ph.D. in economics from the University of Zurich.

Discussants

HENRY AARON is a senior fellow at the Brookings Institution.

RITA RICARDO CAMPBELL is a senior fellow at the Hoover Institution.

GEORGE GREENBERG is with the Office of the Assistant Secretary for Planning and Evaluation, Department of Health and Human Services.

WARREN GREENBERG is an associate professor in Health Services Administration at George Washington University.

ROBERT HELMS is a scholar in health policy at the American Enterprise Institute.

MARVIN KOSTERS is director of economic policy studies at the American Enterprise Institute.

FREDERICK R. WARREN-BOULTON is senior vice president of ICF Consulting Associates.

Regulating Doctors' Fees

1
Overview of Policy Issues

H. E. Frech III

Radical changes in the way physicians are paid under Medicare have been begun by Congress, though these changes have been debated little by experts in health economics and health policy. This volume provides the first major opportunity for the public to analyze such proposals. To put the changes in context, we must first examine the market for physicians' services and the history of Medicare.

The Market for Physicians' Services

The casual observer might conclude that the health care industry and especially the market for physicians' services are almost perfectly competitive. After all, a large city might have fifty hospitals and thousands of physicians. Consumers have many choices to seek out competitive combinations of price and quality. But competition is far from perfect even in large cities with many sellers.

Two related problems prevent real competition. First, entry into the marketplace is limited, largely by restricted acceptance into medical schools. While this limitation raises costs for U.S. medical care and constrains competition among physicians, it is not the focus of this analysis.[1]

The second problem and the root of the imperfect competition among physicians is poor consumer information and weak incentives caused by most health insurance. Because consumers are poorly informed about alternative physicians, they must rely heavily on the advice of friends and relatives. A consumer is not usually well informed about more than a few physicians. Further, even recommendations from trusted friends or relatives are not perfectly reliable, especially for primary care. The value of a particular physician to a particular consumer is idiosyncratic.[2]

Thanks are due to Paul Ginsburg, Paul Gertler, Mark Satterthwaite, Marvin Kosters, and Joseph Newhouse for helpful comments on earlier drafts of this chapter.

1

Given imperfect consumer information, physicians can raise their price above marginal costs or reduce quality below competitive levels without most of their patients switching physicians. The poorer consumer information is, the more like isolated monopolists the individual physicians are.

Most types of insurance undercut consumer information. The insurance also weakens the incentives for consumers to change to low-priced physicians, even if they know about them.

The worst type of insurance is 100 percent first-dollar coverage. The insurance subsidy causes moral hazard—that is, the insurance-induced overuse of medical care. Further, consumers have no incentive to search for low-cost providers or even to use them when they become aware of them. The consumer cannot benefit from such a switch; they will simply select the best physician from their viewpoint, regardless of price. It does not matter if a far less expensive physician is only slightly less convenient. For consumers with this type of insurance, price competition is nonexistent.

Insurance that pays a fixed percentage, typically 80 percent, is better. At least the consumer receives 20 percent of the benefit of finding and switching to a low-priced physician.

The best type of insurance for encouraging better consumer information and using low-priced providers is indemnity insurance. With this type of plan, the insurer pays a fixed dollar amount (typically below the average price) per unit of service. In a pure indemnity system, consumer copayment operates entirely through the bills exceeding the insurance allowance. The difference between the physician's bill and the insurer's allowance is called the balance bill. With this type of insurance, the consumer receives the entire benefit of his choice of a low-priced physician. Furthermore, whatever the degree of consumer information, indemnity insurance leads to a lower price than coinsurance with the same copayment requirement.[3] Thus, this form of insurance promotes the most competition.

Indemnity insurance results whenever insurance benefits include a maximum dollar amount per unit of service, such as in Medicare. Further, indemnity incentives to choose low-priced physicians can be replicated or even exceeded in preferred provider organizations (PPOs) by rewarding consumers for choosing from the preferred list.[4]

Because actual insurance is a mixture of all these kinds, competition among physicians is imperfect. Consumers switch physicians in response to price and quality changes but not in enough numbers to enforce perfect competition. This situation is what economists call monopolistic competition. Aside from health care, it prevails in most other services and in many product markets (for example, law, auto

repair, restaurants, and wine). Monopolistic competition is intermediate between perfect competition and perfect monopoly. Several
chapters in this volume use explicit models of markets for physicians'
services. They all use the model of monopolistic competition.[5]

Since competitive imperfections are based on informational and
incentive problems, rather than inherent economies of scale, they can
be reduced by lowering information costs and by redesigning insurance benefits. Indeed, for the private market, health maintenance
organizations (HMOs) and PPOs are doing just that.

One may think that the imperfect nature of competition argues
in favor of less competition: I believe the reverse is true. Large gains
in efficiency and cost control are possible from improving competition, even if it can never be perfect. As Nobel prize-winning economist Robert Solow is reported to have said, "Just because we cannot
have perfectly sterile conditions is no reason to perform surgery in
the gutter."

Further, consumer choice is important in health care, for consumers are not machines patiently waiting to be repaired. The consumer alone can weigh subjective values with financial and physical
risks. Rational allocation of care requires active consumer choice.

How Monopolistic Competition Works. As the name implies, monopolistic competition has features of both monopoly and competition. Individual physicians have some monopoly power; this is the
monopolistic feature. Like a perfect monopoly, prices in a particular
specialty and locality depend on costs, mostly subjective, and on how
responsive consumers are to price difference among physicians.

Underlying the competitive aspect of monopolistic competition
is the ability of physicians to move about geographically and among
specialties. This mobility, which allows reasonably free entry into
different localities and specialties, has some implications for competition.

Under monopolistic competition, market forces in the long run
roughly equalize physicians' incomes in various specialties and areas.
While in this way monopolistic competition is similar to perfect
competition, in another way it is different. The market forces do not
equalize the relationship of fees to costs. The ratio of fees to costs can
vary because of differing consumer information and insurance coverage. In particular, more complete insurance coverage of surgery can
lead to higher fees relative to costs.

To the extent that income adjusted for training costs varies across
specialties, only a few explanations are possible. First, artificial barriers may block entry to the attractive specialties. Second, subjective

costs may deter physicians from some specialties, especially those with little human contact like pathology and surgery.[6] Third, and perhaps most important, the ability of physicians may differ.

Paying Physicians under Medicare

Most Medicare beneficiaries purchase their medical care in the fee-for-service market. Historically, Medicare has paid insurance benefits based on physicians' charges. Medicare's allowed charge, or allowance, for a particular physician for a particular service was originally determined with the customary, prevailing, and reasonable (CPR) system. In the CPR system, the allowance was the minimum of the physician's actual charge, his own individual customary charge, or the charge prevailing in his area. Medicare pays physicians 80 percent of the allowance; the consumer is expected to pay the remaining 20 percent. Since they are based partly on the individual physician's customary charge, Medicare allowances can vary from physician to physician.

Recent modifications to the CPR system have constrained Medicare payments so that the allowance averages about 30 percent below market price. The prevailing-charge screens for some procedures considered overpriced have also been reduced in the past two years. That discount is roughly constant across various procedures and types of care so that payments are still roughly aligned with, though below, market prices.

The size of the discount shows that the current system effectively obtains physicians' services at a good price. This discount compares favorably with those provided by PPOs and HMOs. High and growing volume and intensity of services are the problem, not excessive prices.

Further, for most physicians, the Medicare allowances do not constitute price control. Doctors may charge more than the Medicare-allowed amount, subject to some restrictions.[7] As noted above, the practice of charging the patient all or part of the difference between the physicians' fees and Medicare allowances is called balance billing.

Problems with the Current System for Paying Physicians

Physicians' payments under Medicare were higher than Congress expected in the beginning, and they have been growing rapidly ever since. The growth has substantially exceeded the growth of the economy almost every year since the program's inception in 1966. While some of this growth reflects rising prices for medical services, most of it results from the rising volume of services per beneficiary.

Some of this growth in volume, in turn, comes from technical progress. Medicine can help people now where it could not before. The treatment of cataracts by removing the clouded lens and implanting a clear plastic one is an example.

Most policy makers, however, believe that much of the increase is of little medical value and therefore not worth the additional cost. Indeed, this increase illustrates the moral hazard of insurance that subsidizes health care. Furthermore, the higher the proportion of the bills paid by the insurer, the worse the moral hazard is. Indeed, as Medigap insurance has expanded in recent years, one would expect the overuse of care to worsen.

Growing Medigap Insurance. Economists have pointed to the large expansion of private supplementary insurance (Medigap) since the inception of Medicare as one of the main causes of the increases in expenditures. By filling in the deductibles, coinsurance, and balance bills planned by the founders of Medicare, Medigap insurance has destroyed the only cost controls of importance in the system. Consumers covered by Medigap insurance grew from 0 in 1966 to over 75 percent in the mid-1970s. This expansion explains both the rapid growth in expenditures and the belief that the increased spending on medical care benefits the consumer little or not at all. Thus, as Thomas McGuire notes in his chapter, most economists have suggested either prohibiting or taxing Medigap insurance.

Policy makers are also concerned with perceived unfairness of payments across medical specialties. The payment per hour is higher for surgical and other procedures than for the evaluative and management services (cognitive medicine) that are billed primarily as patient visits. Physicians' incomes also differ across specialties in the same direction, but not as much. Many policy makers seem to believe that these differences are unfair or inefficient.

Finally, some are concerned about the access of Medicare beneficiaries to care: that is, freedom from nonprice rationing. It is important not to confuse access with the degree of consumer copayment or financial risk. Access is excellent now, because Medicare allows almost unlimited balance billing. For the highest-priced physicians, balance bills may be high, but this is a separate issue. Almost all physicians, no matter how high in quality or in price, are now willing to treat Medicare beneficiaries. As will become clear, the proposal of the Physician Payment Review Commission (PPRC) threatens access.[8]

Many are also concerned with reducing, or not increasing too much, the financial risk facing Medicare recipients. The financial risk is the negative side of higher copayments by consumers; the benefits

5

of higher copayments by consumers include cost control and enhancement of competition.

Much of this concern with raising copayments is misplaced, caused by ignorance of current out-of-pocket payments. Studies have vastly overstated the true out-of-pocket responsibilities of Medicare beneficiaries.

Policy Alternatives

Some policy options for reforming Medicare's payments for physicians' services focus on prices. Examples include reforming the CPR system or introducing fee schedules, which could be, but need not be, cost based. Reducing Medicare allowances, tried since 1972, does not address the root problems of increasing volume and intensity of services.[9]

According to Joseph Antos, most in Washington see a fee schedule that differs greatly from current market charges as vital to reform. That this should have become the dominant view can only be considered bizarre, considering that only a limited amount of serious research is consistent with this view and some conflicts with it.

Some options are also aimed at quantity or intensity of services, including increased beneficiary cost sharing. Although this is the only policy guaranteed to cut costs and raise efficiency, Antos states that this is politically unpopular in Washington.

I believe this unpopularity derives from two reasons, one an erroneous assumption and the other an ideological stance. The inaccurate belief holds that Medicare beneficiaries now face significant out-of-pocket payments for physicians' services, while some are ideologically committed to removing "barriers" to health care.

Out-of-Pocket Payments for Physicians' Services. Since Medicare was founded in 1966, consumer responsibility for deductibles, coinsurance, and balance bills has been greatly eroded by Medigap insurance, which now covers over 75 percent of beneficiaries. Not only does Medigap usually cover deductibles and coinsurance, but also it often covers balance bills. From the massive National Medical Care Expenditures Study, Gail Cafferata estimates that over 70 percent of Medigap plans covering physicians' services pay balance bills.[10] Perhaps relying on more recent evidence from smaller surveys, the PPRC estimates it at much less, 20 to 30 percent.[11] Even if the lower estimate is accepted, however, since physicians accept assignment for over 80 percent of charges, most balance bills are either not charged at all or covered by supplemental insurance. Physicians also are far more likely to balance bill if the beneficiary has Medigap insurance or if the bill itself is small.[12]

Moreover, even on the 20 percent of bills where the physician does not take assignment, the balance may not be collected in a high percentage of cases. Another 10 percent of beneficiaries have their copayment paid entirely by Medicaid and cannot legally be balance billed.

As for the coinsurance and deductible, because of Medigap and Medicaid only about 20 percent of Medicare beneficiaries are potentially liable. Of these, many, perhaps most, have their coinsurance and deductible waived by their physicians. A 1976 survey found that between 36 and 45 percent of physicians always waived the Medicare deductible, while between 34 and 46 percent always waived the coinsurance. A substantial percentage sometimes waived the payments.[13] A 1983–1984 survey found the percentage waiving copayment had fallen but was still large. The percentage of physicians who always waived the deductible was between 25 and 35 percent. Between 15 and 16 percent reported always waiving the coinsurance. Again, a large percentage sometimes waived the payments.[14]

Lumping together insurance premium payments, payments for uncovered services and supplies (for example, drugs and home nursing), and true out-of-pocket payments for hospital and physician care adds to the confusion and to the overstatement of consumer copayment. The figure of $1,700 per beneficiary in out-of-pocket payments, for example, is cited in a PPRC report. But that figure includes Part B insurance payments and payments for uncovered supplies and services and does not subtract Medigap benefits or copayments that were waived by physicians.[15] Thus this figure grossly overstates the copayment for physician and hospital costs.

Ideological Commitments to Availability of Health Care. Many are ideologically opposed to putting "financial barriers" in the way of obtaining medical care. In this view, all medical care should be available with no out-of-pocket payments by consumers. The concept that medical care has a quasi-religious or metaphysical nature underlies the conviction that consumers and society should not have to economize on it.

In reality, medical care is a service, produced with capital, labor, and other materials. In practice, the absence of consumers' copayments leads to overconsumption or to excess demand, resulting in denial of access to consumers (nonprice rationing). It also hinders competition among providers. The ideology opposing financial barriers to medical care guided the Blue Cross and Blue Shield plans in the formative years of American health insurance, leading to irrational 100 percent, first-dollar coverage. Recently, consumers, employers, and unions have realized the destructiveness of the idea. Coverage of private groups has thus moved quickly away from this approach, so that deductibles of several hundred dollars and 20 percent coinsurance for physicians' services and hospital costs are now common.[16]

Medicare, in contrast, has inadvertently gone in the opposite direction. It was started with reasonable cost sharing, 20 percent coinsurance for physicians' services and small deductibles for services of both physicians and hospitals. Since then, however, the explosive growth of Medigap insurance has increasingly destroyed the cost controls built into the original system.

Because Medigap insurance is so widespread, a serious attempt to improve cost sharing must somehow limit or prohibit it. Enlarging the official deductible, for example, would be mostly offset by larger payments from Medigap plans and Medicaid, with little impact on actual cost sharing.

Another policy approach is to expand administrative review of use of services. Unfortunately, given the lack of knowledge about medical effectiveness, this policy would have limited impact. Further research on medical effectiveness would be important for this strategy.

The final category is the one Joseph Antos calls market-oriented options. They introduce more choice and competition in the management of insurance and care for Medicare beneficiaries, including capitation, where a single payment is made to an organization for each beneficiary. For the individual, this corresponds to the HMO option under current Medicare, chosen by only 3 percent of the beneficiaries, probably because Medicare rules and incentives are unfavorable to HMOs.

Closely related to the HMO option is an arrangement with a PPO or other managed care system in which the contracting organization seeks discounts from certain providers and also imposes controls on use. Since the entities would be in competition, they would have incentives to impose controls on use in a way that accommodates the diverse preferences and values of consumers.

Another possibility for some surgical procedures would be a single payment to a physician for certain procedures and diagnoses, a system similar to Medicare's apparently successful diagnosis related group (DRG) payments for hospitalization. The final policy option is the resource-based relative value scale.

The Resource-based Relative Value Scale

The resource-based relative value scale (RBRVS) proposal would create a Medicare fee schedule based entirely on measures of costs or resources used in the production of physicians' services. Since the main resource used in producing these services is the time of the physician, the relative prices are largely based on that time, adjusted for certain factors.

Further, the proposal submitted to Congress by the Physician Payment Review Commission suggests surprisingly drastic limitations on balance billing, effectively imposing price control on many procedures. While this limitation on balance billing has gotten far less attention than the determination of the relative prices, it may affect the health care system more dramatically than the RBRVS itself.

The History of the Cost-based Relative Value Scale

The cost-based relative value scale was first proposed by William Hsiao and William Stason in a 1979 journal article.[17] Making little attempt to justify their idea, Hsiao and Stason put virtually all their effort into measuring effort and constructing a relative value scale. The idea attracted little interest, debate, or analysis among health economists or policy experts, with only one serious analysis in the literature. In a 1987 journal article Jack Hadley and Robert Berenson argued that basing fees solely on some measure of costs would be a mistake.[18]

The idea of a cost-based relative value scale was rejected by the Department of Health and Human Services. When Hsiao asked the Health Care Financing Administration (HCFA) to support a large grant to construct a workable cost-based scale, it declined. Hsiao got favorable attention for the idea in Congress, however. In an extraordinary action, Congress mandated that HCFA fund the study proposed by Hsiao. A congressional mandate for a research project on a particular topic is unusual, let alone an orientation of the project to a particular researcher.

Most of the responsibility for congressional micromanagement of Medicare payments to physicians lies with the recent history of weak presidential leadership in domestic policy. The action also illustrates the isolation of congressional health policy specialists from the greater community of health economists and health services researchers.

Completed in September 1988, the Hsiao study has been evaluated by many government agencies. The most important of these has been the Physician Payment Review Commission, a creation of Congress that examined and modified Hsiao's RBRVS. The commission suggested very strict limits on balance billing and made other recommendations. The PPRC's proposal is being phased in by Congress. It has a great deal of political support, despite the lack of serious intellectual discussion of the matter.

Debate on the RBRVS and the PPRC Proposal

This volume results from a conference designed to stimulate public consideration and debate on the merits of the RBRVS and the PPRC's proposal. To this end, the country's leading experts on the market for physicians' services and health insurance gathered. Some chapters discuss the nature and problems of that market and of Medicare. Others analyze the work of Hsiao and its modifications by the PPRC, and the effects on physicians' fees and income, on consumers' out-of-pocket payments, and on the volume of services consumed. The book concludes with a wide-ranging policy discussion.

One goal of the volume is to broaden the range of ideas under consideration, to loosen the shackles of "political feasibility." Too few options are considered politically feasible when Washington policy analysts dominate discussion, especially those analysts in Congress or the executive branch agencies.

Whatever their intellectual outlook, economists and others in the hothouse political environment often adopt the narrow viewpoint and short time horizon associated with either Congress's or their agencies' perceived interest. That has been an especially serious problem in the case of the RBRVS, since almost all discussion and analysis have been held within the agencies and much has been confidential.

Of course, analyses within the agencies should sometimes be confidential, and the work of the employees should reflect the immediate concerns of their employers. Indeed, how could it be otherwise? But a wider perspective from the universities and other independent institutions is often helpful, especially for radical changes such as are proposed here.

The Chapters

The Policy Background. In an overview Joseph Antos, acting associate administrator for management of the Health Care Financing Administration, explains the ideas and concerns of those in the Washington policy circles. They appear to believe that Medicare's steep increases in payments for physicians' services can somehow be stopped by limiting allowed fees. At the same time, they believe that much money is spent on medical services of little or no value to consumers.

The Market for Physicians' Services and Medicare. A number of the chapters present vital theoretical, empirical, and historical background on the market for physicians' services and Medicare. This perspective is especially important because Washington policy and political discourse has a naturally narrow focus. The actual market and historical context within which policy is made is too often ignored. Policy discussion tends to be ahistorical and atheoretical.

Behavior of physicians and consumers. A conceptual model of consumers' choice of physicians (location, specialty, and price) is presented in the chapter by David Dranove and Mark Satterthwaite. Using the monopolistically competitive framework, Dranove and Satterthwaite stress the causes for differences in physicians' income and price-cost margins across specialties.

Paying particular attention to the possibility that surgeons may be, on average, more able, they suggest that surgery might provide a higher payoff to ability. If so, surgery may attract more high-ability physicians. Because of their higher abilities, surgeons would earn higher incomes even if the market were perfectly competitive or if there were perfectly free entry.

Jack Hadley's chapter focuses on the RBRVS proposal and its intellectual rationale. Supporters of the RBRVS believe that prices relative to costs are far higher for surgery and other procedures than for cognitive medicine. Hadley considers the traditional reasons given: higher insurance coverage and inferior competition for surgery. Although the literature contains no good rationale for the RBRVS, Hadley first attempts to provide the missing rationale and then to criticize it. He notes that at the equilibrium in monopolistic competition with free entry, all prices are equal to average cost but exceed marginal cost. If entry is limited, as by licensure, then all prices will exceed average and marginal cost. The extent of the excess will vary according to the individual demand and cost for each physician. It is unclear whether charges or measurable costs will better mimic the minimum average costs that are the prices under perfect competition.

Hadley cites empirical studies bearing on the rationale of more complete insurance for surgery for the RBRVS. If that rationale were true, more insurance coverage would distort relative fees, as well as raising their level. A recent study of prevailing Medicare fees across

11

states showed that higher insurance coverage did not distort relative fees.[19]

Licensure, fees, and quality. Lee Benham's chapter stresses the limitations on entry and competition caused by licensure. Licensure raises all fees above the competitive level, although it does not necessarily raise fees for surgical procedures more than for cognitive medicine. He also makes the case that quality has not been protected by licensure, noting the enormous variation in mortality rates for specific surgeries.

In part, this variation occurs because the medical schools do not weed out poor performers: total attrition for medical students for all causes is only about 3 percent.[20] Moreover, very little is known about the effectiveness of most medical procedures, a failing Benham attributes to the poor training of physicians in statistics.

In the general discussion, William Hsiao criticizes the authors for using standard monopolistic competition theory but does not offer an alternative model or theory. Satterthwaite sharply distinguishes the monopolistic competition model from the perfectly competitive model, defending it as reasonable, usable, and realistic.

The Value of Physicians' Time. In their chapter William Marder and Richard Willke analyze data on physicians' incomes, hours, and training to focus on differences in pay for time across specialties. Marder and Willke were also able to correct a mistake in the way William Hsiao adjusted his work measures for specialty training.

Marder and Willke found that the internal rate of return to training varied greatly across specialties, from 1.3 percent in pediatrics to 39.1 percent in anesthesiology. Generally, the higher-paid surgical specialties, which required more years of costly investment, had the higher returns. Physicians' time in certain more highly-trained specialties was more than twice as valuable as in others.

Medicare Benefits. Background on Medicare benefits is very important. It may be unwise to apply drastic measures to mend a system that may not be broken or is broken in ways completely unrelated to the "solution."

Medigap insurance destroys cost controls. Thomas McGuire's chapter notes the growth of Medigap insurance from nothing in 1966 to covering over 75 percent of the Medicare population now. McGuire says that while a rational argument might have been made for permitting it in the past, since Medicare's coverage of long hospital stays was inadequate, if catastrophic coverage is finally enacted, any possible rationale will disappear.[21] Over the years, many economists have called for taxing or prohibiting Medigap coverage, and McGuire adds some possible new policies to discourage it.

Pauly noted that current Medicare payment policy may be quite reasonable. It has been successful in obtaining a substantial discount from market fees, comparable to what the best HMOs and PPOs get.

Balance billing is essential. John Holahan and Steve Zuckerman argue in their chapter that balance billing is an important safety valve for fees that are accidentally set too low for certain procedures in particular areas. Balance billing also allows beneficiaries to use the highest quality and highest priced physicians, if they so choose. Another benefit, often overlooked, is that balance billing is an important form of consumer copayment and therefore of cost control.

Jesse Hixon points to economic literature showing that a lower fee allowance, coupled with more balance billing, is the ideal form of consumer copayment. It puts the marginal cost of more expensive care squarely on the consumer, thereby providing the best possible incentives for consumer search and choice of price-competitive providers.[22]

The RBRVS. In their chapter William Hsiao and Daniel Dunn summarize their work in constructing the RBRVS, justifying the whole cost-based approach on the grounds of imperfect competition and differential insurance coverage. Several interesting points emerge.

First, instead of surveying separately the technical skill necessary for each procedure, they combined the skill with the physical effort. Skill, as distinct from physical effort, however, is relevant for some difficult surgery, such as delicate back and neck work, where very few surgeons have the necessary ability even to attempt it.

Second, Hsiao and Dunn argue that the higher payments for surgery led to too much volume. No scientific basis supports this belief, however, no matter what model of the behavior of physicians and consumers one uses.

Third, the authors note that the actual services provided in the key cognitive procedure codes are ambiguous, a problem undermining the RBRVS enterprise.

Time, complexity, and charges. Janet Mitchell, Jerry Cromwell, Margo Rosenbach, and William Stason performed an analysis like that of the Hsiao group. In their chapter they surveyed physicians in a simpler way for time and complexity of procedure and then related these measure to charges. They found quite a good fit, which they

13

interpret to mean that a charge-based fee schedule with some adjustments would be better than the RBRVS.

Finis Welch expresses dismay at the idea of the RBRVS, stressing the impossibility of properly measuring the difference in work or even fees themselves if cognitive services are not well defined. He argues that the apparent implicit model of market behavior used by the RBRVS proponents and by Hsiao and Dunn does not make sense. Finally, Welch believes that one way or another both Hsiao and Mitchell et al. were fitting curves to scatters of fees. That being so, there will always be outliers, especially far away from the mean. This does not mean that they are over- or underpriced in any sense, only that our statistical models and data are limited.

Fee schedules and volume. To investigate the effect of doctors' fees on volume, Mark Pauly spells out, in his chapter, an explicit monopolistically competitive model of market behavior with and without physician-induced demand. The result is conceptual ambiguity and practical uncertainty, as higher or lower fees can either raise or lower use. Pauly suggests that no net effect at all is perhaps the most likely. At the same time, volume may greatly increase or greatly decrease. He sees no scientific basis for the optimistic view of the RBRVS's proponents.

The effects of the PPRC's version of the RBRVS. In their chapter David Colby and David Juba, staff members at the PPRC, summarize their simulations of the effects of the PPRC's RBRVS, based on the assumption of a budget-neutral implementation. For simplicity and because of lack of knowledge, they ignored the effects of volume. The estimated impacts are dramatic because the RBRVS proposal of the PPRC radically changes fees and strictly limits balance billing.

The chapter highlights the effects of some of the PPRC's specific recommendations. They project, for example, a fee increase of 14 percent in rural areas and a decline of 14 percent in very large metropolitan areas (over 5 million population). Much of this change occurs because the PPRC decided not to adjust the value of physicians' time for cost-of-living differences, although all other costs, including wages for nonphysician manpower, are so adjusted. Another predicted result of the proposal is a large decline in balance bills because of the strict limits suggested by the PPRC.

The PPRC recommendations. Paul Ginsburg presented the PPRC's recommendations and their rationale. Like the one by Juba and Colby, Ginsburg's chapter is drawn from the PPRC's report. Ginsburg's chapter mentions fairness among physicians, suggesting that even the PPRC has been attracted to this idea.

One neglected part of the PPRC's proposal is the expenditure target, which is supposed to motivate the medical profession to reduce both use of services and expenditures. I believe that this idea plays nicely into the hands of the American Medical Association, as it would strengthen its role as the bargainer with the government and as the organizer of physicians' efforts to reduce supply. Both roles are natural for a trade association or labor union. The danger, as I see it, is that the AMA will use this power to suppress competition or that organized medicine's method of reducing the supply of medical care will conflict with the beneficiaries' values and preferences.

After supporting the principle of the RBRVS for years, the AMA opposed the expenditure target, some version of which has long seemed inevitable. Perhaps some internal politics explains this behavior.

The specialty societies have become more politically influential than the AMA. Indeed, many specialty societies clearly believe that the AMA does not legitimately represent them. These societies' incentives to reduce output in accordance with consumer tastes seems no better than the AMA's, however.

General Discussion

The volume closes with a discussion of the policy issues by economists, a lawyer, and a physician.

Roger Noll argues that constructing a relative fee schedule that mimics a perfectly competitive one is impossible, because (1) any allocation of true overhead costs is arbitrary; (2) we have no way of separating opportunity costs from rents, since we do not understand income differences across specialties; and (3) we have little idea about the effects of fees on quality. Noll concludes that the only possible explanation for the political support of the RBRVS is that a small, short-term saving can be eked out by temporarily extracting income from the physicians who specialize in treating Medicare beneficiaries. Then the real problem can be passed on to future Congresses and administrations.

Jim Rogers believes that analysts were being too constrained by what appeared to be politically feasible. Instead of tinkering with fee allowances, we should be considering reforms of fee-for-service coverage with more potential. He recommends taxing Medigap insurance and structuring cost sharing to eliminate the coinsurance and increase balance billing.

Rogers also criticized the idea of an expenditure target, noting its similarity to the limitations on Medicare allowances that have forced

15

them below the market level since 1972. Rogers is not optimistic that, if an expenditure target somehow motivates doctors and their organizations to reduce volume, their decisions will be good ones.

Robert Berenson notes that the RBRVS, based on policy decisions and thus not verifiable, is not nearly as objective and scientific as it seems. He criticizes the PPRC's tight limits to balance billing, underscoring the uncertainty about how cutting fees would affect the volume of services. He mentioned several disquieting trends in the responses of physicians to low incomes. Still, he favored the RBRVS.

Applying lessons from other recently deregulated industries, Robin Allen notes that prices declined, as economists have long predicted. Another and unexpected benefit of deregulation is the great expansion of types and qualities of services. Because price control requires careful legal description of the nature of the services, both the prices and the services that result may not be what would most benefit consumers. Thus she favors some form of contracting for HMOs, PPOs, and other private organizations with incentives to provide cost effectively what consumers want.

Glenn Hackbarth, agreeing with the RBRVS proponents that surgeons were overpaid relative to primary care physicians, believes some good might eventually come of the RBRVS. He argues, however, that it is a distraction, taking up too many political, analytical, and administrative resources in relation to a small expected benefit. Any substantial improvement in Medicare requires moving to competing HMOs and away from fee-for-service medicine. Hackbarth believes that the recent administrative cost controls for Medicare's fee-for-service side have been harmful.

Other discussion addresses the slow growth of Medicare's HMO enrollment, the tendency of medical price controls in Europe to stifle innovation, the poor historical record of price controls in general, and the unfortunate results of Medicaid. Low Medicaid fees have caused terrible access problems. After Congress's planned changes take effect, Medicare's fees, including balance bills, will be as low as many Medicaid fees.

Conclusions and Interpretations

Basic Economic Issues. This volume considers a number of basic economic issues relevant to the broad policy problems of Medicare and the RBRVS proposal put forth by the PPRC.

Are surgeons overpaid? Contributors generally assent that surgeons, or some subspecialties among them, might be overpaid. Several note that if surgeons were overpaid and entry into surgery

16

were not too restricted, there should be excess capacity among surgeons. Surprisingly little research has been done on this key issue. The only such research, performed by Victor Fuchs and others in the early 1970s, found low and highly variable surgical work loads.[23] The situation has probably not changed since. The Fuchs work, however, was limited to nineteen surgeons at a single suburban New York hospital and is somewhat dated. More work on this subject should have a high priority, especially among those who favor the RBRVS.

Does the demand side or the supply side control Medicare volume? All analysts have a mental model of the market for physicians' services that guides their work and informs their views. In this context "model" means the analyst's basic understanding of how the market works and how it responds to changes. Models, in this sense, are rarely formal and all too often are not explicit. This causes confusion and is the subject of frequent criticism.

A key conceptual or modeling issue is whether demand or supply is the main limitation on the volume of Medicare services. The following experiment is helpful in answering that question. If demand increased, would most physicians happily take more Medicare patients and provide them the services they seek at current fees? If the answer is yes, then consumer demand is constraining volume. If, in contrast, most physicians would be not willing to treat additional Medicare consumers or would not be willing to provide the services they seek, then supply would be constraining volume.

Without explicitly saying so, proponents of the RBRVS seem to believe that volume is constrained on the supply side. This assumption justifies ignoring the demand side of the market. If the supply side controls, the behavior of physicians will predict effects of changing fees or other reforms.

The authors in this volume, however, generally take the view that utilization in the current Medicare system is constrained most often by demand, not supply. A supply-constrained system would create many access problems for Medicare beneficiaries, which would be easy to observe and generate political pressure for change.

If the system is demand constrained, predicting the effect of fee changes on volume requires examining changing demand resulting from coinsurance and balance bills. Since a reduction in allowed fees cuts coinsurance but could raise balance bills, the effects on demand are ambiguous. Of course, large enough cuts in fees could reduce the willingness of physicians to supply their services to the extent that the system became supply constrained. While some favor such an outcome, I believe that this would impose undesirable burdens on

17

Medicare consumers by restricting access to doctors' services. Further, I believe that political pressure would be put on Congress to undo any change that led to this result.

Policy Suggestions. A number of policy suggestions receive substantial support in this volume. Of course, some support the RBRVS, including Hsiao and the participants from the PPRC. Some favor fee schedules that are not cost based, and some, sometimes the same people, proposed far more sweeping policies. I will take up the most sweeping reforms first.

Encourage HMOs and PPOs. Many of the authors favored greatly expanding the incentives for Medicare consumers to join HMOs and PPOs to harness the private sector's innovative methods for controlling costs while responding to differences in consumers' tastes and values.[24] Interestingly, shortly after the conference, the Department of Health and Human Services announced some reforms in the Medicare HMO option designed to encourage HMOs to compete for Medicare beneficiaries.

Tax or prohibit Medigap insurance. Increasing consumers' copayments substantially cuts spending; it is the one policy change that is guaranteed to work. Furthermore, analysts have long suspected that raising consumers' copayments in a large proportion of the market would redirect research and development toward cost-effective treatments rather than cost-increasing quality improvements. In Medicare, however, directly raising consumers' copayments would be largely defeated by Medigap insurance. In addition, Medicare insurance, without Medigap, has a reasonable degree of cost sharing for consumers in its 80 percent coinsurance for physicians' services. (Of course, further reforms could add coinsurance to the hospital coverage and raise the small deductible.)

The biggest obstacle to improving copayment is Medigap insurance. The main effect from increasing copayments is that Medigap insurance and Medicaid would pay more and Medicare less, with little impact on demand, research, or competitiveness. Further, eliminating or strongly reducing Medigap insurance would be a huge improvement in cost sharing. Ever since the theoretical work of Mark Pauly, we have known that Medigap insurance created a severe externality.[25] Most of the increase in expenditures caused by Medigap insurance is paid for by Medicare, a shift of the insurance burden to the taxpayer. Thus most regulation-oriented economists have suggested prohibiting Medigap, while the more market-oriented ones have favored taxing it. An efficient tax would offset the increase in

Medicare costs that results from Medigap insurance. Research suggests that this would be a very large tax, perhaps over 100 percent, which might eliminate most Medigap insurance.

McGuire brings to our attention another unnoticed disadvantage of Medigap insurance. By imposing extra costs on Medicare, Medigap insurance disguises the true cost of 100 percent coverage under fee for service. From the viewpoint of the beneficiary who wants 100 percent coverage, Medigap insurance makes it appear cheaper than it truly is, therefore reducing consumer demand for HMOs and PPOs.

Eliminating or taxing Medigap insurance would simultaneously reduce Medicare expenses and improve economic efficiency. There are not many such opportunities. Certainly, no tampering with fee schedules could possibly reduce expenditures as much as taxing or prohibiting Medigap insurance.

Are costs a better basis than charges for a fee schedule? A narrower look at the possible fee schedules led to criticism of the RBRVS and the PPRC's proposal at several levels. I will discuss the more general ones first.

Criticism of the construction of the actual Hsiao and PPRC fee schedules aside, a more fundamental question is, Are fees based on costs, however measured, superior to ones based on the market or on charges? Is there an intellectual rationale for a cost-based RVS versus a charge-based RVS? The failure of RBRVS proponents to address this question seriously has caused a perplexing gap in the small literature of the RBRVS proposal. No one has ever actually made the intellectual case for it.[26]

Among the chapters in this volume, the one by William Hsiao and Daniel Dunn at least considers the question, although too casually. Noting that the market for physicians' services is not perfectly competitive, the authors then claim that the elasticity of demand differs by type of service and thus that the ratio of price to marginal cost also varies by type of service. They claim that more complete insurance coverage of physicians' inpatient services than outpatient ones lead to higher markups over costs for inpatient services.

David Dranove and Mark Satterthwaite in their chapter and Hadley in his take up the issue more carefully and thoroughly. While they agree that differential insurance might lead to a bigger markup of price over costs in surgery, some features lead the other way. In particular, Dranove and Satterthwaite argue that it is probably easier to determine the quality of a surgeon than a primary care physician. Further, the fit between consumer and surgeon is more objective for surgery than for office visits. The relationship is not so idiosyncratic

19

as that between the primary care physician and a patient. Research on consumer behavior also leads us to expect consumers to search more for large items than for small ones. All these considerations suggest that competition in surgery might not be so imperfect.

The actual ratios of prices to marginal costs depend on the relative shapes of marginal cost and demand (to the individual physician) curves. There is no logical reason to think that average costs will be closer to the ideal relative fees than will charges.

Finis Welch argues that measured cost would be far less accurate than the imperfect charges for determining a fee schedule. In particular, he noted that some market fees are always unexplainable statistically. He cautions against the assumption that these fees are therefore wrong or unjustified.

Similarly, Roger Noll believes that the model used to predict the value of physicians' work time ignores too many important variables, like the relative scarcity of physicians with different skills, the necessary training, and the psychic costs of certain specialties. Thus the resulting relative fees will be seriously less accurate than fees based on admittedly imperfect market charges.

Perhaps showing how important subjective elements are in coming up with a judgment on this, Mitchell and her colleagues performed a statistical exercise similar to Hsiao and Dunn's. Yet they concluded the exact opposite: that market charges are quite reasonable as a basis for a fee schedule.

Any possible fee schedule would be imperfect. The question is, Which approach gets us closer to the ideal? Are imperfectly measured costs better, or are imperfectly competitive charges better? Or is a combination the best of all?

An alternative fee schedule. While a purely charge-based relative value scale may do less harm than a cost-based one, is it optimal? Can we improve on a charge-based fee schedule by modifying it? The answer given by most of the authors is yes. Most suggest a simple alternative: base a fee schedule primarily on charges but reduce them for a few important procedures that appear to be overpriced. This way, the information from studies like Hsiao's or Mitchell's could help identify overpriced services. But it would not be the sole or even primary basis of any actual Medicare allowances.

Moreover, by selecting only a few important services for which to reduce fees substantially below market levels, the necessary monitoring of quality, quantity, access, balance billing and assignment rate could be done. The RBRVS approach requires large changes in prices for thousands of procedures, making monitoring the impacts needlessly difficult and costly.

Reducing the Medicare allowances for a few services that are believed to be overpriced can be and is being done within the current customary, prevailing, and reasonable system. The fees for several important services judged by the PPRC to be overpriced have been reduced in recent years. Since 1987, fees have been reduced for thirteen families of procedures.

The Effect of the RBRVS on Volume. Implicit in many discussions of the RBRVS, especially that of Hsiao and Dunn, is the idea that reducing the relative payment for surgery and other procedures will reduce the number of them performed, while raising the fees allowed for physician visits will cause more of them to be performed. Pauly's chapter and Newhouse's commentary should raise doubts about any such belief.

The RBRVS's proponents appear to believe that the Medicare market is supply constrained. This seems highly unlikely. But even if the existing market were supply constrained and therefore demand changes could be ignored, how suppliers would respond to fee changes is ambiguous.

If we ignore the possibility of physician-induced demand, a fee cut exerts two opposing forces on the supply of physicians' services. The lower price leads to what economists call the substitution effect that reduces the quantity of the services. At the same time, the loss in income leads to pressure to increase the quantity. The effect of these opposing forces on the willingness of the average physician to supply services is unknown.

Broadening the model to allow a meaningful amount of physician-induced demand, as Pauly shows, compounds the ambiguity; it does not eliminate it. Many who favor the inducement model say that lower fees and concomitant lower income and wealth lead to more inducement and more services. If so, the RBRVS would increase surgery and reduce visits. Lower fees, in contrast, might lead to fewer services, not more. Pauly says that something like this belief must underlie the prediction that the RBRVS will reduce volume. The effects of the RBRVS on volume might range from near zero to very large, but we do not know even their direction.

The Construction of the RBRVS. As many of the chapters show in detail, the RBRVS is not the objective, mechanical, scientific creature that it appears to be. In fact, it requires many value and empirical judgments. Many of these necessary judgments made by Hsiao and the PPRC are criticized in this volume.[27]

21

The vignettes. The starting point for the measurement of physician work was the vignette of treatment. In telephone interviews, physicians were read one- or two-sentence descriptions of symptoms and treatment and were asked to rate the amount of work done. Later, the vignettes were placed into common procedural terminology (CPT) classifications. This approach was criticized for arbitrarily choosing one of many possible situations to stand for the average of the procedure classification. It was as if people were asked the cost of a chicken dinner and the value they gave was later used as representative of the average of all dinners.

In contrast, using the CPT codes directly in the survey ran the risk of simply picking up the physicians' memories of their own actual relative prices, since their prices are defined over CPT codes. This was the reason for using the vignettes in the first place.

Interestingly, Mitchell and her colleagues did use the CPT codes themselves in their survey. Although I understand the reasoning behind the Hsiao and PPRC use of vignettes, I believe that relying on the CPT codes directly is superior.

The physicians surveyed. Hsiao's study was criticized for the physicians it surveyed on two grounds. First, the sample was attacked as unrepresentative and, second, for relying on the answers of physicians for procedures that they did not or could not do. Over half the chest surgeons who answered questions on the work required in open heart procedures, for example, did not do them at all. In my view the physicians were selected in a reasonably representative and random manner, but I question the answers on procedures that few of the physicians actually performed.

Internal consistency of measures of work. The Hsiao group asked physicians for a numerical rating for work, relative to a starting point of 100 for a standard procedure. They also asked the same physicians for what they called the components of work—time, mental effort, judgment, technical skill and physical effort (combined), and stress due to risk. Then, they related the total work answers to the answers for the components of work. The components explained most of the variation of the total work. But the relative weight of the components varied greatly across specialties, undermining the argument that any of these answers measures anything objective or comparable across specialties.

Extrapolation of work to unmeasured services. Limited by time and money, Hsiao's team studied only about 400 of the 7,000 procedures. The work values were extrapolated to the rest by relying on market charges within families of related procedures, largely performed by the same specialty. In effect, the relative work measures simply follow market charges within these families. They diverge from charges mostly across specialties, where the procedures for determining relative work or values are most questionable and arbitrary.

One may think of the resulting fees as following the market, except for depressing some specialties relative to others. Since this was widely viewed as the goal of the project, one can hardly be surprised at the result. Nor can one view the results of the Hsiao or the PPRC studies as independent evidence that some specialties are actually overpaid.

The adjustment for specialty training. Hsiao's adjustments for specialty training are analyzed in the chapter by William Marder and Richard Willke. The Hsiao team ignored the great variations in rates of return to training in different specialties and the larger rates of return generally accruing to the specialties that require longer training periods, largely the surgical and hospital-based specialties. Some of the difference in rate of return across specialties reflects differences in doctors' ability and the psychic costs across specialties. These differences should be reflected in fees.

To the extent that the new relative fees fail to reflect the legitimate differences in ability, training, and psychic costs, they will cause unnecessary problems. In the long run, the differences in income and value of time across specialties will reemerge through market forces. But in the meantime, the disruption of the health economy could be substantial.

The Hsiao group used a 3 percent real rate of return, far less than the roughly 10 to 20 percent actual average real rate of return. The 3 percent rate also tends to reduce the payments to high-investment specialties. Furthermore, they made an algebraic mistake in amortizing the extra training costs, further reducing the difference between the high-investment surgical specialties and the low-investment primary care ones.[28]

The cumulative effect of these judgmental decisions and mistakes is to reduce the fees for the surgical and other procedural specialties relative to the primary care specialties. The PPRC's recommendations are even more extreme.

Much criticized by Finis Welch and other specialists in labor economics, the PPRC recommends that the extra investment in training by certain specialties be ignored completely. Paul Ginsburg's defense was that the subjective rating of work values by the physicians includes skill, which is the return to extra training. By this

23

argument, paying separately for training, as Hsiao proposes, is double counting.

But the human capital literature suggests that learning increases productivity per unit of time. For many procedures, this means that quality is higher. An operation performed by a specialist with several years of extra training is a different and superior product to one performed by a general practitioner, no matter how finely the physical tasks are defined in the CPT codes. Even an office visit to a physician with more and different training is a different product.

Clearly, a full adjustment for the differences in returns to specialty training would lead to smaller relative cuts for surgeons, an outcome that conflicts with both the goal of the Hsiao team and the congressional demands.

The PPRC's recommendation substantially reduces the relative fees of the surgical and procedural specialties. Perhaps the intellectual rationale suggested by the PPRC is not so important. As is reflected in earlier PPRC annual reports, PPRC (and the Congress) had a preexisting view that surgical fees should be cut relative to fees for visits. The PPRC might have simply recommended reducing the fee allowances for procedures, without the RBRVS study, on the basis of market-tested fee schedules from private, competing HMOs and PPOs. The relative value studies, with their statistics, formulas, and learned discussions, lend a misleading air of scientific precision and objectivity to the political proceedings.

The relative scarcity of different specialties. The RBRVS did not actually measure costs at all, because it does not use the cost of the physician's time. By converting from relative physician work per service adjusted for training and other costs, into a relative value scale, the RBRVS treats the adjusted time of all physicians as if it had equal value. In effect, this approach ignores the relative scarcity of different types of medical manpower. Thus the relative value schedules diverge, potentially a great deal, from competitive relative prices.

Economies of scale and scope. The costs of different procedures are subject to economies of scale. Equally important are economies of scope, where costs of a procedure depend on how many related procedures are performed. None of these considerations are reflected in the RBRVS.[29] Somehow, by assigning a single value for work per procedure, physicians have implicitly simplified the problem. The only way to interpret their answers is that they are giving the average for some implicit and unknown hypothetical scale of practice and distribution of procedures.

Noll notes that the RBRVS measures the subjective disutility (or

24

dislike) of work from the viewpoint of the physicians. This probably varies in complex ways with changes in hours of work and type of work.

In response, Hsiao claims that the total work appears to be roughly linear in its measured components but that we have no way to examine the hours-of-work question. Hsiao and others, notably Henry Aaron, defend the RBRVS measurement as perhaps crude but as a rough approximation of average costs, which they asserted were, in turn, a rough approximation of marginal costs.

I find this view hard to credit, since the main input is the physician's own time. I would expect the value of time in particular procedures to vary greatly as hours of work vary. Thus average costs and marginal costs would diverge widely. Furthermore, many office inputs, such as space and machinery, cannot be divided or continuously increased. This cost also varies with the quantity produced.

Nonphysician practice cost. The Hsiao group's estimate of general overhead costs in proportion to measured work effort seems inaccurate. This method seriously overstates the cost of visits to physicians, which use only a few chairs and a pencil, and understates the costs of procedures that require supporting personnel, equipment, and space.

Noll and Newhouse stress that true overhead costs cannot be rationally allocated to different services: overhead costs simply cause average cost to exceed marginal cost.

By treating general overhead as if it occurred in fixed proportion to work, the Hsiao study assumes these costs are perfectly flexible in the following sense. If the measurement of work for a particular procedure accidentally comes out too low, then costs would be arithmetically forced to shrink proportionally. This is illogical, since the actual nonphysician costs for a particular procedure depend mostly on the technology, not on the amount of work the physician does or on variations in the measurement of the amount of work done. Perhaps worse, this method compounds the original measurement error. The PPRC recommends modifying the treatment to a more empirically based approach where measurement errors in the relative work will not be compounded in the nonphysician costs.

The definition of visits. What actually happens in visits to physicians and other cognitive activities is poorly defined. The great variation within each CPT visit code, Finis Welch notes, undermines the entire RBRVS. If we do not know what services we are pricing, then the price itself is meaningless, and the relative prices between it and other procedures are equally meaningless. Even if all the other

25

problems were solved and all the necessary judgments made in a reasonable and unbiased way, this extreme variation might be judged a fatal flaw in the cost-based system.

Indeed, the PPRC regards reform of the visit codes as essential to using the RBRVS to change relative prices among visits. But since the problem lies in distinguishing among various types of visits, one can group the visits and their prices. The result, though far from perfect, can be used as a basis for changing the prices of procedures relative to visits.

The Implementation of the RBRVS. Whether the RBRVS per se is a good idea or not, this volume contains many suggestions on how to implement the RBRVS to do the most good or the least harm. Some of these also predict how generous the fees would actually be.

Implementation of a balanced budget. Many people predict that the RBRVS would, on average, cut fees. With the appearance of objectivity and fairness, the RBRVS would make it politically easier to cut fees in general. If so, some fees would probably be cut drastically. The AMA's apparent belief in budget-neutral implementation is wishful thinking and naiveté.

Indeed, the coupling of the RBRVS with the idea of an expenditure target by the PPRC suggests that cuts will occur. Some policy makers appear to believe that primary care allowances cannot be cut further but that allowances for surgical and other procedures can be cut. In this view, the RBRVS, whatever other problems it introduces by its poor tracking of market or hypothetical competitive fees, does result in cuts for procedures, while keeping allowances for cognitive medicine from being cut.

The budget-neutral simulations reported by David Colby and David Juba show huge average fee increases, as large as 38 percent, for primary care physicians. Most of the authors in this volume argue that primary care allowances were too high, not too low, and were generally opposed to raising allowances for them. Only Robert Berenson argues for actually raising fees for cognitive medicine—and he appears to be joking.

The importance of balance billing. Balance billing performs many important functions in all insurance schemes and especially in Medicare. This would be even more important if the RBRVS cut some allowed fees drastically, as both the Hsiao and the PPRC versions suggest. Without more or less unlimited balance billing, nonprice rationing and quality declines might be serious, particularly in certain specialties and locations where the RBRVS fees would be set especially low.[30]

Unfortunately, the actual recommendation from the PPRC to Congress drastically reduces balance billing. It recommends that balance billing be limited to a percentage of the new allowed fee but does not recommend a percentage. The effects of the rule, however, are simulated for only a narrow and low range, 10 to 40 percent. For many of the more complex simulations, only a narrower range of limits, 15 to 25 percent, were used. The plan approved by Congress cuts balance billing to less than 10 percent by 1993.[31]

The stated reason for limiting balance billing is to protect the consumer from having to make a large out-of-pocket payment to cover the balance bill. The real purpose may be to use the monopoly buying power of the government to depress the prices charged by physicians, especially those who serve mostly the elderly. The result could easily be prices below the competitive level for some procedures and some physicians.

Whatever the true motive, the limit simply transforms what would have been an insurance package into a system of price control.[32] The controlled price is the allowed fee, plus whatever balance billing is permitted. If many physicians are willing to provide good quality service at the controlled price, this price control imposes little harm on consumers. This is more likely if the controlled price is high, relative to market charges. It is also more likely if the market charges are more monopolistic or if Medicare has more market power over the physicians. If the controlled price is set too low, however, consumers will not have access to the best physicians, and the quality and convenience of the service will be degraded.

One scheme that offers the best of both worlds is to identify the physicians willing to take the Medicare allowance as payment in full. It would make sense to publish widely the list of physicians who agree and even to offer them higher allowances, faster claim processing, and other advantages. Then unlimited balance billing for the remainder allows consumers to use their insurance to help pay for care from all physicians, even the very most costly, if they are willing to pay the difference. Except for some limitations on balance billing of nonparticipating physicians, this describes the existing Medicare Participating Physician Program. An expansion and refinement of this program, coupled with lifting the limits on balance billing for the nonparticipating physicians, would be the ideal policy. This scheme also describes the very successful way PPOs generally pay their physicians.

If policy makers are determined to limit balance billing in some way, however, tying the limits to the RBRVS fee is a bad way to do it. The danger, for which balance billing is an important safety valve, is precisely that of setting the RBRVS too low. If so, tying the limit to the RBRVS would make the balance billing limit too low as well. Far better would be to link the limit to the actual market charges.

The balance bill could be set, for example, so that the allowance plus the balance bill would be at the fiftieth percentile of the actual charges for each service in each locality. This would guarantee access without nonprice rationing to at least half the physicians. For services where the RBRVS was far below charges, the limitation would be very loose, as it should be. Where the RBRVS was very generous, balance billing would be more limited.

The actual range of limits on balance billing suggested by the PPRC and adopted by Congress can be described only as surprisingly drastic. Such limits would cause some total fees, including the small allowed balance bill, to be far below the current market. In fact, the fee received by the physician could easily be below Medicaid levels in many localities. It is well known that Medicaid has a serious access problem. In many areas, most physicians will not take Medicaid patients.

The extreme nature of the proposed PPRC limits on balance billing is also apparent in the simulations presented by David Juba and David Colby. Making the analytically useful but very optimistic budget-neutral assumption, they report a national average reduction of between 9 and 31 percent for seven selected surgical procedures with an average reduction for surgery of 18 percent. Obviously, some procedures would be cut more, some less. These are also averages across all physicians in all areas.

On top of this relative price cut for procedures, physicians in very large metropolitan areas (populations over 5 million) would be cut an additional 14 percent. So if we just add the percentage changes, average surgical fees over the seven selected procedures would be cut by 23 to 45 percent, with a mean of 34 percent in very large metropolitan areas. A realistic implementation would not be budget neutral, so cuts would actually be much larger, at least after a few years.

The Medicare fees facing these large cuts already average about 30 percent under the market. Again, for some market areas and some physicians, the existing discount is larger. Thus the average surgical discount in very large metropolitan areas, under the budget-neutral PPRC version of the RBRVS, would be about 50 percent. Obviously, the discount for many procedures and many physicians would be substantially more.

If balance billing were essentially unlimited, this would not create an access problem, although it would expose Medicare consumers to more financial risk than they face now. Therefore, it might not be a very sensible policy.

In any case, a limit of balance billing to 10 percent of the Medicare allowance implies that the total amount the physician could receive would average, under the generous assumptions of the Juba and Colby simulations, more than 45 percent below market fees for surgery. Many procedures for many physicians would be discounted even more deeply. For some beneficiaries in some local areas, this would cause severe access problems.

The radical nature of the PPRC's proposed limits to balance billing is illustrated another way by the Colby and Juba simulations. Without new limitations on balance billing, one would expect a budget-neutral change in Medicare allowances to be budget neutral with respect to balance bills as well; that is, it would have almost no effect on balance bills. The strict limits of 15 percent of the RBRVS, however, are projected to reduce total balance bills by about 73 percent. Even the 40 percent limit, coupled with the dramatic cuts in allowances, would drop balance bills by 38 percent.[33]

More or less unrestricted balance billing also provides better information to Medicare. High levels of balance billing for a particular service in a particular market area show that the Medicare allowance has been set too low and also reveals information on how much too low.

One can only hope that actual limits on balance billing, if any, will be more liberal than those contemplated in current law and will be based on market prices or on the spread between the RBRVS values and market prices.

Monitoring and adjusting fees. Because the proposed changes in Medicare allowances are historically unprecedented, many authors in this volume stress monitoring and quick adjustment for allowances accidentally set too low or too high. Indeed, a thoughtful and rapid feedback and decision-making system could quickly undo the damage caused by inaccurate RBRVS fees. In the long run, whether the original fee schedule was based on costs, charges, or a mixture would not matter. No one seems opposed to this idea, which over time would lead to a market-based fee schedule.

The monitoring would focus on price and especially on nonprice signals from the market. Unfortunately, the planned severe restrictions on balance billing would jumble the price signals. Using the nonprice signals would require Medicare to formulate some idea, even if only implicitly, of how much of each service of what quality it wants its beneficiaries to buy and how much, if any, access problem it is willing to tolerate. Mark Pauly has long argued that Medicare's managers should answer these questions.

If the quantity or the quality were too low, if too few physicians were willing to treat Medicare patients, or if balance billing were too high, Medicare would adjust by raising the allowance. The opposite indicators would lead to reducing the allowance for that procedure in that area. While a rational system requires such a mechanism, the level of monitoring vastly exceeds what Medicare and the PPRC are now doing, especially if the entire RBRVS were to be implemented, changing the prices for 7,000 procedure codes. Further, monitoring and quick response require a degree of managerial independence from political intervention. Perhaps Congress would permit this, perhaps not.

Little or no money can be saved. Many authors suggest that the RBRVS would not save Medicare much money. Roger Noll, in particular, stresses that the political economy of Medicare would guarantee this result. He believes that only very low fees that would lead to a supply-constrained, heavily nonprice rationed system would save a noticeable amount. Some commentators like Thomas McGuire favor this, while Noll and others argue that this system would be unacceptable to the elderly, resulting in political pressure to raise allowances and thereby undo any savings. It is possible, however, that a small amount of savings could be realized in the short run at the expense of those with large, specialized human capital investments—the surgeons.

What Is the Political Attraction of the RBRVS? The scientific underpinnings of the RBRVS are weak. Several of the authors call the whole enterprise ludicrous, an attempt to measure the unmeasurable. Even its proponents defend it primarily by arguing that market charges are even worse. Thus, the question arises, Why does this idea have such an apparently strong political attraction? This, of course, is a question in political economy. This volume contains many fascinating attempts to answer the question.

Peter Zweifel suggests that the AMA leadership may favor it for several reasons: first because it represents a large step toward a negotiated fee schedule, with the AMA the key negotiator, and, second, because the proposal appears to redistribute income from a few highly paid surgeons to many primary care physicians, a sort of redistribution typical of labor unions. Such a plan might engender the support of a majority within the AMA.

While some increases for primary care doctors would be likely, at least for a few years, the idea of much possible redistribution is based on the naive idea of something close to a budget-neutral change. The most likely outcome is reduced fees for doctors as a group.

The drastic restrictions on balance billing would also ensure physician incomes measurably lower than current levels even if the implementation were budget neutral with respect to Medicare's own spending. While sharp limits on balance billing have gotten less attention, they might have a larger and more adverse impact on consumers and physicians than the RBRVS itself would have.

There is probably some room for a small redistribution from specialized surgeons to taxpayers, at least for a few years. This redistribution might occur at the expense of long-run efficiency and costs, however; but perhaps Congress is less concerned about long-run problems. Noll also stresses that the RBRVS would require a great deal of analysis and regulation, thus raising the demand for economists and bureaucrats with knowledge in this area. Indeed, he could point to this volume as one of the first examples.

Separately, Glenn Hackbarth and I believe that intellectual causation also seems to be at work. Hackbarth notes that a small number of active and interested congressmen and staff members dominate congressional health policy making. Holding that current relative fees and incomes of different specialties are unfair and unjustified, they see any scheme like the RBRVS that reduces the incomes of surgeons relative to internists as good on ethical or aesthetic grounds. Needless to say, these individuals are not experts in health economics or health policy or in labor economics. More seriously, they appear to be isolated from the best analysis of these issues.

Perhaps the policy makers have somehow come to believe that the economic analysis available at the universities and think tanks is mere mathematical doodling, unrelated to the actual world and its policy problems. While this may be an accurate criticism of some academic work, particularly in mathematical economic theory, it is certainly not true for the work of the top independent health economists in academia and in research institutes, many of whom are authors in this volume. For the policy makers to ignore these analysts, as they appear to have done, is a serious mistake.

While agreeing with Hackbarth on the importance of intellectual causation, I suggest a slight extension to his theory. The RBRVS appears to be favored by influential Washington policy makers even over a charge-based scheme that would accomplish a similar redistribution with less dislocation. These people believe that the RBRVS is

31

somehow an objective, scientific, and mechanistic black box that does away with the necessity of empirical and value judgments. Thus it is seen as fair.

Our long history of seeking such mechanistic solutions to scientific and practical economic problems has resulted in various mistakes and irrelevancies, from the internal rate-of-return rule for investments to the old-fashioned mathematical growth theory of the 1960s.

A key theme of this volume is that the RBRVS is not objective: it requires many empirical and value judgments, from the beginning vignettes of care to the extension of the schedule to procedures not studied. Furthermore, these judgments have to be skewed against the highly trained surgical specialties to give the politically desired result. Reasonable treatments of the amortization of specialty training and nonphysician practice costs, within the general framework of the Hsiao study, could easily lead to a RBRVS that did not much reduce surgical and other procedural fees relative to cognitive service fees.

Conclusion

The RBRVS has been enacted and is scheduled to phase in over the next few years, even though it has gotten almost no public attention from the country's top health economists and analysts. I can only hope that the questions raised in this volume will reduce the political momentum behind the RBRVS to allow time for a fuller and more public discourse on this and other Medicare reforms.

PART ONE

Physician Markets and Medicare Benefits

2
The Policy Context of Physician Payment

Joseph R. Antos

There is a widely held perception that the cost of providing medical services, including physician services, to the American people is too high and is spiraling upward rapidly. Too much of this spending is considered to be wasteful and the services potentially unnecessary or even harmful to the patient. At the same time, many believe that our health care system is not providing basic services to perhaps 33 million Americans. The hope is often expressed in Washington policy circles that we should be able to halt or reverse the expenditure spiral, extend health coverage to everyone in this country, and improve the effectiveness of medical care—usually with the sentiment that "it's high time we took care of this problem."[1] Should anyone express pessimism about the success of such an undertaking, current folklore about the Canadian or European experience is offered as evidence that "it" can be done. After all, if they can do it in Canada, Britain, or Germany, why can't we do it here?

This is the broad context in which Medicare physician payment

Since this chapter was written, the 101st Congress passed legislation that established a number of changes for physician payment under the Medicare Part B program. Under the Omnibus Budget Reconciliation Act (OBRA) of 1989, a four-part physician payment reform package was enacted that established (1) a fee schedule based on resource costs, (2) service volume performance standards, (3) limits on physicians' balance billing, and (4) increased support of effectiveness research and practice guidelines. The fee schedule, based largely on the relative value study of William Hsiao and colleagues at Harvard University, will be phased in over a five-year transition period beginning in January 1992. Fees will also vary from one locality to another based on a geographic adjustment factor. Despite these legislative changes, debate continues over a number of issues and approaches surrounding longer-term physician payment policy and reform. In this context, this paper provides a continuing framework for discussion and analysis. I wish to thank George Schieber, Ira Burney, Bob Kazdin, Jack Langenbrunner, Stephen Jencks, Terry Kay, and Ted Frech for their helpful comments. The section describing policy alternatives relies greatly on the work of Terry Kay. The views expressed here do not represent the policies of any agency of the U.S. government.

reform is being considered. The Medicare program costs $100 billion a year and covers 33 million elderly and disabled beneficiaries. Roughly one-fifth of total U.S. expenditures for health is covered by Medicare. Because Medicare is the largest health insurance program in the country, significant changes in Medicare policy will have repercussions throughout the health care system. And because Medicare is a federal program, the political dialogue more frequently revolves around budget deficits than around medical considerations.

In recent years, the target of policy and budget reform has shifted away from hospitals toward physicians. The introduction of the hospital prospective payment system (PPS) in 1984 has proved to be a powerful tool in controlling Medicare's hospital expenditures. No such sweeping policy change has been adopted for physician payment in the more than twenty-year history of the Medicare program. We may now be on the verge of such a sweeping change. Publication of the Harvard study of resource-based relative value scales (RBRVS) in the fall of 1988 has served as a catalyst for wide-ranging policy development in this area.[2] Policy actions that may shake the foundation of the business of medicine could be taken by the end of 1989. This essay provides a background for interpreting the coming debate.

The discussion focuses on the most important factors that have converged to promote physician payment reform, particularly those that relate to the explosion of Medicare expenditures for physician services. The forces at work are integral to the structure of the medical marketplace in this country and therefore cast doubt on the efficacy of proposals that do not alter that basic structure. Several policy options are described in the following pages, along with some collateral issues that will be important in implementing any payment reform.

Pressures for Reform

The pressure for payment reform has grown as physician spending has soared upward. In fiscal year 1990 Medicare spending on physician services will be in excess of $30 billion. Between 1984 and 1987, Medicare spending for physician services per beneficiary increased at an annual rate of about 15 percent, which is twice the comparable figure for per capita gross national product. This is in contrast to the growth of spending for hospitals, which, since the introduction of the prospective payment system in 1984, has averaged about 6 percent.

Rapid growth in physician expenditure is not a new phenomenon. Table 2–1 shows that Medicare physician spending has been

TABLE 2-1
ANNUAL INCREASES IN MEDICARE PAYMENTS FOR PHYSICIAN SERVICES, 1976–1987
(percent)

	1976	1977	1978	1979	1980	1981	1982	1983	1984[a]	1985[a]	1986[a]	1987
Physician payments	18.8	21.3	17.5	18.6	22.4	18.8	19.5	18.2	10.3	11.2	9.8	16.9
Consumer Price Index	5.8	6.5	7.6	11.3	13.5	10.3	6.2	3.2	4.3	3.6	1.9	3.6

NOTE: Calendar year basis.
a. Physician fee freeze: July 1984 to April 1986 for participating physicians and July 1984 to December 1986 for nonparticipating physicians.
SOURCE: HCFA Medicare Statistical System and *Economic Report of the President, 1989*.

increasing at double-digit rates for more than a decade. Even during periods of high general price inflation—such as 1979–1981, when the Consumer Price Index (CPI) grew at more than 10 percent per year— Medicare physician spending has increased at nearly twice the general rate of inflation. During periods of low inflation, such as 1983– 1987, program costs have grown at two to five times the general rate of inflation.

Even if there is no further expansion of Medicare benefits, spending for physician services is likely to triple over the next ten years. In part because of the anticipated increases in expenditures in physician services, total Medicare spending is expected to exceed spending on social security by about the year 2003, and to make Medicare the country's largest entitlement program. In the absence of policy changes, Medicare spending will be greater than social security *plus* defense spending by about 2012.

Another important issue spurring interest in physician payment reform is the medical effectiveness of Medicare expenditures. A variety of studies have questioned the scientific wisdom of some medical treatments, noting, for example, that 17 percent of coronary angiograms and 32 percent of carotid endarterectomies may be unnecessary.[3] The extent of medical inappropriateness appears to be about the same whether a particular service is used frequently or infrequently. This suggests that medical inappropriateness invites two significant risks: treatment might be received when it is unwarranted, and treatment might *not* be given when there would be real benefits for the patient.

The question is, Are we spending our health dollars wisely? Clearly, that is a question of great concern to many people: patients, physicians, private insurers, and the government. A considerable amount of work is going on now to push forward our systematic knowledge of what works and what doesn't work in the practice of medicine. For the foreseeable future, however, it is unlikely that scientific analysis of medical practice will be able to keep pace with the rate of innovation there.

The issue of payment equity across medical specialties has been perhaps the area of greatest emphasis in Professor William Hsiao's work on the RBRVS. Disparities in incomes between the evaluative and management specialties (such as internal and family medicine) and the procedural specialties (surgery, anesthesia, radiology, and pathology) are widely recognized and have persisted for many decades, predating the enactment of the Medicare program. One of Hsiao's contributions to the debate is his detailed quantification and analysis of these payment differentials. Although policy makers accept that the observed differentials do reflect serious distortions in the structure of medical prices, what price structure is analytically appropriate remains an open question.

Any distortions (and inequities) that are present in the payment structure persist over time, providing an incentive to overperform certain kinds of services. In turn, those payment incentives draw medical students into higher-paid specialties. Thus, although payment structure distortion is most often cast as an equity issue, it has equally important implications for economic efficiency.

Still another concern has been access to care and financial protection for beneficiaries. On the whole, Medicare beneficiaries have excellent access to care. The assurance of payment has by and large solved what was once a serious problem for the elderly, although access to some types of medical care can be difficult in rural areas or the inner city. Again, this distribution of physicians is influenced by the payment structure, and some see payment reform as a way of reducing remaining access problems.

The ultimate question for Medicare beneficiaries is how their basic costs will be affected by physician payment reform. Medicare pays 80 percent of allowed charges for physician services, after the $75 deductible is met. For most beneficiaries, the remainder is covered by supplemental insurance (either through private Medigap insurance or state Medicaid programs). Less than 20 percent of beneficiaries have no supplemental coverage. Even those with supplemental insurance, however, are often subject to out-of-pocket costs if the physician's charge exceeds Medicare's allowed charge, a phenomenon known as balance billing.[4] As physicians' charges have risen, beneficiary costs have increased, through higher Medigap insurance premiums or direct payments (for those without Medigap coverage) and higher balance billing. In 1987, Congress introduced restrictions on balance billing by instituting a maximum allowable actual charge (MAAC). The comprehensive physician payment reform may incorporate explicit mechanisms for protecting beneficiary finances.

For all these reasons—costs, effectiveness of care, payment equity, access to care, and beneficiary protection—a consensus has developed that the way we now acquire and pay for physician services is not working and must be reformed. Whatever reform is undertaken, it must take into account the factors that have contributed to the growth in physician expenditures.

Growth in Physician Expenditures

What is causing the overall increase in spending on physician services? Contrary to conventional wisdom, the central problem is not the growth or aging of the Medicare population, which explains only about 15 percent of the increase over the past ten years.[5] About half of the increase is related to greater volume and intensity (including the growth of new services and technology) and the remainder to higher prices.

Medicare's current method for paying physicians is the customary, prevailing, and reasonable (CPR) charge system. The payment for a service is an amount that is equal to the least of three charges: the submitted charge, the physician's customary charge, and the prevailing charge for similar services. Year-to-year growth in the prevailing charge is limited by the Medicare Economic Index (MEI), which reflects the physician's cost of doing business. CPR is, in essence, an extremely complicated two-tier fee schedule, with increases in Medicare payments for some (but not all) services limited by the MEI.

Past federal policies have focused almost exclusively on constraining prices as a way of controlling costs, primarily through the MEI introduced in 1972 to constrain the growth of charges, the freeze on charges starting in 1984, and selective price cuts for "overpriced" surgical procedures. Predictably, these policies have at best only temporarily slowed down the rate of increase of Medicare expenditures. Moreover, they have done little to improve the effectiveness of medical care, payment equity, or access to care and beneficiary protection.

These policies have been unsuccessful largely because the medical market in the United States contains strong incentives to encourage growth in the volume and intensity of services. The factors contributing to the growth are well known.

1. *The structure of the payment system.* The fee-for-service system that dominates the market pays for individual services on a piece-rate basis. Clearly, this system rewards the provision of more services. Although much of the increase in volume and intensity does provide real medical benefits, the question remains, where is the dividing line between appropriate and inappropriate care? Under current Medicare payment practices, physicians have some discretion to assign more remunerative codes to services ("upcoding") or to bill separately for services previously billed under one code ("unbundling"). There are no incentives for physicians to reduce their charges, even if their costs go down. Medicare often pays more for specialists than for nonspecialists who provide the same services. As a result, there is a growing proportion of specialists in the Medicare program.

2. *Technology.* Technological growth has given rise to new services

and methods of treatment. Medical progress has been rapid, but expensive. As medical practice has improved, we have been able to save many who, a decade ago, would not have survived. But few institutional changes have occurred to enhance society's ability to weigh the opportunity costs of treating very ill patients in the context of resource constraints. As dramatic (and dramatically expensive on a per case basis) as treatment of severe trauma patients or dangerously premature births or the most complicated cases may be, even greater total costs are incurred for what has become, with technological improvement, routine care. The expanded use of diagnostic and elective procedures—made possible in part by medicine's growing ability to perform those procedures safely, efficaciously, and with less patient discomfort—is driving up U.S. health costs.

3. *Physician supply responses.* The increasing numbers of physicians per beneficiary and the growing competition for patients puts downward pressure on the price of medical services. As the real price drops, there is a financial incentive for the physician to treat patients more intensively, and thus increase billed charges. The risk of malpractice litigation has also encouraged the practice of defensive, and probably wasteful, medicine.

4. *Patient demand.* There have been distinct improvements in medical care—conditions that were formerly untreatable can now be treated, and the discomfort of many procedures has been reduced. This is indeed a positive development, but it has increased the demand for care. The same effect has been produced by the availability of higher supplemental insurance coverage and greater physician acceptance of Medicare charges as payment in full, both of which reduce financial disincentives.

These are strong forces in today's medical market, and they are not transitory phenomena. The environment they have formed around physicians and payers will clearly persist in the years to come. Any reform proposal must, in some way, address these important factors.

Policy Alternatives for Medicare Payment Reform

According to the Health and Human Services 1987 report to Congress on paying physicians, the goals of payment reform could be to: control expenditure growth, ensure continued access to quality care, prevent the transfer of financial burdens to beneficiaries, be clinically reasonable and equitable, simplify the system, establish Medicare as a prudent agent for the government and for beneficiaries, create incentives for efficiency and competition, be implementable soon,

41

respect the diversity of the current system, promote decentralization and deregulation, and minimize disruption.[6] Although each of these goals is laudable, many of them are in direct conflict with each other and some are more feasible than others. Nonetheless, the coming policy debate will have to establish a balance among them. Systematic reform will require a political consensus to determine the trade-offs among competing goals.

For purposes of analysis, it is useful to sort the policy alternatives into types of strategies according to their primary focus, whether it is prices, quantities of services, or the underlying market structure. These are all important concerns of any reform effort, of course, although policies that deal with prices or quantities may be more effective in permanently changing the market than policies that intend to do so directly.

Price-oriented Options. As mentioned earlier, Medicare's CPR system of payment for physician services is based on whichever of the following amounts is lowest: the submitted charge, the physician's customary charge, or the prevailing charge in that locality for similar services. This system has been widely criticized, and some proponents of reform would like to see it either modified or replaced with a fee schedule.

CPR reform. Of the many technical difficulties cited, a particular problem under CPR is how to define localities for payment purposes and determine what procedures should be bundled together. In addition, the system encourages the physician to keep upward pressure on charges, since future payments are tied to past levels. As new procedures are introduced, any special skills or effort expended in providing the new service results in high charges. Even if improved techniques reduce the costs or skills required for the service, charges are not reduced. Under CPR, the charge distribution has become skewed across medical specialties and has created an inflationary trend in the overall level of charges. Although public discussion has emphasized replacing CPR with a new fee schedule, CPR reform could achieve some of the same goals and would perhaps be the least disruptive price-oriented option. It is, however, a short-term measure at best and, like any other attempt to regulate prices alone, does not get at the problems of volume and intensity. Moreover, it may not even correct the inappropriate incentives of CPR.

Fee schedules. Replacing CPR with a fee schedule provides an opportunity to establish in one fell swoop a more understandable, more uniform, and perhaps more acceptable price structure for physicians. A new fee schedule can be developed in many ways, for example, by relying on current charges or by using information on the economic inputs to medical services (as in the resource-based relative value scale).

Whatever approach is used, a fee schedule represents an administrative attempt to reproduce the information about supplies and demands for services that would be generated in a competitive market. This is difficult enough when attempted once; the complexity increases exponentially as the fee schedule is updated and modified over time. Nonetheless, a fee schedule can directly address current pricing inequities and inefficiencies, and ways can be found to moderate the administrative problems of implementing the system. Like other price-oriented options, this policy does not address the problems of increasing volume and intensity.

The Harvard proposal for a resource-based relative value scale is the starting point for the other reform proposals now being discussed in Congress. It is important to remember what the Harvard RBRVS is, and what it is not. First, it is not a self-contained fee schedule. Other statistical components must be developed to turn the RBRVS into a fee schedule. The RBRVS is simply a set of relatives, whereas a fee schedule is a set of prices. Second, it is not the only, and perhaps not even the best, way to develop a resource-based fee schedule. The Physician Payment Review Commission (PPRC) has already proposed a variety of methodological changes in the Harvard model. Third, it is not easily implemented and administered. Fourth, it is not a way of changing the fundamental incentive to expand the volume and intensity of services inherent in the current fee-for-service system. The RBRVS is only a way of setting the prices for a fee-for-service system. And fifth, it is not an easy solution to the many political problems inherent in reforming physician payment. There is no easy solution.

In spite of these limitations, the Harvard RVS is a significant policy proposal. It reflects the dominant view in Washington that an overall reform of physician payment should include a price schedule that deviates substantially from the current structure of charges. It is frequently argued that if current charges are inappropriate and market imperfections prevent a realignment of these charges, starting fresh with a better set of relative prices is a critical step toward reform.

Quantity-oriented Options. Two of the quantity-oriented options, beneficiary cost sharing and second surgical opinions, are directly concerned with consumer demand for services. The remaining options are aimed at influencing physician incentives and decision making.

Beneficiary cost sharing. Medicare beneficiaries are responsible for the first $75 of covered services. After the deductible is met, the beneficiary is responsible for 20 percent of the allowed charge per service and, for unassigned claims, any amount by which the actual charge (as limited by the MAAC) exceeds the allowed charge. The goal of cost sharing is to give beneficiaries an incentive to select less costly providers and to question the necessity of services. The idea of increasing beneficiary costs has not garnered much political support. Recent complaints from Medicare beneficiaries about the costs of the catastrophic benefit and congressional reaction to those complaints are ample testimony to that. In addition, this approach might have little effect because so many of the elderly purchase Medigap insurance, which covers the deductibles and coinsurance.

Second surgical opinion programs (SSOPs). Surgery has accounted for about 40 percent of the total increase in physician spending since 1984. In an attempt to reduce unnecessary risk to patients and to control surgical spending, Medicare and many private payers and Medicaid programs use SSOPs to ensure that the surgery performed is medically necessary. SSOPs are limited by the state of scientific knowledge about the effectiveness of alternative treatments. As more knowledge is gained about effectiveness, there will be a stronger clinical basis for the recommendations of such programs.

Clinical guidelines and effectiveness research. The primary purpose of clinical guidelines and effectiveness research is to provide physicians and others with information that can assist them in determining the type of care that should be rendered to a particular patient. Nonetheless, effectiveness research may affect decisions regarding what services will be covered. The argument for this research strategy is that there is little consensus on when procedures should be done because not enough hard data are available to establish guidelines. Note, however, that neither guidelines based on consensus nor effectiveness research will necessarily reduce the volume and intensity of services; effectiveness research could even lead to the increased use of some services.

The effectiveness strategy has also given rise to some political and policy concerns, such as the appropriate role of the payers, including the Health Care Financing Administration (HCFA), and the providers in approving effectiveness research, how research results are to be used in administering federal and private health financing programs, and how the research will affect individual physician behavior. Debate has also revolved around practice guidelines versus practice standards. Although effectiveness research is in an early stage, this strategy is likely to have long-term implications.

Utilization review and coverage policy. Medicare carriers, peer review organizations (PROs), insurers, and medical societies all attempt to change physician behavior through education, withholding payment, or other sanctions. Still another approach is utilization review, which may operate in three ways: (1) prospectively, before a service is rendered, through preadmission screening or second surgical opinions; (2) concurrently, through the monitoring of care during treatment or after a service is rendered, but before payment is made; and (3) retrospectively, through reviews of claims and medical records, either before or after payment is made. It might be possible to better target utilization review activities on physicians with large increases in Medicare volume and intensity, or in geographic areas where the number of procedures per beneficiary is largest.

The coverage policy approach is closely related to utilization review, although it is administered differently. Coverage policy is the method by which Medicare defines the services it will pay for and the circumstances in which it will pay. The huge number of existing procedures and the rapid growth in new procedures make coverage policy difficult to administer, with the result that it is not widely used in dampening the volume of medical services. In the case of new technologies, Medicare coverage requires assurance of the safety and effectiveness of the treatment, but the tests used are very general and can only be used to a limited extent to discriminate among treatments. Except in rare cases, existing procedures are covered by Medicare.

Expenditure targets. This option attempts to control Medicare expenditures directly by establishing an acceptable rate of increase in aggregate Medicare expenditures for a given geographic area and time period. One could set an expenditure target for the year for a group of services, all physician services, all Part B services, or even all Part A and Part B services. This method would not attempt to control volume and intensity directly, but it would control the growth of expenditures regardless of what happens to volume and intensity if the policy was successfully implemented.

Medicare could recapture expenditures exceeding the predetermined target in one of two ways: by recapturing excess expenditures through lower payments for services in the next time period, or by withholding a percentage of the payment until the end of the time period, when actual expenditures could be compared to the target amount. If expenditures exceed the target, the withheld amount can be reduced by the excess expenditure amount before being distributed to physicians.

Because this option is a departure from past practice, it has numerous implementation problems that would have to be worked out. To the extent that expenditure targets are enforced by controlling prices, this policy could be as ineffective in controlling service utilization as current pricing strategies. Another factor to consider is the economist's fallacy of composition. Individual physicians, under expenditure targets, would have a strong incentive to increase their own billings as rapidly as possible to get a larger piece of a now-fixed pie. Expenditure targets will probably require new kinds of group negotiations among doctors and between groups of doctors and the federal government. Such developments could alter the nature of competition in the medical marketplace.

Market-oriented Options. The following policy alternatives would bundle together various medical services for payment purposes in order to provide incentives to control costs and reduce the variability in payments that is frequently seen when services are purchased separately. Because a single payment is made for a bundle of services, physicians have less financial incentive to perform services that only marginally affect the patient's health outcomes.

Capitation. Under a capitated approach, Medicare makes a single payment in advance for all covered services for each beneficiary. In contrast to fee-for-service systems, capitated systems provide incentives for providers to control both price and utilization and so create a mechanism for controlling Medicare outlays. Capitated systems have a number of related advantages; federal regulation could be reduced, for example, because the capitated system could handle the details of payment. Although capitated care is widely available in the United States, only 3 percent of Medicare beneficiaries are enrolled in capitated systems. Even if it showed strong growth, other strategies would be necessary for the short and medium term.

Geographic capitation. Under a geographic capitation system, the insurer is at risk for the physician services available to all Medicare beneficiaries living in a particular geographic area, such as a state or carrier service area. In effect, the federal government agrees to buy the Medicare benefit package at a fixed price from a single underwriting entity on behalf of all Medicare beneficiaries in the area. Competition could be encouraged by permitting beneficiaries to enroll in other capitated plans in the same area. Under this approach, Medicare might be able to take advantage of the benefits of dealing with capitated entities without having all beneficiaries enroll in health maintenance organizations or other capitated plans.

Physician capitation. Another alternative would be to make a capitated payment to physician groups for some or all Part B services, instead of all Medicare services. Services covered could include all physician services or a package of selected services, such as primary care along with outpatient laboratory tests and X rays. The individual primary care physician or group practice could receive a capitated payment for the primary care of each enrolled beneficiary. The obvious advantage of physician capitation is that it provides direct control over Medicare's physician expenditures without restricting the capitated group to full-service providers.

Preferred provider organizations (PPOs) and other managed care arrangements. A PPO is a network of providers who agree to provide health care services at lower than usual fees in exchange for expected advantages, such as prompt payment and an increased volume of patients. The savings from PPOs are generally achieved through efforts such as utilization review, hospital precertification, concurrent review of inpatient days, discounted fees, and the use of preferred providers.

PPOs, prepaid plans, and other insurance programs often employ case management techniques to control expenditures for particularly expensive patients. For example, they may manage the use of services directly, offer special benefits, and direct patients to particular sources of care.

HCFA is developing a PPO demonstration to test the feasibility of offering Medicare beneficiaries the option of receiving managed health care services on a fee-for-service basis.

Bundling physician and facility payments and physician diagnosis-related groups (DRGs). At present, Medicare makes a separate payment for each physician's service and also makes a payment to the facility providing the services, such as a hospital or ambulatory surgical center. The volume and intensity of some physicians' services might be controlled by making a single payment for all associated physician charges. This payment could be combined with the payment to the facility, or could be made separately to a physician group or to medical staff. There are many possibilities for developing prospective, per case payments for physician services, which might include selected services performed in inpatient (for example, "physician

DRGs") or hospital outpatient departments and ambulatory surgical centers. In general, bundled payments encourage providers to reduce the use of marginal procedures and reduce the opportunity for the discretionary billing of services.

Other Policy and Implementation Issues

The Harvard study, coupled with other HCFA research, has provided empirical insight into some of the issues that must be addressed in the coming months of political debate.

Budget neutrality. Some have argued that a budget-neutral fee schedule (or some other reform) is needed to gain the acceptance of the physician community. This idea is debatable, although it is certain that payment reform will not seek to increase Medicare expenditures.

Even budget-neutral implementation might require an expenditure cut in one sense. Physicians whose fees have been cut are likely to increase the volume and intensity of the services they provide. The response is likely to depend not only on the physician's ability to recoup losses by inducing volume, but also on many other factors, such as the ability to substitute other services, the amount of discretion the physician has over billing for services, the degree of physician dependence on income from Medicare, the ability to recapture Medicare losses from non-Medicare patients, and the degree to which other payers also adopt payment reforms. HCFA actuaries would estimate how much volume might increase with the introduction of a fee schedule. Budget neutrality would require an appropriate reduction in the amount of money *per service* going into the system, in order to maintain a constant total expenditure. Budget neutrality does mean an expenditure reduction to those physicians who maintain a constant volume of services in the face of reduced fees.

Degree of income redistribution across specialties or among physicians. Under a RBRVS fee schedule, fees for evaluation and management services could rise by as much as 70 percent, while some surgical fees could drop by as much as 60 percent.[7] Although some have questioned whether the redistributions will necessarily be that large, sizable redistributions across specialties are predictable. Are changes of this magnitude politically acceptable? Would they have an impact on access to care? This issue is already part of the debate and a phase-in period or some other softening of the impact of payment reform is likely to be implemented.

In discussions of the Harvard RBRVS, attention has focused primarily on income redistribution across specialties, but geographic redistributions may be more politically significant. Congress has asked the HCFA to develop an index to adjust for differences in practice costs across geographic localities. There are numerous ways to develop such an index, just as there are numerous ways to develop a national fee schedule. Without going into the technical details of index construction, some examples can be cited to illustrate the kinds of redistributions possible. According to the HCFA's estimates, implementing RBRVS nationwide would increase total physician payments in Columbus, Ohio, by roughly 1 percent.[8] Instituting RBRVS in a budget-neutral way with a full geographic adjustment could reduce physician payments in Columbus by as much as 5 percent. Since Columbus is a somewhat lower-cost place to practice than the rest of the country, a geographic adjustment reduces payment. In contrast, average expenditures in New York City would drop 39 percent. Given the high costs of doing business in New York City, however, a full geographic adjustment reduces that cut to 22 percent, which amounts to a 17 percent differential. These examples are based on only one form of geographic practice-cost index, but they illustrate how any such index could work.

It would be difficult to justify a fee schedule that did not account in some way for obvious differences in practice costs across localities. But it is also clear that the impact of even the most logically developed fee schedule could be contentious. The case of rural physicians may be instructive. Specialists and surgeons are less prevalent in rural than in urban areas, and for that reason one might expect rural physicians to fare better financially under an RBRVS fee schedule than under the current charge structure. Again referring to HCFA estimates, if RBRVS is implemented without a geographic practice-cost adjustment, physician payments in rural west Texas would increase 3 percent. With a practice-cost adjustment, however, payments could decline 15 percent. Although the size of the redistribution could be reduced by using a different statistical formulation, the point is that such a result is possible. With extremely low real estate prices and other costs in many rural areas, physician incomes may be redistributed away from rural areas, even though such areas are often medically underserved.

Political mechanisms will develop to "correct" such anomalies. If a fee schedule is justified, a method of reclassifying physician localities could develop. Note that Congress has requested similar urban-rural reclassifications for hospitals under PPS.

Another factor that influences the pattern of redistribution is the level of charges prevailing in an area in relation to the national average. California, for example, has high prevailing charges for physician services, and consequently the institution of an RBRVS fee schedule would reduce allowed charges by 19 percent. Illinois, in contrast, has low prevailing charges, and would gain 9 percent with an RBRVS. These estimates are clearly not the result of skewed distributions of physicians by specialty in these states.

Who wins and who loses under physician payment reform ultimately depends on the dispersion around the average payment for any group of physicians. For example, internists gain an average of 15 percent with an RBRVS fee schedule, but 18 percent of all internists would *lose* 10 percent or more in allowed charges. Similarly, thoracic surgeons lose an average of 27 percent with RBRVS, but 7 percent of these surgeons *gain* 10 percent or more in allowed charges. This dispersion reflects both the mix of services provided by individual physicians and the distribution of physicians in areas with relatively high or low prevailing charges. This kind of dispersion about the mean is also seen across different geographic areas and across specialties within a given area. The unavoidable complexity of the impact of a systemwide change like RBRVS certainly makes political choices that much more difficult.

Balance billing and mandatory assignment. Some might argue that an RBRVS-based fee schedule is scientifically determined and is so accurate that it represents the "right" prices and for that reason should be considered payment in full for medical services. Others would point out that the fee schedule simply reflects averages— average patients with average conditions treated by average doctors in the average American town—and that actual situations are seldom "average" and require some flexibility in billing. It is true that a fee schedule would raise the fees for some services, and therefore would also increase the beneficiary's liability for copayments. Whether or not a type of fee schedule or some other reform is implemented, balance billing is an important issue. Numerous proposals dealing with balance billing are already under discussion. They range from no limits on charges of any kind, to controls on the rate of charge increases, to caps on the balance billing amount, to assignment for the low-income elderly, to full mandatory assignment. Restrictions on balance billing could lead to unacceptable reductions in access to care in those cases where a fee schedule sets too low a price. Furthermore, the high percentage of physicians who accept Medicare charges as payment in full suggests that balance billing restrictions may not provide much additional beneficiary protection. Assignment rates vary from state to state, however, and streamlining of the current MAAC limits is high on the Congress's agenda. Consequently, a new policy to limit balance billing is likely to receive careful consideration.

Concluding Remarks

Wholesale reform of Medicare's physician payment system is needed, and circumstances have made policy changes inevitable. What kinds of policies will be enacted and whether they will truly constitute systemwide reform remain to be seen. No single policy option can, by itself, provide the desired changes. As a result, most proposals now under discussion combine several strategies. The PPRC, for example, supports a modified RBRVS fee schedule with national expenditure targets and continued restrictions on balance billing. PPRC also supports the development of medical practice guidelines, enhanced utilization review, and the encouragement of capitated systems and physician group practices. The American College of Surgeons (ACS) proposes a fee schedule for surgical services that is based on both resource costs and demand-side factors, expenditure targets for surgical services, practice guidelines, and assignment for low-income Medicare patients. The ACS approach to a fee schedule would substantially reduce the redistributive effects of an RBRVS fee schedule. The American Society of Internal Medicine supports RBRVS and effectiveness research, but rejects expenditure targets. Other groups will undoubtedly develop additional alternatives.

The final decision on payment reform rests with Congress. As Congress considers the issues, the political ramifications of each alternative will loom large. Which groups favor a given option and the financial impact of an option on constituents are important. Equally important are the new incentives that each option would create in the medical market. From an economic perspective, the best policy will be the one that provides incentives for prudent and appropriate medical care in a cost-effective way. Let us hope that Congress can find such a reform option in the months to come.

3

The Implications of Resource-based Relative Value Scales for Physicians' Fees, Incomes, and Specialty Choices

David Dranove and Mark A. Satterthwaite

Fees that Medicare pays to reimburse physicians for their services, translated to an hourly basis, vary considerably by specialty. As Hsiao et al. document, for example, surgeons' fees are substantially higher than internists' fees even after corrections are made for differences in the length of training, office expenses, and malpractice coverage.[1] A resource-based relative value scale (RBRVS) is intended to adjust fees so that (1) all specialties are compensated at about the same hourly rate (after correcting for intensity of work and costs of training, office operations, and malpractice coverage) and (2) with the new fee structure the aggregate amount paid by Medicare to all physicians remains essentially unchanged. Such a change, Hsiao et al. assert, would ameliorate noncompetitive distortions in physician fees that exist because of the pervasiveness of insurance, imperfect information of consumers, and legal restrictions on competition.[2]

To evaluate the desirability of basing payments on RBRVS, one needs to understand the sources of the observed pathologies in the current system of fees. If, on one hand, the current differences are an equilibrium result, then attempts to undo them through the imposition of a new fee schedule may ultimately fail through market responses to it. If, on the other hand, the pathologies result from historical practice in the administration of Medicare, private health

Ted Frech and Frank Sloan both made useful comments that have materially improved this chapter. This material is based upon work supported in part by the National Science Foundation under grant SES 8705649. Any opinions, findings, conclusions, or recommendations expressed in this publication are those of the authors and do not necessarily reflect the views of the National Science Foundation.

insurance, and the medical education system, then a new fee schedule has a reasonable prospect of achieving its goals over both the short and long run.

This chapter, first, presents a theory of physician fee determination that explains the observed discrepancies in the rates at which current fee schedules compensate physicians and, second, works out this theory's implications for a world in which Medicare payments to physicians are set on the basis of an RBRVS. Payments based on an RBRVS are assumed to change dramatically the distribution of Medicare reimbursements across specialties while remaining almost budget neutral for the federal government.[3] In the short run this tends to lessen existing differences in compensation rates and average incomes earned by physicians in different specialties. This theory, however, implies that in the long run the self-interested specialty choices of physicians may tend to restore existing income differentials among specialties even if the partial equalization of compensation rates that an RBRVS is designed to achieve is permanent.

Fee Determination in the Short Run

Physician fees are not set competitively by supply and demand. If physician fees were competitively set, a physician of given clinical skill, personal attentiveness, office setup, and hospital affiliation would have no discretion in the fee charged. Each physician would first select qualitative attributes, read from the market the fee schedule those attributes implied, and then select a quantity. Patients would regard all physicians of the same price and qualitative attributes as perfect substitutes. A competitive market with price determined by supply-and-demand considerations implies that if (1) physician i and i' both charged the same fee and had the identical qualitative attributes and (2) physician i decided to reduce patient load by a given amount and physician i' decided to increase patient load an exactly compensating amount, then the required number of patients would without protest switch from i to i'.

This and other implications of perfect competition are, of course, absurd in relation to the reality of the physicians' services markets. Consumers generally care about the personal identities of their physicians. If physicians i and i' appear to have identical fees and skills, some patients idiosyncratically prefer physician i whereas others prefer i'. Because there is idiosyncracy in consumer preferences, each physician faces a downward-sloping demand curve. A physician who either charges a higher-than-average price or possesses lower-than-average skills still attracts some patients. Each physician sets fees

FIGURE 3–1
Demand for Physician Services under Monopolistic Competition

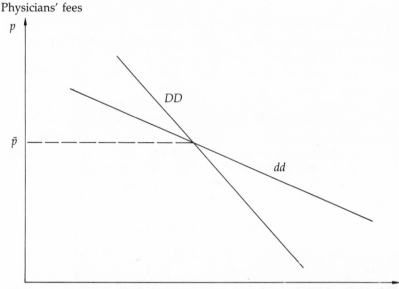

partly in response to these demand considerations and partly in response to cost considerations. That is, each physician has monopoly power to exploit in setting fees. Consequently in all but the smallest metropolitan areas or rarest specialties the appropriate model of physician fee determination is monopolistic competition.

For the purposes of this chapter the essential aspects of monopolistic competition are as follows.[4] Figure 3–1 diagrams the demand function facing a monopolistically competitive physician. The curve labeled DD, the market demand curve, is the demand physician i would serve if all physicians in that specialty coordinated their prices as if they were a cartel. (More properly this is the fractional market demand curve because it is the physician's fraction of the market demand for care in a specialty.) Its price elasticity of demand is just the price elasticity of consumers' demand for services of that specialty. (This is the elasticity that the RAND health insurance experiment measured.)[5] The curve labeled dd, the physician's individual demand curve, is the demand physician i faces if all other physicians in the community fix their fees at $\bar{p}$ and physician i varies his individual price p. It is more elastic than DD because it reflects the

54

tendencies of consumers both to consume less as price rises and to switch away from high-priced providers to lower-priced providers. (This is the elasticity measured by Lee and Hadley and McCarthy.)[6] By definition the individual demand curve cuts the market demand curve at $\bar{p}$.

All physicians i are assumed to maximize net income.[7] In the short run they do this by taking $\bar{p}$ as fixed and adjusting p. They take $\bar{p}$ as fixed because all but the smallest communities have many competing physicians. Therefore when physicians change their price, they have only a negligible effect on competitors, who do not react to the changed price; this vindicates the assumption that $\bar{p}$ is fixed. The solution to this pricing problem is to set the price so that marginal revenue equals marginal cost. This condition simplifies in this context to the well-known formula

$$p = \frac{MC}{(1 + 1/\alpha)} \tag{3-1}$$

where $\alpha < -1$ is the price elasticity of the physician's individual demand and MC is the physician's marginal cost. (The interpretation of α, the price elasticity, is that if p_i is increased 1 percent, then the quantity demanded increases α percent. If $\alpha = -2$, then a 1 percent increase in price results in a 2 percent decrease in demand, for example.) Thus if either marginal cost increases or demand becomes less price elastic (that is, α increases toward -1), then a physician has a tendency to increase price.

Determinants of Individual Demand Elasticities

If the physicians' services market is indeed monopolistically competitive, then a key to understanding variation of fees across metropolitan areas and across specialties is understanding the determinants of physicians' individual demand elasticities. Satterthwaite and Dranove and Satterthwaite have developed such a theory based on consumer search:[8] consumer preferences are idiosyncratic, and the information that each consumer obtains about each physician is noisy in the statistical sense. The greater the idiosyncracy relative to the noise, the smaller is the individual demand elasticity facing each physician.

The premise of the theory is that each consumer who needs a physician searches among the physicians in a community for one who offers an acceptable match in quality, price, personal manner, and location. This matching process is quite idiosyncratic: one consumer may prefer physician i over physician i', while another consumer with objectively similar needs may prefer i' over i. Consumer search for a physician is likely to be indirect through the solicitation of recommendations from relatives, trusted friends, and knowledgeable acquaintances. This type of search takes substantial time and yields noisy information.

Such a conception of how consumers search implies that each physician has market power in the sense of a downward-sloping individual demand curve with respect to price. Some consumers find physicians who match their idiosyncratic needs and preferences extremely well, probably much more than a physician in the community chosen at random. A consumer so fortunate becomes a loyal patient. If the physician raises the price marginally, the match remains sufficiently good that such a patient still selects that physician. Some patients of the physician are less loyal because their match is barely adequate. If the physician raises the price marginally, then these patients are likely to continue their search because the higher price converts the barely adequate match into an inadequate match. Thus a physician loses some, but not all, patients each time the price increases. The responsiveness of demand to changes in price depends on the costliness of search, the degree of idiosyncracy in consumer preferences, and the noisiness of their estimates of the physicians' actual price levels.

Search Costs. Searching for a physician is a time-consuming and anxious task. A consumer who has an extended family living nearby may find it much easier to obtain useful recommendations than does a consumer who has no relatives in the area. Similarly people in communities that are growing rapidly or have rapid turnovers of residents may find a search more expensive than do people in more static communities. Satterthwaite shows that if the difficulty of consumer search decreases, then individual demand with respect to price becomes more elastic, provided reasonable assumptions about the underlying probability distributions are satisfied.[9] As the search becomes cheaper, consumers can make finer distinctions among physicians.

Accordingly in communities where search is relatively easy, physicians' individual demand functions tend to be relatively elastic. Physicians in such communities have an incentive to set relatively competitive prices. Physicians in communities where search is hard, by contrast, have an incentive to set relatively high prices. Not only may search costs vary across communities, they may also vary across specialties. It seems plausible, for example, that families with young children may find search for a community pediatrician cheaper than a search for pediatric cardiologist, as they are likely to have many friends and relations who can provide information about the former but not the latter. To the extent this is true, then pediatric cardiologists have an incentive to set their price so that their markup above marginal cost in percentage terms is greater than that of community pediatricians.

Noisiness of the Estimates. An evaluation of a physician is never perfectly precise, particularly if the evaluation is based on the physician's reputation rather than repeated experience. The accuracy of the evaluation may vary according to the aspect of physician practice being evaluated. The recommendation may be accurate, for example, about the amenities of the physician's office, less accurate concerning the physician's pricing, and almost noninformative about technical skills. Dranove and Satterthwaite show that as a consumer's observation of price becomes less precise and noisier, demand becomes less elastic.[10] In making a choice between two physicians, a consumer cannot make the choice on the basis of prices that cannot be observed. Observability may vary across both communities and specialties.

Idiosyncracy of Consumer Preferences. Consumers search for physicians who provide good idiosyncratic matches to their particular needs. The idiosyncracies may be as simple as location but may also relate to style of practice and even skill. A prospective mother, for example, may seek out information from friends to identify a good obstetrician but for personal reasons may idiosyncratically prefer an obstetrician who supports Lamaze deliveries. Dranove and Satterthwaite show that greater idiosyncracy in preferences decreases the individual price elasticities of demand.[11]

Without idiosyncracies patients may have little reason to choose between physicians. Idiosyncracies in preferences create loyalties that enable physicians to set high prices. Once a mother has had one successful Lamaze delivery, she is likely to prefer strongly the same physician to assist in the next one. If other expectant mothers have similarly idiosyncratic preferences, then obstetricians face relatively inelastic individual demand curves and have an incentive to set a large price-cost margin.

Insurance. Since insurance reduces the out-of-pocket cost consumers bear, it makes less elastic the demand the individual physicians face and thus increases the fees that they tend to charge. Variability of insurance coverage exists across specialties and across communities and induces variability in fees. There are many possible reasons for variability in insurance coverage. Surgical specialties may be better insured than nonsurgical specialties both because surgery tends to involve greater financial risk to the consumer than do most medical therapies and because the completion of surgical procedures is more easily verified than is the delivery of cognitive services such as diagnosis. Market demand for surgery may be less price elastic; moral hazard is less of a concern. A particular community may have fuller insurance coverage across all specialties than is typical, for example, because of the historical strength of a large union in the community.

Physician Supply. The supply of physicians in a community is not included as a determinant of physicians' individual price elasticity because no direct causal relationship is apparent between the number of physicians in a community and the demand elasticities they individually face. Indirect relationships, however, may exist. Satterthwaite, for example, has proposed that increasing the number of physicians in a community raises consumers' search costs.[12] As the number of physicians increases, each physician's reputation becomes more diffuse; that is, physicians are relatively anonymous in large cities. Thus increasing the number of physicians may actually lead to higher fees. Conversely, increasing the number of physicians in a community may lower marginal cost, and thus prices, because each physician tends to see fewer patients than previously. Consequently, increasing the supply of physicians has an indeterminate effect on the fees they charge.

Summary. Price in the physicians' services market is determined jointly by marginal cost and the individual physician's price elasticity of demand through the formula $p = MC/(1 + 1/\alpha)$. This price elasticity α is determined by a host of influences: the cost of the consumers' search, the noisiness of consumers' price observations, the degree of idiosyncrasy of consumers' preferences, and insurance all appear to be important. The model has been applied in Pauly and Satterthwaite, as well as Satterthwaite, to explain price variation within a particular specialty across communities.[13] The model can equally well be applied to explain price variation within a particular community across specialties.

Effects of Medicare on Demand and Short-Run Equilibrium Price

To understand how an individual physician's selection of a fee would be affected by a relative-value scale, one must first examine the

FIGURE 3-2
KINKED DEMAND CURVE FOR PHYSICIAN SERVICES TO
MEDICARE RECIPIENTS

Physicians' fees

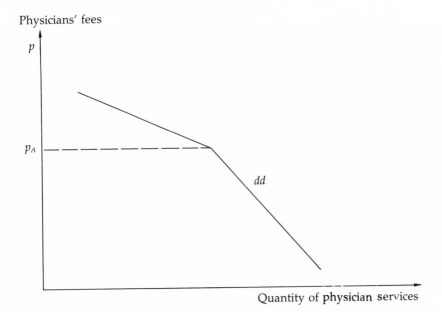

Quantity of physician services

decision each physician faces regarding acceptance of assignment and balance billing.[14] The decision to take assignment depends on at least four factors: the physician's customary fee to non-Medicare patients, the Medicare prevailing fee, the fee the physician would charge Medicare patients in the absence of assignment, and the costliness in office expenses and payment delays of not accepting assignment. In electing not to accept assignment, in all likelihood a physician prefers to charge a price to Medicare patients that exceeds the Medicare prevailing rate; that is, the physician wishes to balance bill.

Figure 3-2 shows the individual demand curve dd that an individual physician faces from Medicare recipients; this figure is a simple modification of the individual demand curve in figure 3-1. Let p_A be the lesser of the Medicare prevailing fee and the physician's customary fee; it is the price the physician receives if assignment is accepted. The physician's individual demand is kinked at p_A. If the physician does accept assignment, the fee charged is no greater than p_A and the Medicare patients bear out-of-pocket at most 20 percent of that fee. If the physician balance bills, the fee charged is greater than p_A, and the

Physicians' fees

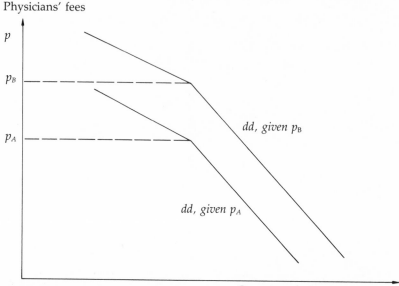

Quantity of physician services

patients bear 20 percent of p_A plus 100 percent of the balance greater than p_A. This kink at p_A creates a discontinuity in the physician's pricing response; for a wide range of marginal costs up to some critical value, the physician maximizes income by choosing price p equal to p_A.[15] For marginal costs above this critical value, the physician prices above p_A and balance bills.

Changes in the Medicare Prevailing Fees. If Medicare increases its prevailing fee from p_A to p_B, three cases must be considered. First, the typical physician in the specialty has been accepting assignment and setting the fee p equal to p_A. Figure 3–3 shows the effect of such an increase in the Medicare prevailing rate from p_A to p_B. The kink shifts up, and the slopes of the segments of the individual demand curves remain unchanged. The slopes are invariant because they are determined by consumers' search behavior, which is not affected by the level of the Medicare prevailing fee. Because of the changed location of the kink, the physician almost certainly finds it advantageous to increase the fee to the new prevailing fee p_B and to continue accepting assignment.

Second, the typical physician has not been accepting assignment initially, which means that fee p is greater than the initial Medicare prevailing fee p_A. The new Medicare prevailing fee p_B is increased sufficiently so that it exceeds the physician's fee p. In this case the physician will certainly raise his fee to at least p_B and may raise it further. If p is raised only to p_B, then the physician will begin to accept assignment; otherwise balance billing will be continued.

Third, the typical physician has not been accepting assignment and has been setting fee p both above p_A, the original Medicare prevailing fee, and above p_B, the new prevailing fee. In this case the physician continues to balance bill but at a price higher than p. The price is raised because at price p the individual demand is less elastic when the prevailing rate is increased to p_B. In a manner analogous to that shown in figure 3–3, raising the prevailing fee shifts out the physician's individual demand curve so that at price p a greater quantity of services is now sold. Specifically each consumer's out-of-pocket cost is reduced at least 80 percent of the difference $p_B - p_A$, which causes the consumer to demand a greater quantity. This increased quantity, with no change in the slope of the dd demand curve, implies that this demand becomes less elastic at the original price p. The pricing formula (equation 3–1) then implies that the physician increases price.

In this third case the amount of the price increase depends on the amount of the quantity increase at the original price p when the Medicare prevailing fee increases to p_B. The increase in quantity is determined by the slope of the market demand curve. Market demand for some specialties may be more elastic than for other specialties; specialties with more elastic demands tend to increase their fees more. Nevertheless market demand for most specialties is not particularly elastic; the price increase in response to an increase in the Medicare prevailing fee is likely to be small, and the actual out-of-pocket costs to consumers probably decrease.

Conversely, if the Medicare prevailing fee is reduced from p_A, then the story reverses in the obvious manner. The physician who accepts assignment at p_A most likely reduces his fee to the new Medicare prevailing fee and continues to accept assignment. Some physicians who have accepted assignment stop accepting assignment and begin balance billing. The physician who balance bills reduces his fee (but probably not as much as the Medicare prevailing fee was reduced) and continues to balance bill. Out-of-pocket expenditures for patients of balance-billing physicians may therefore increase.

This analysis raises an interesting and perverse possibility: an RBRVS that is budget neutral from the viewpoint of Medicare may

61

significantly increase cost to Medicare recipients. Such a scenario has a certain degree of face validity. Those specialties that would experience reductions in fees with the imposition of an RBRVS could have the most inelastic market demand. To the extent these specialties balance bill, their response to RBRVS would be to make only slight reductions in the fees at which they balance bill their patients. Conversely specialties that would experience increases in fees with the imposition of an RBRVS could have the most elastic market demand. To the extent they balance bill, their response would be to increase their fees. The net result could be an increase in consumers' total out-of-pocket expenditures (and an increase in physicians' gross income), despite the RBRVS's budget neutrality for Medicare.

Change in Marginal Cost. Over time the marginal cost of a particular procedure could fall substantially, and demand for that procedure could come predominantly from Medicare recipients. The presence of a kink at the Medicare prevailing fee, p_A, in each physician's demand for that procedure implies that even as cost falls, the physician's maximizing strategy is to reduce price no further than p_A and to begin accepting assignment if not already doing so. As a consequence profit margins may increase rather substantially over time.

Balance Billing. Balance billing adds considerable uncertainty to predicting the ultimate effects from any reform of Medicare fees such as an RBRVS. Nevertheless balance billing serves two important roles within the Medicare system. First, balance billing can reward quality. The possibility of securing a higher-than-average price is an important incentive for the physician of superior ability to invest the effort needed to translate ability into exceptional service.

Second, balance billing provides a safety valve that essentially guarantees access to care for most Medicare patients even if serious errors are made in the setting of Medicare fees. If balance billing is forbidden and if for a particular specialty Medicare fees are set too low relative to the fees that practitioners can obtain from serving non-Medicare patients, then a proportion of physicians may refuse to serve Medicare patients. Access would be compromised. To the extent that Medicare fees are noncompetitive with non-Medicare fees, physicians will balance bill to make up the difference and access will not be as seriously compromised, except among lower-income elderly.

Summary. Instituting an RBRVS such as the one proposed by Hsiao would generally decrease Medicare payments for surgical specialties and increase Medicare payments for cognitive specialties.[16] Physicians in surgical specialties would be able to undo partially the economic effects of the RBRVS, however. Surgical specialists who are already balance billing tend to reduce their full price less than the amount by which the RBRVS reduces the Medicare prevailing fee. Surgical specialists who are accepting assignment are more likely to begin balance billing. Similarly, cognitive specialists who are balance billing tend to increase their full price less than the amount by which the RBRVS increases the Medicare prevailing fees or begin to accept assignment. The effect on aggregate gross physician income is thus indeterminate, even if the RBRVS is budget neutral for Medicare.

Location Decisions in the Intermediate Run

"Intermediate run" means a period long enough for a physician to move to a new location if that new location promises a better package of income and satisfaction but too short to abandon the current specialty and either to enter a new specialty or to quit medicine entirely. Marder finds that a substantial percentage of physicians change their county of practice each year.[17] This coupled with the location decisions of new physicians suggests that substantial location adjustments are made in the intermediate run. Each physician tends to select the community in which to practice at least partially on the basis of the income likely to be earned.

This tendency implies that in the intermediate run physicians of given ability within a particular specialty will earn about the same real income in whatever community they locate. Suppose community k has M members of a given specialty, and community k' has M' members. Further suppose a freshly trained physician in that specialty can earn more income by locating in community k. The physician tends to locate there. When located there, the physician reduces the average income of physicians in that specialty in that community k because price tends to stay unchanged and demand for the specialty's services is now split among $M + 1$ physicians instead of M. This reduces the differential in incomes between the two communities because income for specialists in community k' remains unchanged. This process continues until incomes for physicians of the specialty in question are equalized in communities k and k'. As implied by this tendency for incomes of physicians in a particular specialty to be equal across communities, a community with demand conditions such that the specialty's fees are above average compared with fees in comparable communities tends to have more specialists per capita than average.

Cross-sectional Correlation of Fees and Physician Supply. This ten-

63

dency for the locational decisions of physicians in a specialty to equalize their incomes across all communities in which they locate explains a well-known conundrum within health economics: regressions of physician fees from a cross section of communities invariably obtain a significant positive coefficient on the physician-population ratio. (This argument was apparently first made by Satterthwaite.)[18] This is strange if one thinks of the physicians' services market as perfectly competitive: if the market is competitive, an increased supply of physicians should drive price down sharply. A recent example of such a regression is found in Cromwell and Mitchell:[19]

> Certainly, the most dramatic finding is the strong, positive influence surgeon density has on equilibrium surgical fees. . . . If the coefficient for surgeons per thousand in eq. (4) is attributed solely to physician inducement, then a 10 percent increase in surgeon density results in a fee inducement of 9 percent per operation, or a long-run elasticity of 0.90. This would imply only a marginal decline in net incomes from surgery with increased competition.[20]

We suggest that the regression is more appropriately interpreted as a semireduced form location equation.[21] Our alternative interpretation is that, if, for reasons of consumer information and insurance, surgical fees in a community are 9 percent above average fees nationally, then the number of surgeons per thousand is expected to be 10 percent above the national average; otherwise the high fees would put surgeons' incomes in that community above the national average for surgeons.[22] More crudely put, high fees attract surgeons: surgeons do not cause high fees.

Effect of RBRVS on Location. A switch to RBRVS would tend to reduce geographic variation in reasonable fees.[23] With balance billing, in markets where the RBRVS reduces fees, the demand curve for individual physician services would shift in. Without balance billing, lower fees would further constrain physicians' pricing. Either way, incomes would fall. Some physicians would migrate to local markets where fees and incomes have risen. New physicians would similarly show stronger preferences for such markets. These migration and entry patterns would persist until once again there is equality in incomes across markets. Unless the RBRVS completely does away with geographic variation in prices, the existing equilibrium relationship between fees and the geographical locations of physicians would persist in attenuated form.

Specialty Decisions in the Long Run

"Long run" means a period long enough for physicians to alter their specialty choice if a new specialty promises a better package of income and satisfaction. As only a small percentage of physicians change specialties, any force for equilibrating incomes across specialties must come predominantly from the specialty choices of new physicians. Consequently income disparities across specialties may persist longer than disparities across location. Nevertheless, if entry into the specialties is free, in the long run the tendency should be for physicians of a given ability to earn about the same income in whatever specialty they choose.

A simple baseline model illustrates this tendency for incomes to equalize across specialties. Average incomes may not equilibrate even in the long run for at least three reasons, which can be illustrated by slightly reformulating the baseline model: (1) compensating income differentials among specialties may be necessary to equalize the attractiveness of the several specialties, (2) high-income specialties may be the beneficiaries of entry barriers such as restrictions on residencies, and (3) average ability may vary across specialties as a result of varying rewards to ability across specialties and self-selection by graduating medical students.

Baseline Model. The model has two specialties. Physicians in specialty 1 are surgeons and produce surgical services; physicians in specialty 2 are internists and produce cognitive services. Competition among physicians within each specialty is characterized by monopolistic competition: each physician sets a markup (price minus marginal cost) according to the elasticity of demand faced. The demand elasticity can vary across specialties; prices and markups can vary across specialties. If consumers, for example, have better information about the prices charged for cognitive services than for surgical services, the price elasticity of demand facing internists is bigger in magnitude than the elasticity facing surgeons. Thus, the markup for cognitive services is less than the markup for surgical services.

A strong tendency exists to equalize incomes in the long run because physician specialty choice is determined in part by the income that physicians can expect to earn in each specialty. Specialties offering higher-than-average incomes over time attract disproportionately many new physicians; this reduces the average income in the specialty. The converse is true for relatively unprofitable specialties. To the extent physicians are free to choose their specialties, these choices tend to equilibrate incomes across specialties, regardless of the prices per unit of service in each specialty.

In the long run a relatively high price per unit of surgery serves to attract more physicians to surgery and reduces the volume of surgery each surgeon provides. Excess capacity in surgery results: each surgeon's volume may be considerably less than capacity. Similarly, relatively low prices for internists means fewer internists, each having high volumes. The incomes of surgeons and internists, however, are identical. Within limits, manipulating the relative fees of surgeons and internists through either market forces or government edict affects the overall income level of physicians and distributes excess capacity between the two specialties but in the long run does not cause any income differential between specialties or any shortages for consumers.

The exception to this occurs when the price for cognitive services is so low relative to the price for surgical services that an internist, to earn what a surgeon earns, must produce such a large volume of services that the capacity constraint is reached. Equilibrium then takes the form that each surgeon has excess capacity and each internist produces at capacity. Surgeons and internists continue to earn identical incomes.

The important feature of this latter equilibrium is that shortages persist in the long run for cognitive services. The number of internists is insufficient to meet the total demand for cognitive services: internist's fees are too low relative to surgeons' fees. As a consequence young physicians choosing their specialties elect surgery; this choice exacerbates the specialty's oversupply and drives down surgeon's incomes, even as a shortage of internists persists.

If prices get too far out of line, this can cause severe problems in the form of shortages. Any reform of fees should be concerned about this possibility. Nevertheless, casual empiricism suggests a good bit of excess capacity exists in the physician services market as a whole. If so, then prices can be altered within some range without causing shortages in either the short or the long run.

Compensating differentials. One plausible explanation of persistent income differentials across specialties is that some specialties may be intrinsically less pleasant than others. Thus a physician entering the less pleasant specialty must be rewarded with premium pay. Manipulating prices cannot eliminate income differentials that result from a compensating differential.

Compensating differentials, however, are certainly idiosyncratic among physicians. To physicians the differential between two given specialties may be positive or negative. Therefore unless the compensating differential happens to be large for the marginal physician (that is, the physician who in equilibrium is indifferent between the two specialties), the income differential between the specialties is small.

Entry barriers. The force behind the equalization of incomes across specialties is the specialty choice decisions of medical school graduates. Suppose, however, a surgical specialty board could somehow restrict the number of surgical residency slots so as to be less than the demand for those slots. This would produce a long-run income differential in favor of surgeons. Seeing the high incomes in surgery, medical students would try to enter residency programs but some qualified students would be excluded because of the supply restriction.

In this case, manipulating prices either through the market or by edict could eliminate the income differential between the two specialties in both the short and long run. Again, a policy that reduces surgeons' fees to the point where their incomes are equal to those of internists completely eliminates the benefits the surgeons obtain from their entry barrier. This also clears the market for residency slots in the sense that the number of students seeking surgical residencies equals the number of residencies available.

Entry barriers may not be a satisfactory explanation of income differentials, especially in the long run. In the long run one expects large queues of potential entrants to lead to relaxation of entry barriers. Noether has shown that this characterized the medical profession as a whole during the period 1965–1984.[24] It is unclear how this characterizes individual specialties. Possibly the costs of training residents in some specialties is much higher than others; this may cause hospitals to be unwilling to expand the supply of slots in those high-cost specialties even when facing excess demand. Additional empirical work is needed to document the existence and nature of entry barriers in specific specialties.

Heterogeneity of ability, returns to quality, and self-selection. An alternative explanation of the persistence of income differentials across specialties is the heterogeneity of physician ability resulting in high-ability physicians earning higher incomes. This by itself does not guarantee income differentials since high-ability physicians may distribute themselves equally across specialties. But if the financial returns to ability differ across specialties, then high-ability, high-income physicians concentrate in the specialty offering the highest returns to ability (low-ability, low-income physicians concentrate in other specialties). In equilibrium, the specialty in which high-ability physicians concentrate has a higher average income than other specialties.

The financial returns to ability may differ across specialties in a number of ways. Of the two discussed here, one is based on the technological characteristics of specialties, and the other, on imperfections in consumer information. This discussion considers a world with two specialties, internal medicine and surgery, and two types of physicians, high-ability and low-ability. High-ability physicians, no matter which specialty they enter, on average produce better outcomes for patients than do low-ability physicians. We finally suppose there are many more low-ability physicians than high-ability physicians, so that in equilibrium there are low-ability physicians in each specialty. Without compensating differentials and entry barriers, free entry guarantees that in equilibrium low-ability physicians earn the same income irrespective of their specialty.

First, the possibility of technological differences across specialties can be considered. For the sake of argument, suppose the incremental difference in outcome that a high-ability physician is expected to produce is smaller in internal medicine than it is in surgery. This could follow from the different technical natures of their practices. As an extreme example, suppose the principal activity of surgeons is transplanting hearts, and the principal activity of internists is providing innoculations before foreign travel. Ability clearly matters more in the former activity than in the latter. Consumers therefore are much more concerned about the surgeon's ability than the internist's ability and are less willing to trade ability for convenience in selecting a surgeon.

As a consequence, high-ability surgeons have much greater demand than do low-ability surgeons. In contrast, high-ability internists have only slightly greater demand than do low-ability internists. The income differential between high- and low-ability physicians must be greater in surgery than it is in medicine. Since incomes of low-ability physicians are the same in both specialties, high-ability physicians in making their specialty choice maximize their income by choosing surgery.

Second, the possibility of asymmetric information can be considered. Physicians know their own abilities, but patients have only noisy estimates of physicians' abilities.[25] Moreover the noisiness of these estimates differs by specialty. The greater the precision with which patients observe ability, the greater are the returns to ability.[26] When patients search for a physician, they get an estimate of ability that is correlated with true ability. High-ability physicians systematically have more patients select them than do low-ability physicians. Consequently, for any given price, the quantity of services demanded from a high-ability physician exceeds that demanded from a low-ability physician. Suppose consumers can observe the ability of surgeons more easily than the ability of internists. Then high-ability surgeons have much greater demand than low-ability surgeons, but high-ability internists only slightly greater demand than low-ability internists. The implication, as before, is that high-ability physicians concentrate in surgery.

The behavior of this market is closely related to Akerlof's "lemons" analysis of used car markets. The inability of consumers when shopping for internists to recognize and reward physician ability drives all high-ability physicians out of internal medicine and into surgery. In Akerlof's model it is the inability of consumers to recognize good-quality used cars that drives all good-quality cars out of the used car market.[27]

It is intuitively plausible that consumers could have less difficulty in observing ability for the high-income specialties such as surgery, radiology, anesthesiology, and pathology than for medical specialties providing cognitive services. First, these high-income specialists are usually based in hospitals, so that their work is more often evaluated by other physicians than by patients. Physicians can likely make sharper distinctions between the quality of other physicians than can patients. Second, the nature of their work lends itself to more objective evaluation. The relative ease of evaluating the outcome of open heart surgery can be contrasted with the difficulty of evaluating the decision to recommend surgical versus medical intervention for heart disease. In general the activities of physicians in the low-earning specialties, which include substantial amounts of diagnosis and treatment of minor problems, as well as health maintenance and prevention, appear less susceptible to objective analysis. The relatively high earnings of dermatologists, a specialty that one might associate more with internal medicine than with surgery, seems to be the exception that proves the rule: their output is easily observable!

If the source of income differences across specialties is differential returns to ability, then changing fees according to the RBRVS may affect the distribution of incomes across specialties. The short-run effect is an obvious change in the relative incomes of physicians in each specialty, regardless of each physician's ability level. In the long run this induces changes in the specialty choices of new physicians; eventually the proportion of high-ability physicians in each specialty will change so as to restore income equality for each ability across specialties. Except by coincidence this will not restore income equality across specialties when income in each specialty is averaged over all physicians of both ability levels.

Conclusion

One of the principal motivations for RBRVS is that the extreme variance of rates of compensation across specialties makes them unacceptable as a guide for public reimbursement. In the short run an RBRVS can achieve some success in eliminating this perceived inequity, although the presence of balance billing may attenuate the effects of the RBRVS. In the long run the entry decision of medical students choosing their specialties may further undo the RBRVS's effect in the sense that current income differentials may be restored, even if current differentials in rates of compensation are somewhat narrowed. Hard predictions as to these long-run effects cannot be made because of poor understanding of the causes for the current income disparities. Nevertheless these negative conclusions should not be regarded as an endorsement of the status quo. The current sets of prices that different specialties charge result from an obscure process of monopolistic competition that has been influenced by factors such as consumers' abilities to observe prices accurately. No reason exists to think that the resulting prices are even close to optimal in any reasonable sense.

The Relativity of Prices to Medical Care

A Commentary by Frank A. Sloan

The basic issue considered here is how much to pay physicians for the various types of services they provide. Since, at least for the time being, the fee-for-service system will be retained, the discussion centers around how much physicians should earn for performing various tasks per unit of time. The task is determining more the right set of wages than the right set of incomes. Of course wage rates and incomes are related. Because of the focus on relative values, this commentary is limited to relative prices for medical care, without a discussion of issues related to the determination of the price of a relative value unit. Ideally the market would provide a guide for relative prices. But there is widespread unease about using prices for various physicians' services as a guide because such prices may be distorted. Potential sources of distortion include differential insurance coverage for various types of services and perhaps varying degrees of market power for various services for other reasons as well, such as different degrees of consumer ignorance for different types of services. Hernia repairs are rather common, but complex treatment modalities for certain cancers are not.

To establish relative values, one would like to preserve legitimate sources of variation in the existing price structure while eliminating the variation from illegitimate sources. This is difficult.

Legitimate sources include nonphysician input price differences and compensating physician wage differences because of risk (medical malpractice insurance does not fully indemnify physicians), wear and tear (some specialties may be more stressful than others), prestige, regularity of work hours, locational amenities, training cost, amount of attention needed for a task (the cost of a mistake varies across procedures), ability (some types of work require rare talents, for example, microsurgery), and effectiveness of a procedure (if a

71

diagnostic procedure results in a quicker and more certain diagnosis, for example, it should be priced higher).

Illegitimate sources of variation in existing prices include: entry barriers, perhaps from binding limits on the slots in certain residency programs; inadequate information flows, abetted by restrictions on information flows; and insurance-induced distortions, produced, for example, by imbalances in coverage for various procedures. It is not easy to ferret out effects on existing prices from these illegitimate sources. Moreover, as a long-run strategy, it is preferable to deal with these illegitimate sources of variation, such as entry barriers or impediments to the flow of relevant information, directly rather than to rely exclusively on a pricing policy based on a relative value scale. Such policies as antitrust counter guildlike practices of the medical profession.

Although relatively high ability merits a high relative price, a relative value scale is likely to be a blunt instrument. One would like to pay the talented hand surgeon a high price and the blundering hand surgeon a pittance. As a practical matter, a relative value scale cannot make this type of distinction. Other policies are needed: good information flows, meaningful peer review, and the like.

Dranove and Satterthwaite, in chapter 3, always seem to offer new insights. This chapter is no exception. These comments reflect a perspective from the empirical side of the discipline of economics, although the comments are conceptual as well as empirical.

The chapter carefully develops models of physician behavior under the standard assumption (for economists) of profit maximization as well as other assumptions, such as constant marginal cost (for quantity). Predictions are derived when possible. When this is not possible, the authors clearly identify the source of ambiguity in prediction.

The chapter could be strengthened in three areas. First, the chapter treats Medicare as the only buyer of physicians' services. When the creators of Medicare designed the program, they saw Medicare beneficiaries competing with other patients for physicians' time. If Medicare did not pay enough, physicians and other providers would not spend enough time with Medicare beneficiaries. This worry led to acceptance of usual, customary, and reasonable reimbursement for physicians' services under Medicare part B. If at the present time Medicare were to reorient its fees in a major way, Medicare beneficiaries might be placed at risk. This is less of a concern now than when Medicare was adopted, but it is more of an issue in specialties in which physicians are not highly dependent on Medicare patients for revenue. A short-run choice not considered by the authors is the physician choice of patient by payer source. This is probably the first response that the analyst should examine.

Crucial to analysis of effects of a Medicare relative value scale are possible pricing responses of other payers, private insurers, and state Medicaid plans. Would these other payers also realign their fee structures? These other payers might realign their prices in a counter-vailing fashion. The supply of a certain category of physicians could become "inadequate" because of mispricing on Medicare's part. A payer would pay more to "bribe" physicians to keep serving its insureds. Under the Medicare Prospective Payment System, private payers believe that they are paying more as a consequence of Medi-care "tight" pricing policy. That is, hospitals are thought to be raising charges to make up for the shortfall from Medicare. It might be useful to apply various models of strategic behavior to analyze the "game" that may be played by various major payers.

Second, the chapter uses standard models of physician behavior. The use of such models is acceptable for empirical work. The model sometimes generates predictions that can be refuted by statistical analysis. In this chapter, however, there is no empirical work. Conclu-sions follow from the assumptions. One should be told how sensitive these conclusions—and policy recommendations—are to the under-lying assumptions. In their defense one can say that the authors are properly modest about their conclusions because even with the standard assumptions, the direction of effects of policy changes they consider cannot be determined.

Noneconomists and some economists like models in which the physician or hospital has unexploited monopoly power. When the government or private payer (such as a Blue plan) takes an action that hurts the financial interest of the provider, the provider responds by raising price to other payers toward the profit-maximizing position. (This type of behavior was discussed above in the context of Medicare PPS.) According to these models, a surgeon facing RBRVS might raise charges to patients under age sixty-five. To the extent that a surgeon can recoup a loss from Medicare, he or she may not move or leave the specialty. All this goes to show how little can be deduced from a theoretical argument alone.

Third and finally, some of my comments fall under the general heading of empirical. The authors should have referred to the empir-ical literature on physician location and specialty choice. There is also more literature on physician pricing than the authors note, for exam-ple, empirical evidence on the effect of generosity of payer reimburse-ment on fees. Much of this evidence is ambiguous, like the theoretical work. But if it had been considered, it may have yielded some useful insights.

The discussion of physician ability in the chapter is provocative, but again reference to the literature could have been helpful. Even twenty years ago there was literature, based in psychology and in medical education, on the types of persons who enter various physician specialties.

4
Licensure and Competition in Medical Markets

Lee Benham

On October 25, 1983, U.S. Marines landed on the island of Grenada and rescued 650 American students who might have been at some risk from revolutionary conflict. The students were not vacationing there. They were not studying local culture or tropical plants. They were studying to become licensed physicians in the United States. Licensing laws in the United States have limited entry into medicine and have generated high relative earnings for physicians, leading in turn to excess demand for medical education. The St. George University School of Medicine on Grenada was founded in 1977 in response to such excess demand. By paying $6,000 per year for tuition to study in Grenada, individuals whose applications to U.S. medical schools were rejected had a chance of circumventing the usual barriers to becoming a licensed U.S. physician. The military invasion was neither a simple nor an inevitable consequence of licensure. Nevertheless, without the existing system of medical licensure the American students would not have been on Grenada, and without the students the invasion was less likely.

Licensure has important and unappreciated consequences. This chapter addresses an issue less dramatic than marines landing on a beach, but one that is significant to the current concerns: the impact of licensure on strategies followed and on innovations developed to reduce the variability and to improve the quality of medical care.[1] The current policy debate concerns alternative regulation of physicians and the associated consequences for the cost and quality of their services. Through licensing, physicians have been heavily regulated for most of this century. It seems appropriate to explore some of the consequences.

Previous studies have established that effective licensing restricts the entry of new practitioners, raises the earnings of licensed members, and raises prices. Issues about quality, the subject of this chapter, have received less attention.

The emphasis of previous research on earnings and prices likely results more from the analytical neatness of economic theory concerning barriers to entry and the comparative simplicity of the tests required than to the longer and more complicated chains associating licensure with innovation, quality, or organizational structure. Clear tests of the impact of licensure on these less direct consequences are difficult since a licensed environment cannot usually be compared directly with a similar unlicensed environment. Furthermore no theory of licensure indicates with any precision when licensure will be introduced or eliminated; what system might replace licensure is unsure; the relative impact of various anticipated consequences of licensure on many features of the medical marketplace is unknown; and many consequences are unanticipated.

Rationale for Licensure

Medical licensure is usually rationalized on the grounds that medical service is too complex for consumers to make a wise choice, that patients are dependent upon the providers for information and are vulnerable to opportunistic behavior by providers. According to this view medical licensure raises the quality of medical services and reduces the uncertainty of outcome by limiting consumer choice to licensed practitioners who are in turn constrained by professional codes of ethics and by legal limits on the practices permitted. Both the ethical rules and the regulations have traditionally restricted the use of commercial practices such as advertising, brand names, and specialized management accountable to stockholders, auditing, and hierarchical control. Such commercial practices have been anathema to the guild values of professional autonomy and self-regulation and have frequently been viewed as prima facie evidence of poor quality.

The medical licensure system, it is argued, protects consumers by inculcating a code of ethics, by limiting entry to selected high-quality practitioners, by monitoring licensed practitioners through state boards, and by limiting commercial practices. If these methods are successful, low variability in quality should be observed. If variability is low by "reasonable" standards, then little improvement along this dimension can be anticipated from encouraging alternative approaches or other innovations. If, however, the variability is high, the potential for successful innovation in this area is increased.

The practice of medicine involves a heterogeneous mix of patients and problems, with uncertainty of outcome. For this reason, it is frequently alleged that comparisons of quality of care cannot be made across physicians or hospitals, and in fact few comparisons have been made. The small number of studies on this issue reflects the incentives in this market to undertake the appropriate studies. It is useful to review some existing findings: they suggest highly variable outcomes.

Over a four-year period from 1959 through 1962, the National Halothane Study examined 856,000 operations in thirty-four hospitals. An important by-product of this study was the finding of large differences in postoperative mortality among the participating institutions. After adjustments for sex, year, occurrence of a previous operation, physical status, age, and type of operation, a threefold variation in death rates remained for "middle death rate" operations. The authors of the study conclude that "the evidence for 'real' institutional differences in the six operations [examined] is strong. . . . About half the [1,750] positive excesses in death came from three institutions and about half the negative excesses in death came from three institutions."[2] If the patients treated in the three worst hospitals had gone instead to the three best, these data suggest that *ceteris paribus* about 1,750 fewer deaths would have occurred.

A second study, by the Stanford Center for Health Care Research, examined the observed incidence of in-hospital deaths after surgery among 314,000 patients in fourteen surgical categories in 1,224 hospitals.[3] Significant differences in mortality ratios across hospitals were found for five of the surgical categories. The standard deviation of mortality ratios for these five procedures ranged from .36 to .77; in-hospital death also varied substantially across hospitals.

In the same study, in a separate analysis of 8,493 patients in seventeen hospitals, the observed and the expected incidence of death within forty days or of severe morbidity at seven days was calculated for fifteen surgical categories. The ratio of observed death or severe morbidity to expected death or severe morbidity was almost twice as high in the worst hospital as in the best.

A third study, by Luft, Bunker, and Enthoven, examined mortality rates for twelve surgical procedures of varying complexity in 1,498 hospitals during 1974 and 1975. "The mortality of open-heart surgery, vascular surgery, transurethral resection of the prostate and coronary bypass decreased with increasing number of operations. Hospitals in which 200 or more of these operations were done annually had death rates, adjusted for case mix, 25 to 41 percent lower than hospitals with lower volumes."[4]

In a subsequent analysis of these same data, variables other than surgical volume were considered.[5] Hospitals with large house staffs had higher death rates than expected, and hospitals in the western region had lower rates. Volume remained the most significant variable related to mortality rates, but only a small proportion of total variance was related to the variables examined. The main point again is that standardized death rates varied substantially across hospitals.

Other observations on the variability of quality were provided by experts in the field. The executive director of California's Board of Medical Quality Assurance, Robert Rowland, argued that "10 percent of the physicians who are practicing now should not be practicing without some kind of restraints—either a rehabilitation program, limits on surgery, or some other oversight of practice."[6] The New York state commissioner of health, David Axelrod, said, "As many as ten percent of the state's 45,000 practicing physicians are either mentally or physically impaired or incompetent at some point in their careers."[7]

In response to these allegations concerning the percentage of physicians who should not be practicing, William Rial, president of the American Medical Association, said that the courts and the Federal Trade Commission are responsible for the problems of medical discipline. One implication of Dr. Rial's argument is that the monitoring and disciplining procedures were satisfactory before recent court decisions to increase due process and FTC interventions into the self-regulation process.[8] I have seen no evidence to suggest that the problem of variability is greater today than in the past when the profession had more regulatory autonomy.

Ethical Standards

Why was this high variability observed? High ethical standards, controls over entry, and self-regulation are usually assumed sufficient for adequate quality control. This chapter examines each in turn. The variability in quality would not necessarily diminish significantly even if all practitioners adhered to strict ethical standards.

In an idealized world ethical professionals would consider the pecuniary element incidental to their medical decisions and would never sacrifice their patients' interests to their own. Even this idealized world, however, would retain aspects that adversely affect innovation, quality, and costs. Goods and time are not free, even to the totally self-sacrificing. The day contains only twenty-four hours. Physicians' time available to diagnose and patients' time to be diagnosed and treated are limited. Tests cost money. The problem of scarcity remains. Choices must be made among options.

These ideal practitioners would decide what to do and how on the basis of their training and experience. They would abide by their perception of the norms of good practice. They would decide how much time and how many resources to spend educating themselves on new techniques. They would decide on the effort to be spent on auditing their own performances and on quality control. They would decide how much specialization is appropriate and what procedures are better accomplished by another medical specialist or manager.

For many such decisions, however, high ethical standards do not provide useful guidelines. These professionals have been trained to provide medical services; they are not generally trained in management, auditing, or decision analysis. Even for physicians with appropriate training in these areas, the opportunity to practice and develop skills is limited. They lack time to become fully expert in all these areas; hence some decisions are better than others.

Even if one of these practitioners were sufficiently wise to know the appropriate division of labor and wished to subcontract services, including managerial decision making, when appropriate, a major obstacle remains. Licensed practitioners are constrained by the rules of their professions from subcontracting many procedures. The collective decisions of the licensed profession limit the division of labor. Consumers are thus dependent not only on the ethics and wisdom of the individual practitioner but also on the ethics and wisdom of the collective profession. Is a consensus on all aspects of ethical practice to be expected? If not, then not only must the practitioners be wise and ethical concerning what is to be done, they must be wise and ethical concerning issues of collective choice.

Organizing a profession, or any set of individuals, in a way to promote good policies through collective decisions is a formidable task. The collective decisions depend not only on the constitutional rules under which they operate but also upon the information produced in the market. Thus ethical practitioners must know about the implications of alternative constitutional procedures and the appropriate level of competition to produce the necessary information with which to make both personal and collective decisions, even in a world of highest ethical standards.

Selection and Training

A second method of quality control often proposed is careful selection and intensive training of practitioners. Similar problems arise here. What are the appropriate criteria for selection? What kinds of training enhance performance? What should practitioners know to reduce their variability of performance? To deal with these issues, the possi-

79

bilities of variation in quality must be recognized, and the techniques needed to measure that variation must be understood. Since these depend significantly on statistical techniques, practitioners who make personal and collective decisions should be well informed on statistical matters. Some features of the incentives to learn and apply statistics should be considered.

First some specifics of medical and premedical education can be examined. For the entering medical class of 1987, 28,123 students applied for 17,027 positions. There is considerable competition at this stage, but once admitted, few students fail. The total attrition rate for all reasons is less than 3 percent.[9] Compared with other forms of graduate and professional training, this rate is extremely low. Medical students who are not performing satisfactorily are usually given repeated opportunities to pass. This does not imply that most medical students are lazy or incompetent but simply that the competition for the physician's license is largely concentrated in the premedical years.

Therefore the forms of premedical competition will substantially influence the medical profession's stock of knowledge and the creation and dissemination of subsequent knowledge and innovation. What forms does this competition take? The *Medical School Admission Requirements, 1989–90* states: "College grades are perhaps the most important single predictor of medical school performance . . . the mean undergraduate GPA [grade point average] of first-year entrants for 1987–1988 entering class was 3.44." Only 10 percent of applicants with less than a 3.0 GPA were admitted.[10]

Obviously good grades are important for admission to medical school. If a course is not required for admittance to medical school, prospective applicants must weigh carefully the likelihood of receiving a good grade in that course against its other benefits. Taking even a single demanding course may be risky. Admissions committees argue that grades are only one of several criteria and that diversity and intellectual depth are considered in the admissions decision. A committee faced with 5,000 applicants for 120 places, however, is likely to examine seriously only those transcripts close to the grade norms. Unsurprisingly, few successful premedical students take demanding courses other than required subjects.

Of the total 17,027 members of the entering medical class of 1987, 62.9 percent majored in biology, chemistry, or biochemistry. Only 1 percent majored in mathematics, 0.6 percent in physics, 0.8 percent in economics, and 0.5 percent in philosophy. In addition, medical school requirements for mathematical training are modest. Of the 119 medical schools in the United States, only 47 require any mathematics beyond high school, and only 23 require calculus.[11] Because A's are not easily obtained in mathematics courses, this system discourages mathematical training among premedical students.

In 1989 only one medical school required a statistics course as a prerequisite: the University of South Florida. Few even mentioned statistics as a desirable option. Indisputably, good decision making is central to good medicine. The role of mathematics and statistics in this process is not effectively recognized. A few schools are alert to the possibilities of statistical techniques, for research purposes, but most do no more than require a short course of elementary statistics during medical school.[12]

It can be argued that specialization is appropriate in the modern, complex world and that statisticians should worry about statistics while physicians should concentrate on biology and chemistry. Physicians also make decisions concerning their practice of medicine and concerning the medical policies of hospitals, however. The type of information generated, the interpretation of the evidence, and the approaches to innovation are strongly influenced by physicians' perceptions of what is relevant. These perceptions depend significantly on their knowledge of statistics. To the extent that existing policies discourage mathematical and statistical literacy among physicians, they inhibit innovations in quality control, which depend upon statistics.

State Licensing Boards

A third source of quality control is provided by the state boards of medical licensing. For this control to be successful, adequate resources are required. Yet, few resources have been devoted to monitoring the quality of practice after an individual has been licensed. Applicants to medical school are given close scrutiny. The budgets for the state medical boards suggest that the licensed practitioners are not.

Some comparative expenditures illustrate the contrast between pre- and postlicensing evaluation. For the 1983 incoming class of 120 medical students, Washington University received 5,519 applications. With an application fee of $45, total revenue from applicants' fees was $248,355. This revenue, which is generally spent on the selection process, equals about $2,070 per student ultimately enrolled in that class. If the $2,070 were invested in long-term government bonds with a yield of 9 percent, the investment would produce an income stream of $185.40 per student per year.

Application fees are a trivial part of the total cost to candidates

81

of the selection process. Students spend many years and substantial resources preparing for the selection process. They choose high school and college curricula carefully to achieve high grades and to appeal to the medical school admissions committee. They take special courses to prepare for the Medical College Admission Test. The allocation of a considerable proportion of the higher education resources in the United States is influenced by criteria for medical school admission.

Expenditures of state medical boards made to monitor the quality of licensed practitioners are in contrast to this. The state of Florida, as an example, in 1983 spent about $41.70 per year per physician in monitoring costs.[13] This is less than 25 percent the magnitude of the interest on student application fees.

The budgets of the state boards, however, do not reflect the full resources devoted to postlicensing oversight because medical professionals are charged with monitoring each other. Of 270 allegations of physician misconduct brought to the attention of the Wisconsin Medical Board in 1982, however, only 1 was raised by the state medical society. The defendant in this case was a chiropractor. In another case a physician "had had ten malpractice suits filed against him in ten years, with two awards made to plaintiffs, six settlements out of court, and two suits dropped. Although he was removed from one hospital's staff, no notification was given to others; although the medical society was aware of him, it did not inform the board." A television reporter investigating this matter noted, "I can name right now in our community at least ten pharmacies which refuse to fill prescriptions written by certain doctors. It would be very useful if that information were available to the Medical Board."[14]

The executive director of California's Board of Medical Quality Assurance, Robert Rowland, said in 1983 that California was "one of the few states with a relatively efficient and mature" enforcement system. In 1982, 2,300 complaints were investigated, and approximately 200 formal accusations against physicians were made. From these, forty-four outright revocations or voluntary suspensions of licenses resulted. Rowland noted that although California has a mandatory reporting law, only 11 percent of the complaints came from members of the profession or professional societies. He indicated that the informal approach often used in hospitals of getting "that clown off the staff" was worse than inadequate since such a physician would pose a continuing threat elsewhere. He argued that venal intent on the part of physicians running the program was not the problem. "But the reality is that the positive reinforcement for running an effective program is simply nonexistent." Professionals encounter criticism, hostility, and suspicion from their peers for their enforcement efforts.[15]

The secretary-treasurer of the New Mexico State Board of Medical Examiners, Robert C. Derbyshire, has argued that many offenses warrant a second chance but that some do not. One instance of the latter is trading narcotics for sexual favors. He said this was rare but increasing and cited the case of a physician who had been given a "slap on the wrist" by the medical board after he was found trading drugs for sex. The president of the medical board involved in this case told Derbyshire that "this man lives in my town and I couldn't go back and face my colleagues if we revoked his license." The board president added that the physician in question had a great following and had suffered enough from the publicity, and the board could not deprive him of his means of livelihood.[16]

The New York state commissioner of health, David Axelrod, chastised physicians and hospitals for failure to report misconduct, incompetence, and impairment of physicians. Despite a law that makes disclosure mandatory, he believed that only a fraction of incompetent physicians was being reported. Of the 760 cases reported in 1982, only 12 were referred by the state medical societies.[17]

In one Illinois case a healthy twenty-three-year-old died after exploratory brain surgery. The Illinois Department of Registration and Education and the Medical Disciplinary Board of Illinois did not inquire into the case. Nor did they inquire about the case of a patient who underwent nose surgery and came out a quadriplegic. Nor did the boards pursue other malpractice charges against the surgeon in charge.[18]

These examples illustrate some of the problems associated with the limited resources of the boards and the sparse flow of information to them from practitioners and hospitals. Reforms have been instituted, but the prospects of major improvements in this form of quality control seem limited given the incentives within the system.

The maintenance of quality requires that some set of individuals or some institution have a serious and continuing stake in the matter. The current licensing system severely inhibits the opportunities for specialization in quality control. Under the present system who benefits, other than patients, from systematic collection of the data appropriate to evaluate quality, and who benefits from disciplining a physician?

Licensing Airline Pilots

One could consider the mechanisms of monitoring and quality control in other industries. One major source of control arises from various commercial practices that are proscribed by licensing. In particular, brand-name reputation can be a valuable asset that is at risk if quality varies significantly. A failure of performance by a single employee can adversely affect not only that individual but also the reputation of the firm. If the potential damage is great, the stockholders' and hence the managers' interest is to invest in procedures and managerial systems to reduce that risk.

To illustrate the role of reputation and brand names, the licensing procedures in use in medicine could be imposed on the airline industry. Because consumers are assumed to be incapable of choosing an air carrier and commercial practices are inconsistent with safe and appropriate air travel, an individual who desires to fly would first consult a licensed pilot. The pilot not only would provide advice on the best time of departure and the type of equipment but also would fly the plane or would recommend another flying specialist. The self-interest of the pilot would be assumed not to influence the professional advice given. All licensed pilots would have passed a qualifying examination after many years of preflying training and flying school. The quality of the pilots would be validated by the long and rigorous training program. Commercial practices would be prohibited.

The airplanes would be owned by an individual pilot or by a group of pilots. Sometimes airplanes would be leased, and sometimes local governments would provide planes at low cost to the local licensed pilots. Some pilots would fly regularly, others only occasionally. The pilots would be self-employed and thus not under the control of management or stockholders. They would be regulated by a pilots' code of ethics and by the regulatory structure of the profession. Unethical practices would be monitored by professional boards composed of licensed pilots. The choice of plans, routes, airports, fuel, copilot (if any), speed, takeoff and landing protocol, mechanics, and safety procedures would be made by the pilot.

Since licensed pilots would work alone or in small groups, peer monitoring would be difficult. The pilots' association would collect little systematic information on each pilot. Pilot experience with particular planes would not be systematically collected or distributed, for example. Complaints would sometimes be made by disgruntled consumers or their relatives, and occasionally action would be taken. Every year a few pilot licenses would be suspended or revoked. In some years a flurry of suspensions might be observed, especially after wide publicity concerning drunken flying or planes running out of gas.

Some outsiders might note the accident rate appeared to vary considerably across pilot groups. Prices and travel time would also vary widely. The pilots' association would respond that each trip is unique, that flying is as much art as science, that a crash does not indicate an incompetent pilot, and that higher licensing standards would reduce the incidence of regrettable accidents. The pilots' associations and their licensing boards would examine complaints and check performance. Members of the association and the supervising boards would be committed to quality service and they would try hard. The standards set by the medical profession would be emulated.

If the airline industry were limited to a system of self-regulating licensed pilots, the issues would likely be discussed on the pilots' terms. The pilots might assert that stockholders are interested only in money and not in the safety of passengers; that managers are not pilots and should not interfere with the pilot-passenger relationship; that if pilots were mere employees, they would be constrained from serving the passengers' best interest; that managers would put safety at risk to serve stockholders' interests; finally, that the pilot's reputation and indeed life are on the line in each flight. Who could possibly be better than the pilot at determining appropriate modes of modern complex air transportation?

Given actual experience with commercial airlines, these arguments are likely to be dismissed. Consumers do not want an individual pilot, however well-trained, to decide whether to check the fuel supply before takeoff. Consumers want a system that monitors the pilot's behavior closely. If a pilot drinks and flies, consumers want a system that brings immediate and severe sanctions. Consumers want the likelihood of arrival to be relatively free of the personal preferences or idiosyncratic behavior of the individual pilot.

If a plane crashed under the strict licensing regime, the pilot might be blamed, but what useful conclusions could consumers draw? Since X crashed, one should not fly with X or perhaps even with X's associates. The fact that X crashed would not provide much useful information concerning future flights. Consumers would perhaps become more aware of the variance in pilot quality, but awareness of the problem would not directly promote a system that produced the desired information. Consumers would still be left, as in medicine, with the problem of choosing a pilot for the next trip. They might ask around among acquaintances, but those with the most crucial information might be unavailable, along with their pilot.

If the licensing regime were extremely strict, then systematic information would not be available to compare performances. The cost of collecting such information would be high. Who would have incentive to collect and analyze such information systematically? Certainly not the regulatory boards, which would spend at most a few hundred dollars per pilot per year to monitor and discipline. The pilots themselves would have strong opinions concerning their own ability and the abilities of their fellow pilots. Given the dearth of systematic information available, the probable accuracy of their characterizations is unclear. They would presumably possess some relevant information, but few would publicly characterize themselves or their close colleagues as incompetent. Rarely would they inform the pilots' board of their evidence or opinions.

In contrast to this hypothetical scenario, the present commercial airline system provides a powerful incentive to elicit safe trips from pilots. A principal asset of any airline is its reputation. A crash can have major adverse consequences for the stockholders and employees. Under the present regime a pilot's errors can be costly for many individuals other than the pilot and passengers. Those who are potentially affected find it in their own interest to monitor pilots closely. The resources spent by an airline to monitor and retrain their pilots is vastly greater than would be the case in a strict licensing regime. Procedures are standardized, rules are set, employment contracts emphasize the adverse consequences of pilots' deviant behavior, tests and retraining are given regularly, other employees are encouraged to be alert to and report problems, flight reports are maintained, and accident patterns are explored. If the reputation and assets of the firm are largely dependent upon pilots' performances, then pilots are seriously monitored and provided with technical and human backups.

Some might argue that air safety is a result of federal regulations, but with or without regulations airlines suffer considerable losses from pilot error. Thus airlines that desire survival monitor their pilots closely.

The airline example might be dismissed by some because flying is alleged to be simpler than the practice of medicine. The argument asserts that while each flight differs because of weather, other planes, weight, or mechanical failure, these differences are small in comparison with the differences encountered in the typical medical practice. Even if the argument is accepted that medical practice is inherently the most complex task in the world, the conclusion that strict licensing is the solution does not follow. If flying became more complex, should pilots be more or less carefully monitored by their firms?

Impact of Commercial Practices

More commercial practices in medicine will make the situation worse, it can be argued. What evidence in medicine supports the hypothesis that brand names provide incentive for quality control?

At least one study raises directly relevant issues and illustrates the potential benefits of certain commercial practices.[19] This study is concerned with the quality of contact lenses provided by various professional groups and by commercial sources.

The eye care market is a good place to examine the impact of restrictions on quality because regulations vary across states in the United States. The professional associations expend great efforts to constrain the commercial operations. Regulatory limits are often placed on the type of commercial practices permitted. Limits are placed on the use of trade names, on employer-employee relationships, on relationships between lay individuals or lay corporations and professional corporations, on the number of branch offices a professional may operate, and on practice location (for example, not in drug or department stores).[20] These regulations are generally based on the view that commercial-corporate-nonprofessional practitioners cut corners in the interest of profits and drive even the professional, high-quality practitioners to lower their standards.[21] The stringency of these regulations does vary by state, however, as does the market share of commercial firms. In some states commercial firms have a substantial proportion of total sales; in other states their share is more limited. There is some opportunity in this market to observe quality control practices and innovation in professional and commercial markets.

Three groups provide contact lens services: ophthalmologists, optometrists, and opticians. Licensed ophthalmologists and optometrists are permitted in all fifty states to perform all procedures necessary to prescribe and fit contact lenses. Opticians, who have much less education than ophthalmologists or optometrists, are not licensed in twenty-nine states. Opticians are not permitted to prescribe contact lenses, and they operate under various degrees of restrictions concerning the fitting of those lenses. Some ophthalmologists and optometrists view opticians as having insufficient knowledge to fit contact lenses safely and effectively. Some ophthalmologists doubt the capability of optometrists to provide quality services and vice versa.[22]

The Federal Trade Commission in 1978 undertook a study of the quality of contact lens fitting, with the cooperation of the American Academy of Ophthalmology, the American Optometric Association,

and the Opticians Association of America. The methodology proposed to determine the relative quality of contact lens fitting was
modified in response to criticism from the three groups' representatives. The quality standards were those of the professional associations and do not necessarily coincide with those of informed consumers. After no further objections were offered to the procedures, the
final methodology was set. The respective associations identified
qualified members of their professions to serve as field examiners.

A national sample of 31,219 households was selected in eighteen
urban areas for initial screening. Of 22,512 who returned the questionnaire, 1,871 had been fitted for contact lenses within the previous
three years and were still wearing lenses at the time of the survey.
From this set of 1,871 people, 502 were interviewed by the FTC staff
concerning the source of their lenses, and they were then examined
by representatives of the three groups, using the agreed criteria for
quality. The examiners did not know the source of the lenses. Seven
separate conditions of each eye were evaluated. Generally there was
agreement concerning the scoring of these conditions; when there
was not, a system of averaging was devised. These fourteen quality
scores (seven for each eye) were combined to provide summary
quality scores for each individual. The extent of eye and lens exami-
nations administered to this sample of individuals is impressive.

The quality of lens fitting was summarized for four groups of
providers: ophthalmologists, commercial optometrists, noncommercial optometrists, and unclassified optometrists and opticians. Commercial optometrists were those who worked for large chain firms or
who purchased display ads in local Yellow Pages. Noncommercial or
professional optometrists were those who usually were solo practitioners, who practiced in nonmercantile settings, who did not use
trade names, and who were members of the American Optometric
Association. The unclassified optometrists included those who could
not be placed into one of the two previous categories because of
insufficient information. They also included optometrists who practiced in health maintenance organizations, the military, or other
settings that were neither commercial nor noncommercial.

Several separate tests of quality were undertaken. Statistical
comparisons were made on six of these tests separately and on
weighted and unweighted sums of the seven separate measures. In
none of the sixteen separate statistical tests did commercial optometrists show significantly lower quality than noncommercial optometrists or ophthalmologists. In all four statistical tests that examined the
summary scores of quality, commercial optometrists had significantly
higher quality than noncommercial optometrists. Opticians, who

were unlicensed in some states, did not have significantly lower quality on the overall summary score than ophthalmologists or optometrists.[23]

The representatives of ophthalmology and noncommercial optometry were not enthusiastic about these results, although they had participated in the development of protocols and the tests of quality. The American Academy of Ophthalmology termed the study "incomplete in scope, inadequate for public policy, and insensitive to consumers' medical eye needs" and "out of date."[24]

The American Optometric Association "remains opposed to commercial practice and has been conducting a large media campaign to emphasize the quality care it believes is best offered by private practitioners." President Timothy Kime recently called the FTC study on quality "another example of the reasons AOA feels that Congress should investigate and review the role and responsibility of the FTC to interject themselves into health care matters."[25]

What is most noteworthy about the response of professional organizations is the absence of proposals to undertake other similar studies examining the relationship between source of care and quality. Without additional systematic information concerning the quality of contact lens fitting, the FTC results cannot be rejected. The study stands as perhaps the most careful examination of the relationship between commercial and noncommercial sources of care and quality of service.

The FTC study also estimated the average price for a uniform package of services, including the contact lenses themselves, the eye exam, follow-up care, and initial lens care kit. The results are shown in table 4–1. Opticians are not permitted to prescribe lenses, so their package price includes the prescription price from another source. In relative terms, commercial optometrists charged 14 to 54 percent less than other fitter groups for hard lenses, and 30 to 56 percent less for soft lenses.

Recently Valerie Cheh has undertaken a more extensive analysis of the FTC data. She concludes there is a positive relationship between average health outcomes and commercial competition. She also presents evidence suggesting that fewer patients experienced extremely poor outcomes in areas with more commercial competition.[26]

Summary

Medical licensure is rationalized on grounds of protecting consumers from uninformed choices. Yet a clear consequence of licensure is to inhibit the production of information concerning the comparative

89

TABLE 4–1
AVERAGE ADJUSTED PACKAGE PRICES FOR CONTACT
LENSES AND FITTING, BY SOURCE, FEBRUARY 1980
(in dollars)

Fitter	Hard Lenses	Soft Lenses
Ophthalmologists	183.85	234.54
Opticians	160.66	205.52
Noncommercial optometrists	154.00	195.33
Commercial optometrists	119.21	150.07
Unclassified optometrists	136.41	212.48

SOURCE: Gary D. Hailey, Jonathan R. Bromberg, and Joseph P. Mulholland, *A Comparative Analysis of Cosmetic Contact Lens Fitting by Ophthalmologists, Optometrists, and Opticians* (Washington, D.C.: Federal Trade Commission, Bureau of Consumer Protection, Bureau of Economics, December 1983), p. C-7.

performance of practitioners and hospitals. This in turn reduces the incentive to introduce innovations that would facilitate comparative evaluations and improve quality control. Codes of ethics, even if strictly adhered to, are not sufficient to ensure consistent practice; the elaborate and expensive admissions process provides little training in techniques that would permit practitioners to evaluate systematically their own or others' performance; few rewards exist for managers or quality control specialists to collect and evaluate comparative performances; the state licensing boards, which are the principal mechanisms for monitoring licensed practitioners, have few resources and limited incentives to carry out their tasks; and practitioners do not generally see it in their interest to inform the board of other physicians' deviant behavior. Given the training and incentives, it is not surprising that practices of widely varying quality survive.

This variability will decline when decision makers have a major stake in reducing variability. Licensure rules currently inhibit this process. One potential benefit of increased commercialization of medicine is in this area of quality control. The threatened loss of institutional reputation because of poor quality controls would provide incentives to monitor systematically and to alter practices when appropriate.

Protecting the Medical Profession

A Commentary by Peter Zweifel

In chapter 4, Professor Benham attacks the popular notion that regulation of the medical profession and licensure in particular enhance the quality of medical care. Indeed even a mere reduction of heterogeneity in the quality of service, with its mean level unaffected, would constitute a benefit to risk-averse patients. Unfortunately Benham does not present evidence linking the variation in quality in different states of the United States to the presence or absence of licensure. The door is open to the argument that without licensure, variability would be larger still than it is at present. He does show, however, that licensure does not result in a higher average level of quality in the case of contact lens fitting, based on the Federal Trade Commission study of 1980. Since the seven quality indicators used in that study were developed under the auspices of the professional associations involved, in particular the American Academy of Ophthalmology, its systematic failure to find statistically significant differences in favor of licensed providers constitutes rather strong evidence. Incidentally the data contained in the FTC study would also allow testing of whether licensure is associated with a reduced variability in the quality of care provided.

On balance, however, the case against a relationship between licensure and quality has been established to a sufficient degree by Benham to ask a question that comes to mind quite naturally: If licensure of physicians does not contribute to its prime stated objective, why is it so widespread in the entire world, including all Western countries, even the most market-oriented ones? The remainder of this comment is devoted to a tentative answer to this question. In the

This text draws in part on P. Zweifel and R. E. Eichenberger, "The Political Economy of Corporatism in Medicine," presented at the annual meeting of the European Public Choice Society, Linz, Austria, March 29–April 1, 1989. Helpful comments by R. E. Eichenberger (University of Zurich), H. E. Frech (University of California, Santa Barbara), and J. P. Newhouse (Harvard University Medical School) are gratefully acknowledged.

91

main, licensure is interpreted as the outcome of an exchange taking place on the "market for protection," with medical associations acting on the demand side and politicians on the supply side.

Every worker would like to be protected from competition. Creating a cartel is a first step toward this end, allowing sales prices for goods and services to be maintained above the ever-changing levels of competitive markets. The next step is to get the state to provide even more protection, for example, through immigration laws, as cited at the beginning of Benham's chapter. A necessary condition for activating politicians and public administrators is a powerful lobby, the spearhead of a cartel. Thus one is led to investigate the reasons why physicians are more successful than other professional groups in forming and maintaining an effective cartel. Apparently the benefits derived from it must be particularly great while its costs are particularly low.

On the benefits side, keeping price competition among its members at a minimal level comes first for any cartel. A medical association's chances of successful performance in this respect are greatly enhanced by the presence of health insurance. Because of ample health insurance coverage (or even the existence of a national health service as in the United Kingdom and Italy) in Western countries, patients have no incentive to seek out physicians providing reasonably priced services.[1] Therefore each individual physician realizes that price cutting would contribute little to business volume. With the cartel's discipline going unchallenged, a medical association is especially likely to reach its primary objective of limiting price competition.

Given successful cartelization, the benefits to be reaped through the political process are substantial as an important share of the public budget is devoted to health. Thus members of a medical association can count on their lobby channeling large sums of tax money toward themselves.

Once established, a medical association meets with approval among the general voting public as soon as the redistributive element in health care provision becomes strong enough. Social health insurance schemes with their age-independent contributions constitute unstable intergenerational contracts; in times of rapid demographic change, they even tend to create cohorts of lifetime gainers and losers.[2] A well-organized medical cartel not only enforces homogeneity of price but also establishes certain modes of practice as ethical. Through fostering a certain stability of medical care, it thus contributes to tomorrow's aged population obtaining a share of medical care comparable to their predecessors' of today. Today's contributors to social health insurance thus may gladly accept a well-organized medical cartel guaranteeing an unchanged future distribution of medical services, for example, between different age groups.

There are reasons for believing that the costs of creating and maintaining a medical cartel may be lower than for other professional groups. The first point is the standard argument that price discrimination cannot be easily undermined in the case of personal services. Medical associations in many Western countries are responsible for the negotiation of fee schedules containing a great amount of price discrimination to the detriment of high-income earners. Medical services delivered to members of private health insurance in Germany, for example, are priced about three times higher than those delivered to members of statutory health insurers. The latter category comprises general mutual funds, substitute funds (mainly for white-collar workers), and employer-sponsored funds. All of these funds are subject to a body of regulation that dates back to the old German Reich. The surcharge paid by the privately insured thus amounts to income-increasing price discrimination, whose establishment and maintenance constitutes one of the major functions of many medical associations.[3] Such price discrimination is unlikely to be challenged effectively because of the absence of secondary markets for medical services.

A second and somewhat related fact is the weakness of international competition in the domain of medical care. There is little shopping around for cheap physician services across national borders because of the substantial transaction costs. National medical markets are therefore inherently less open than others and facilitate the successful operation of a cartel.

Finally, a medical association can achieve control of market entry at relatively low cost with an additional instrument. By constraining the delegation of tasks in medical practice, it inhibits the forming of large, corporate medical firms, with consequences for the monitoring of quality that are vividly expounded by Benham. Entry into the medical market remains tied to the single medically trained individual, rendering control over access at the time of educational choice particularly effective. Licensure thus can be seen as one of several elements that contribute to the low cost of maintaining a medical cartel.

Taken together, both the benefits and the cost side of the equation appear to make it comparatively worthwhile and at the same time easy to create and maintain a cartel of the providers of medical services. Thus demand for protection in the political arena is strong.

In what follows, the supply side of the market for protection is analyzed with the focus on the behavior of politicians. Again it is argued that the benefits derived from granting additional protection to physicians compare favorably with the costs.

Allowing physicians to form an effective cartel holds the promise of providing quite a few votes. Physicians are opinion leaders in their communities, and their many contacts in an advisory role permit them to influence a considerable number of individuals. Being older than average, these individuals also tend to participate more than others in political elections. Thus the benefits of the support of physicians can be rather large for a politician seeking election.

While the preceding argument holds before the establishment of medical associations, a second point directly relates to the control over market entry exerted by these associations once they are established. This control, performed by medical schools at admission as a sort of prelicensure, is commonly believed to restrain the total public expenditure on health. Being able to rely on the cooperation of organized medicine in preventing another health cost explosion is a valuable asset to a politician, especially when the electorate is seeking relief from taxes. Keeping a lid on physician stock admittedly drives prices of medical services up unless the state steps in as a monopsonistic purchaser of medical services. Politicians, however, are much more concerned about expenditure. Although the quantity of medical services consumed would be little curtailed by a price hike (estimated price elasticities being in the -0.1 to -0.3 range), reduced physician density might well lower expenditure through its effect on the time cost of medical care.[4] Longer journeys and waiting times to see a physician increase the costs to be borne by the patient. This increase of time cost weighs heavily in a situation where the monetary costs are just about subsidized to zero, as in most Western countries except the United States.[5]

Granting the medical profession the protection afforded by market closure is not without costs to politicians. For one thing, in countries where premiums for health insurance directly enter the labor cost (as in the United States and West Germany but not in the Netherlands or Switzerland, where health insurance is in the main individually contracted), employers have started looking for ways to reduce the health care burden. Since the employers' main objective is to contain medical expenditures rather than prices, however, abandoning professional licensure does not appeal to them. Health insurers themselves have never attacked licensure, probably because they would want to limit the set of eligible providers of services, as shifting the increased medical expenditures forward to consumers through premiums may not always be possible. At the least they would have

94

to face a trade-off between cheaper medical services available from a wider range of providers on the one hand and the wage costs of loss adjusters of the type known in property-liability insurance on the other. These adjusters would determine the class of authorized medical practitioners for the health problem at hand and could be appealed to in cases of questionable success of treatment. In all, a politician favoring the continuation or even strengthening of professional licensure in medicine should meet with little opposition from the business community.

Supplying protection to physicians through licensure may also be costly to a politician for a reason stressed by Benham. Licensure could well have detrimental rather than beneficial effects on the quality of medical care. But even if licensure resulted in a net deterioration of care, politicians advocating it would probably lose few votes. First, much of the excess mortality showing up in the statistics cited by Benham concerns old people, who were expected to die anyway in a few months or years. Second, these deaths are individual cases, occurring here and there, frequently behind the walls of a hospital. Both facts serve to reduce the importance of quality in medicine compared with the issue of safety in the airline industry, at least from the politician's point of view. Most people who die in an airplane crash are of prime working age; their deaths are definitely judged as premature by family members and friends. Moreover the simultaneous loss of dozens or even hundreds of lives almost automatically creates an interest group of survivors that may hold their political representative indirectly responsible for the catastrophe. Because of the mass media, those survivors find it easier to form a pressure group than do people spread across the country who militate against an allegedly substandard quality of medical treatment as the cause of a relative's death.

In all, granting protection to the medical profession seems to be rather attractive from a politician's vantage point. Professional licensure could even be the instrument of choice because its drawbacks tend to be counterbalanced by the relief it provides to the public health budget.

The politicoeconomic analysis of licensure attempted in the previous section focused on the status quo. If approximately correct, it may provide the basis for a look into the future. Are there developments apt to challenge licensure of the medical profession?

The demand for protection in the guise of licensure will not decrease. The recent increase in physician density in most Western countries certainly constitutes a challenge to medical associations.[6] The issue, however, is the integration of a growing number of young

95

members starting their practice rather than the demise of licensure. In France and Germany, for example, the state has taken over the rationing function itself, with the selection of candidates for the fixed total number of admissions left to the profession.

On the supply side it may become more difficult for politicians to provide protection to the medical profession in the form of licensure. The public seems to be aware of growing mismatches between the types of services demanded and supplied in health care. Women preferring childbirth at home frequently notice that obstetricians fail to provide the type of support they could expect from midwives. Psychosomatic illness is considered to be handled less than satisfactorily by general practitioners and psychiatrists alike in many quarters. Finally, the intensive medical care provided to many patients in the last few months of their lives does not seem to correspond to their preferences although such care consumes a lot of resources.

There may be a growing awareness that professional licensure stands in the way of innovations in the organization of health care delivery that would serve both to complement the spectrum of services offered and to limit the cost of their production. But so far the tendency has rather been to license additional groups of health personnel (such as the community health nurse) with narrowly defined tasks. Apparently, increased flexibility in the provision of health care can be expected to come from competition between different systems (such as HMOs and PPOs) operating within the confines of a market for medical manpower that continues to be strongly segmented along present lines.

5
Theoretical and Empirical Foundations of the Resource-based Relative Value Scale

Jack Hadley

Medicare's policy of physician payment is about to change from the customary-prevailing-reasonable system of paying charges to a fee schedule, which is a fixed list of how much it pays for each service physicians provide. Like the Diagnosis Related Group (DRG) price list for paying hospitals, a fee schedule may vary across areas and possibly by specialty, but the basic relationship of one service's fee relative to another will stay fixed for several years.

How will Medicare arrive at its fee schedule? Right now the only train in the station, or at least the one that most people are buying tickets for, is the resource- (or cost-) based relative value scale (RBRVS), created by a team of researchers at Harvard University.

The goal of the Harvard study is to "develop a resource *cost-based* relative value scale by investigating the resource *input* costs of physicians' services and developing methods to measure them." Furthermore, "*to measure resource costs*, we developed a model that measures three resource *inputs* to physicians' services . . . the work of particular services and procedures, . . . specialty-specific practice costs, and the opportunity cost of training."[1]

In particular, for each physician service, the resource-based relative value is defined by the formula

$$RBRV = (TW) \times (1 + RPC) \times (1 + AST)$$

where *TW* is the total work input of the physician for that service, *RPC* is an index of relative practice costs across specialties, and *AST*

I am grateful to Steven Zuckerman, John Holahan, W. P. Welch, Roger Feldman, and H. E. Frech for their comments on an earlier draft of this chapter. They are absolved, however, of any responsibility for the content.

is an index of the amortized value of the opportunity cost of additional training across specialties. "Work is modeled as a function of four dimensions: time, mental effort and judgment, technical skill and physical effort, and stress."[2]

The RBRVS is indeed a most impressive train. Hundreds of physicians participated in the development process. The *Journal of the American Medical Association* devoted an entire issue to the study's results at almost the same time that the *New England Journal of Medicine* published a major article about the Harvard RBRVS by the same research team: unprecedented testaments to the study's importance.

Although the rush to get on board continues, the goal of this chapter is to pause to examine the principles that fundamentally drive the train's engine. What does economic theory imply about the conditions under which a resource-based relative value scale is appropriate, or at least is preferred to a relative value scale based on charges? What does economic theory say about how to construct an RBRVS? How closely does the Harvard RBRVS adhere to these principles? Is there an alternative to the RBRVS, Harvard-style or otherwise?

To put these questions into context, table 5–1 reproduces some of the relative values calculated by the Harvard study. They differ substantially from relative values based on charges. Adopting the Harvard RBRVS at face value means that some services would have their fees substantially reduced while others would be increased dramatically. One cannot help but ask what underlying economic conditions could give rise to fees that appear to be so out of whack relative to their costs.

The usual answers are differences in insurance coverage by type of service and a noncompetitive market structure. One of the objectives of this chapter is to examine the consequences of these factors in the context of simple economic theory and to assess whether the results of the Harvard study are consistent with that theory. This evaluation leads to five main conclusions.

First, if the markets for physicians' services are perfectly competitive or monopolistically competitive with free entry, the fee charged equals the average cost of production, regardless of whether some, all, or no services are insured. Relative values based on accurately measured costs are the same as relative values based on charges.

Second, if markets are noncompetitive and have limited entry, prices indeed exceed average costs. With one exception, however, no services are priced below average cost. Nor is observed average cost the minimum of the average cost function. Furthermore the markup of price above average cost depends on the shapes of the demand

TABLE 5-1
RESOURCE-BASED RELATIVE VALUES AND MEDICARE CHARGES

Procedure Code	Service Description (Specialty)	RBRV	1986 Medicare Mean Charge ($)	Ratio of Medicare Charge to RBRV
90070	Office visit, extended service (allergy and immunology)	126	36	0.29
11642	Excision, malignant lesion (dermatology)	159	220	1.38
90630	Initial consultation, complex service (family practice)	283	86	0.30
49505	Repair inguinal hernia, age 5 or older (general surgery)	476	732	1.54
90750	Initial history and examination, healthy individual adult (internal medicine)	114	20	0.18
90060	Office visit, intermediate service, established patient (obstetrics and gynecology)	101	33	0.33
58150	Total hysterectomy (obstetrics and gynecology)	982	1,542	1.57
90020	Office visit, comprehensive service, new patient (orthopedic surgery)	189	57	0.30
29881	Arthrosocopy, knee, surgical; with meniscectomy (orthopedic surgery)	905	1,387	1.53
90020	Office visit, comprehensive service, new patient (thoracic surgery)	213	64	0.30
33512	Coronary artery bypass, autogenous graft; 3 coronary arteries (thoracic surgery)	2,871	4,663	1.63

NOTE: Medicare Part B submitted charges for 1986.
SOURCE: W. Hsiao et al., "Results, Potential Effects, and Implementation Issues of the Resource-Based Relative Value Scale," Journal of the American Medical Association, October 28, 1988, pp. 2431–32.

and cost functions for each service. Thus for any two services, it is indeterminate whether the ratio of charges or the ratio of measured average costs is a closer approximation of the theoretically ideal relative value, that is, the ratio of the minimum points of the average cost curves.

Third, allowing for differences in insurance coverage by type of service shifts the demand for services, but it also moves the cost of production, so that the basic indeterminacy of preferring relative costs over relative charges does not change.

Fourth, the Harvard RBRVS is not a cost-based relative value scale. It omits the cost or price of the physician's own input to producing services. Rather it is a relative work scale. While some might argue that this approach is appropriate, it is not consistent with economic theory or, as judged from the quotes above, the Harvard study's own goals.

Last, the Harvard study's formula for calculating RBRVS is inconsistent with the economic theory of cost in that it omits both the scale of production and the possible presence of economies (or diseconomies) of scope. Physicians are multiproduct firms: the cost of producing any one service depends on the mix and volume of other services. In addition the Harvard study's method of allocating nonphysician costs to specific services bears no obvious relationship to the way in which economic theory suggests average and marginal costs could be estimated.

Despite these conclusions, the Harvard study's principal premise may be true: some services are overpriced and some possibly underpriced, though not necessarily priced below cost. The critical point is that notions of overpriced and underpriced should be based on more than just price relative to cost. Furthermore using a simple formula to measure resource costs is not enough. No matter how intuitively appealing, a simple formula cannot accurately capture the incredible complexity of measuring the cost of physicians' services. The physician's first maxim, Do no harm, should be followed to guard against a solution that is worse than the problem.

It is not, however, that nothing is wrong with the market and competition should "do its thing." Adopting a fee schedule would be a sensible policy for Medicare and for other insurers. But basing that fee schedule on what at best is a crude approximation of true relative resource costs is a concern.

Rather Medicare, preferably in conjunction with other large insurers, should become an educated and informed consumer on behalf of its beneficiaries. Medicare should base the fees it is willing to pay not only on how much a service costs but also on what a service is worth in terms of its benefit to patients and whether its beneficiaries get too much or too little of that service. These decisions require judgments, not formulas.

Politically formulas are popular. They leave no fingerprints, and the more complex the development of the formula, the less assailable it is by critics. Medicare and other insurers, however, cannot simply pay the bills by formula and then stand back as passive observers. Their beneficiaries' physical and financial health both demand more active evaluation of the services received for the payments made.

Is there an alternative to a resource-based relative value scale? There is one, based on relative charges. Basing relative values on relative charges, however, does not mean that charges have to be accepted exactly as is.

A major contribution of the Harvard study is its demonstration of the fact that large numbers of physicians can be surveyed, assembled in panels, and led to a valid consensus. Physicians, along with insurer representatives, economists, accountants, and patient representatives, could be surveyed and brought together in panels to discuss how to alter charges, based on perceptions and evidence of overservice, underservice, efficacy, excess profits, and rapid technical change.

Making the right judgments is not easy. Thus deviations in the fee schedule from existing charge levels should be small initially, as a practical, political safeguard. Moreover Medicare and other insurers need to develop much better systems for tracking the quality and volume of specific services. The change in Medicare part B quantity, for example, is called "the residual"; that is, what is left over after price changes are netted out of expenditure changes. The Medicare statistical system does not measure quantity directly.

Implementing a fee schedule is only the first step. Maintaining it requires continuous monitoring: by service, volume, distribution, assignment rates, magnitude of balance billing, and other measures of access, such as waiting time for an appointment, acceptance of new patients, and concentration of care to Medicare beneficiaries in a relatively few practices in an area.

The remainder of the chapter is organized around a set of questions. What is a relative value scale, and how does it relate to a fee schedule? What is a resource-based relative value scale? What is an ideal relative value scale? Why does anyone want to replace the current system with a fee schedule? What can be done to fix the current system? What are the theoretical and empirical foundations of the RBRVS? How well does the Harvard study satisfy the underlying theoretical conditions? Finally, what is the alternative to an RBRVS?

Value Scales

Relative Value Scale and Fee Schedules. A relative value scale is a cardinal ordering of the services physicians provide. Each service is assigned a number from the scale. That number indicates its worth, or value, relative to every other service. The unit in which the scale is denominated is completely arbitrary. The base or numeraire service could be assigned any value, for example, 1, 10, or 50, as long as services that are valued twice as high as the base service are assigned values of 2, 20, or 100.

Multiplying the relative value scale numbers by a monetary conversion factor produces the fee schedule. If the monetary value is $1, then the relative value scale is identical to the fee schedule. But a fee schedule could also be created by applying a conversion factor of $1 to some services, $2 to others, and $10 to still others.

Ideal Relative Value Scale. An ideal relative value scale reflects both the cost of providing a service and its benefit or worth to patients. In a system of perfectly competitive markets, the market price has been shown to fulfill this function. Thus relative values based on competitively determined relative prices are an ideal relative value scale. Perfect competition also leads to equality between the price of a service and the minimum average cost of producing that service in an optimally scaled plant or firm.

Early relative value scales developed by the California Medical Society were based on physicians' charges. These seem to have been more a matter of convenience rather than an ideal, however. Most analysts agree that the markets for most physicians' services are not perfectly competitive. Thus a relative value scale that is nothing more than the ratios of existing average charges is not considered an ideal relative value scale.

Resource-based Relative Value Scale. A resource-based relative value scale bases the cardinal ordering of physicians' services on the resources and costs of providing them. It departs fundamentally from a charge-based relative value scale by ignoring totally, it is alleged, the distortions implicit in market fees. As shown below, economic theory establishes an equivalency between the average cost of producing a service and its price in a perfectly competitive market. The Physician Payment Review Commission used this logic in recommending the development of a relative value scale based on resource costs. "A resource cost basis would reflect estimates of what relative values would be under a hypothetical market that functions perfectly. Under such a market, competition drives relative prices to reflect the relative costs of efficient producers."[3]

The logic underlying a resource-based relative scale appears compelling. It rests on two critical assumptions, however. First, the costs of producing services are not influenced by the same factors that allegedly distort market fees. Second, resource costs can be measured with reasonable accuracy on a service specific basis.

Faults of the Current System

The current system of establishing fees for physicians' services paid by Medicare is known as the customary-prevailing-reasonable (CPR) system. Most private insurers use a similar approach, called usual-customary-reasonable. (Medicare's method was explicitly modeled on the method used by Blue Shield plans in the early 1960s.) Under CPR, physicians are free to charge whatever they deem appropriate for a service. This is called the actual charge. As defined by Medicare, the customary charge for a service is the median of the charges submitted by the physician for that same service in the preceding year. The prevailing charge for that service is the seventy-fifth percentile of the distribution of the customary charges of all physicians in the area. Finally, the reasonable charge, which is the amount Medicare pays for the service, is the lowest of the customary, prevailing, and actual charges for that particular claim.

The reasonable charge, the amount actually paid, is often a mystery to both physicians and patients. The prevailing charge screen may be limited by the Medicare Economic Index, which is supposed to constrain the rate of growth in prevailing charges according to a formula based on the growth in general earnings and in physicians' practice costs. Both customary and prevailing charge values are updated periodically as physicians change their billing behavior. In recent years these updates have been either frozen or modified, depending on whether physicians agreed to accept assignment on all claims. Furthermore there can be wide variation in what physicians in the same area receive as payment depending in part on when they located there and how high their initial charges may have been. Charges for new services may be initially quite high and tend to stay there unless market forces drive fees down; this tends not to happen with medical services. Finally, in some areas or for some services where a relatively small number of physicians typically provide the bulk of the volume of that service, those physicians may be able to accelerate consciously the growth of customary and prevailing charge levels through their billing behavior.

Aside from being inequitable, confusing, and mysterious, however, the current system is alleged to have two major problems, which the RBRVS, it is hoped, will help solve. First, expenditures for physicians' services are growing too fast, growing faster than spending for other medical care. How much of this growth is because of price increases and how much because of quantity increases is not at all clear. Physicians' charges, as measured by the physicians' services component of the consumer price index, have been growing much more rapidly than prices in general, although they are not changing differently from other medical care prices. (From 1980 to 1988 both the physicians' services component of the consumer price index and the entire medical care index increased 85.5 percent, while the all-items index increased 49.6 percent.)

Medicare does not pay what physicians charge, however. It pays less, and the discount has been increasing in recent years. The program has supposedly frozen and constrained fee levels for various periods over the last few years. But part B reimbursements per enrollee have grown as much in the last five years, about 75 percent, as they did in the previous five years, when price increases were much larger. Thus Medicare analysts seem to think that expenditure growth is primarily attributable to volume increases (and shifts from less expensive to more expensive services).

The second major problem is that fees in the current system are distorted. The word "distorted" is emphasized because it is not entirely clear what distortion means in this context. One line of argument is that variations in insurance coverage distort fees. In particular, although most physicians' services are insured, some are not. Therefore the prices charged for insured services are higher than they would be in a no-insurance world, or conversely the prices charged for uninsured services are lower than they would be in a fully insured world.

A second form of distortion, perhaps also due to insurance variations, is that prices charged bear an uneven relationship to the costs of providing those services. Some fees are considerably higher than costs, some approximately equal costs, and some allegedly considerably below costs. Why physicians continue to provide those services may be an interesting side question, especially since they can charge more than Medicare pays. It would also be interesting to know whether the assignment rate for services allegedly paid below cost is lower than that for other services.

104

A third form of distortion concerns variations in fees across geographic areas and to some extent among physicians in the same area. The fee for the same service can vary substantially, depending on the geographic location. Consequently, it is believed, distorted fees send physicians the wrong signals about where and what specialty to practice.

These two problems, inflation and distortion, occur in a market for physicians' services that most believe is imperfectly competitive. The basic conditions for perfect competition are free entry and many sellers and buyers with perfect information about the quality and prices of the products being sold. The last of these conditions is most often not satisfied. The physician-patient agency relationship is supposed to compensate for patients' inadequate medical knowledge, though not necessarily for imperfect information about prices.[4] Furthermore, with little repeated buying for many services or little opportunity or time in many cases to shop around, and with a high cost associated with price shopping—one has to evaluate the quality of alternative providers as well as ascertain their price and one risks alienating one's current provider—even a well-functioning agency relationship is unlikely to produce the equivalent of perfect competition.[5] Rather the market for most services is better characterized as monopolistically competitive, which means in effect that physicians face downward sloping demand and marginal revenue functions for most services.

Fixing the Current System

Two basic approaches for repairing the current system have been advocated: make the system more competitive or regulate it more tightly by establishing a fee schedule and setting up various utilization review mechanisms. The competitive strategy rests essentially on two pillars. One is giving patients a greater incentive to shop around and purchase prudently by increasing cost sharing. The other is encouraging people to join insurance-type groups, such as health maintenance organizations and preferred provider organizations, that have the specific medical knowledge to evaluate product quality and price and can use that information to negotiate or establish prices that correspond more closely to prices under perfect competition. In other words the competing groups can more easily obtain perfect information than can any individual member. (Unfortunately the incentives of the group's owners may not coincide with those of its members, especially with short-term exit a very real phenomenon.)

The regulatory approach, or more accurately the fee schedule

105

approach, would still use fees as signaling mechanisms for both providers and patients. The fees, however, would be set by an administrative agency or process. This does not necessarily mean that fees are set arbitrarily or capriciously.

Rather the goal is to set fees such that the desired quantity, mix, quality, and distribution of services is provided at the least cost to payers. If fees are set too low, quality is likely to suffer at first, and in the long run quantity (or access) is reduced as fewer physicians choose to treat Medicare patients and ultimately fewer people choose to become physicians. (This assumes that lower fees mean lower incomes for physicians. Some question this assumption on the grounds that demand inducement can offset any reduction in fees.)

If fees are set too high, people receive services of little marginal benefit, the level of amenities exceeds what people are willing to purchase on their own, and payers spend more than necessary (unless higher fees lead to negative demand inducement on the part of physicians: a novel proposition that follows logically from the demand inducement model).

Theoretical and Empirical Foundations of RBRVS

The theoretical foundation of the RBRVS is one of the most fundamental propositions of microeconomic theory. In a perfectly competitive market, that is, many buyers, many sellers, and perfect information, equilibrium is attained when

$$AC = MC = MR = AR = P$$

average cost equals marginal cost equals marginal revenue equals average revenue equals price. This configuration leads to maximum (albeit zero economic) profits for suppliers, given the input prices they face, and maximum benefit for consumers, given their incomes and preferences.

As argued earlier, however, several alleged distortions may result in price exceeding average cost for some services, while for other services the reverse is true. Therefore, the argument goes, if the efficient average cost can be measured directly, then the relative value of service i to service j can be constructed as

$$RBRV_{ij} = AC_i / AC_j$$

and this resource-based relative value would be exactly the same as, or at least approximate more closely, the relative values that would occur in a perfectly competitive market with its attendant positive outcomes for overall welfare, that is,

$$\text{RBRV}_{ij} = AC_i/AC_j = P_i^*/P_j^* < P_i/P_j$$

where the P^*s are the competitive market prices and the Ps are the actual or distorted prices generated by the current market for physicians' services. What is the validity of this assumption under the conditions that allegedly distort relative prices: differential insurance coverage and imperfect information?

Differential Insurance Coverage with Perfect Competition. Assume initially that there are two services, evaluation-management (EM) and procedures (PR); there is no insurance coverage for either service; and the market for each service is perfectly competitive. That is, the physician is a price taker for both services; therefore the demand curves for each service faced by an individual physician are horizontal, although the market level demand curves are presumably downward sloping.

One of the services, *PR*, becomes insured. Since out-of-pocket price is now lower at every level of output, the demand curve shifts up and to the right. A new equilibrium is established at a higher price and a higher quantity, assuming that the aggregate supply function is upward sloping.

Whether the higher level of output is socially desirable is another issue. To the extent that increased use of services is the result of moral hazard, then the new output level may be too high. If people were underusing services in the uninsured situation, however—that is, people were forgoing use of services that would improve their own and perhaps others' welfare more than the cost of extra care—then the increased use associated with insurance coverage would improve overall welfare. (For the underconsumption argument to be valid, however, one has to appeal to the existence of some combination of inappropriate time discounting, positive externalities, personal income constraint, and imperfect knowledge of the full benefits of care.)

Does insurance distort the relative valuation of the two services? Relative fees will change in the short run since the insurance-induced increase in demand will cause an increase in the fee of the procedural service. The fee for EM may also increase, however, if resources have to be bid away from producing EM to producing PR. Thus one could say that relative fees are distorted by insurance since they may in fact change.

Yet, if the market is competitive, the new equilibrium must eventually satisfy the fundamental equilibrium condition. Relative values based on fees are exactly the same as relative values based on average cost since in a competitive equilibrium price equals average cost. Insurance in and of itself does not make a competitive market noncompetitive, even if it leads to higher quantities and higher fees. Furthermore this conclusion is independent of whether some or all services are insured.

Two implications are that absolute fee levels are higher where insurance coverage is more broad. Relative fees may not change much at all, however, since some resources may be bid away from producing EM, which would raise the fee for EM. In the long run the final absolute and relative fee levels depend on conditions of entry.

There is little empirical evidence on the relationship between insurance coverage and relative fees. One study did find results generally consistent with the argument that relative fees do not vary with insurance coverage.[6] Looking at Medicare prevailing charges for fifty services across states in 1978, the study found that a 10 percent higher level of insurance coverage (measured by total insurance premiums per capita) was associated with absolute fees averaging from 2.4 to 3.4 percent higher, depending on the type of service (surgery, office visits, radiology, or ancillary). In contrast the insurance coverage variable was not significantly related to any of the relative fee values. A 10 percent higher level of insurance coverage was associated with only a 0.3 percent variation in relative fees on average. (An initial comprehensive office visit for a new patient was the numeraire.)

Other studies have shown that insurance leads to higher fee levels and that the prevailing method of determining insurance payments, that is, the customary-prevailing-reasonable system in Medicare, is inherently inflationary.[7] But these results do not in and of themselves imply that relative fees are distorted by insurance.

Monopolistically Competitive Market Structure. Is the market for physicians' services perfectly competitive? If not, does insurance cause distortions in relative fees in a noncompetitive market? What are the implications of a noncompetitive market for relative values based on costs without any insurance effects?

Most of the research pertinent to assessing the competitive structure of the market for physicians' services has been focused on the question of supplier-induced demand (SID). Basically SID, or target income pricing, can take place only in a noncompetitive market because a competitive market causes a physician to lose all patients if that practitioner sets prices above the market-determined level. Therefore, the argument goes, if the market can be shown to be competitive, or at least consistent with the implications of the competitive model, then this amounts to prima facie evidence against the SID theory.

Almost all of the early studies relied on a single variable, the ratio of physicians to population, in single-period cross-sectional analyses of physicians' prices or incomes to "test" whether the market is competitive.[8] For a variety of reasons, especially the endogenicity of physician supply with price or income and the omission of other key variables, these early studies should be disregarded. More recent evidence, using much better data and more fully specified theoretical models, has found relatively strong evidence that the market for primary care services (or for services provided by primary care physicians) has competitive elements.[9]

On a much more simple level, fee dispersion within an area seems to be smaller for office visits than for other services,[10] and according to data from the American Medical Association for 1973–1980, the rate of increase in visit fees was about the same as the increase in the overall physician fee component of the CPI.[11] (The physician fee component increased 88 percent, compared to 80 to 96 percent for office visit fees for general practitioners, internists, general surgeons, and pediatricians. Since physicians' incomes were increasing less rapidly than inflation during the 1970s, which presumably would be high motivation to raise fees faster than inflation, one may conclude that at least for visits the market may be reasonably competitive. Furthermore the increases in fees were similar across specialties, even though their income experiences were much more dissimilar.[12]

For nonvisit services, that is, operations and diagnostic-therapeutic procedures, the empirical evidence is much thinner. On its face, however, it seems highly plausible that the market for these services is monopolistically competitive. The information gap between physician and patient is much greater than for office visits. Once a patient has agreed to initiate a diagnostic or therapeutic course of action, it is difficult to switch to different providers, except on referral. Finally, because most people undergo a major procedure only once, sometimes in an emergency situation, there is no opportunity to build up information through repeated purchase. Nor is there much opportunity to learn from the experiences of other patients, because "every patient is different." At best one might talk to a handful of patients, hardly enough for reliable inferences about quality and outcome in relation to price.[13]

What are the implications of a monopolistically competitive market for insurance distortion and for an RBRVS? The standard equilib-

FIGURE 5–1
EQUILIBRIUM IN A MONOPOLISTICALLY COMPETITIVE MARKET

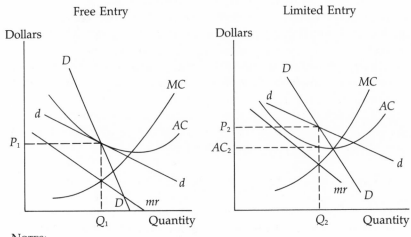

Free Entry   Limited Entry

NOTES:
DD = demand curve under the assumption that all physicians charge the same price for the service.
dd = demand curve under the assumption that other physicians' prices remain fixed.

rium condition without insurance is depicted in figure 5–1, under alternative assumptions about the entry of new providers.

These simple models produce two implications relevant to the above question. First, with free entry, firms do not earn excess profits—that is, price equals average cost—but they do produce a less than optimal volume of output. Therefore the average cost of a unit of output exceeds the minimum average cost of an efficient size firm. The main point, however, is that relative values based on observed average costs are the same as relative values based on fees.

With limited entry, price exceeds observed average cost, which in turn exceeds minimum average cost. If this service is compared with a service sold in a perfectly competitive market, then relative values based on average costs are closer to the ideal relative value, the ratio of the minimums of the average cost functions, than are relative values based on average fees. The difference between the two is the excess profit earned for the service for which P exceeds AC. The competitive product is not underpriced relative to cost, however. Rather the procedural service is overpriced.

Figure 5–2 considers the case of two procedural services pro-

110

FIGURE 5-2
MONOPOLISTIC COMPETITION WITH LIMITED ENTRY: TWO SERVICES WITH IDENTICAL COSTS BUT DIFFERENT DEMAND FUNCTIONS

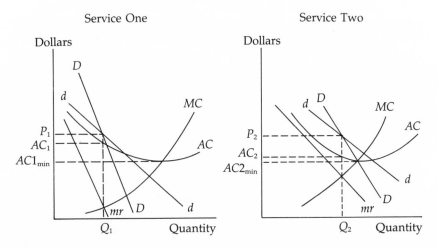

NOTES:

$((P_1/P_2) - 1) < (AC_1/AC_2) - 1)$
DD = demand curve under the assumption that all physicians charge the same price for the service.
dd = demand curve under the assumption that other physicians' prices remain fixed.

duced under the assumption of monopolistic competition with limited entry. For both services, price exceeds observed average cost, which in turn exceeds minimum average cost. Given an ideal relative value equal to the ratio of the two minimum average costs, can anything be said about whether relative fees or relative observed average costs are closer to the ideal relative value?

In general the answer is no as long as the markup of price above average cost is not identical for every service. (If it were, then relative charges would be about the same as relative average costs.) One service may have an average cost close to the minimum of the average cost curve, for example, but a high markup of price above average cost because of the nature of demand for that service. Another service, however, may be produced at an inefficient (high) level of average cost but have a low markup of price above cost. Given nonconstant markups, for any pair of services, the better approximation to the ideal relative value depends on the relative shapes of

111

the average and marginal cost and revenue functions. A priori there is no reason to think that one is always closer to the ideal.

Does the introduction of insurance alter these results? As in the case of perfectly competitive markets, insurance does not fundamentally alter any of these results. The relative positions of the various demand and cost curves may change, presumably in the direction of higher fees and greater quantities. But nothing about the introduction of insurance suggests that markups of prices above average costs change in a uniform or systematic fashion. Thus the answer to the basic question "Which is closer to the ideal relative value, relative average costs or relative fees?" remains indeterminate.

Services Priced below Average Cost. So far the theory implies that no service is priced below its average cost. This seems to contradict the widely held notion, displayed in table 5–1, that some EM services are major money losers. Is there a theoretical counterpart to this impression? Two cases need to be distinguished: systematic pricing below cost and random occurrences of cost exceeding price.

Undoubtedly, for some proportion of EM cases, the value of the time a physician puts into the case exceeds the fee received. One often hears about the brief follow-up visit, with a fee of $18, for example, for which the physician spends two hours in reviewing the patient's history, talking to other physicians, and reading medical journals. One also hears about the physician who walks in to see a hospitalized patient, says "How are you feeling today," walks out, and bills for an intermediate hospital visit of $45. While the latter is probably not typical of every single EM service, neither is the former. Both types of situations probably occur, and since physicians continue to provide EM services with considerable regularity, they are unlikely to be consistent money losers. This conclusion is entirely consistent, however, with the statement that they are not as profitable as procedural services.

These two examples may also be symptomatic of another problem with EM services. Specifically the whole taxonomy of visit codes is imprecise and leaves considerable ambiguity about both the duration and content of an EM service. Nevertheless, although there is considerable concern over the proliferation of codes, the physicians' inability to bill for some aspects of an EM service, such as time spent talking with family members or other physicians, reading the relevant literature, and reviewing medical histories, may be a real problem. From the perspective of third-party payers and patients, however, it is difficult, if not impossible, to monitor how much time physicians might spend in these activities. In an era of great concern over the growth in the volume of services, creating new services whose delivery cannot be monitored even by the patient may be viewed as imprudent, to say the least.

The second case cited, systematic pricing of certain services below their average cost, is possible if physicians treat office visits as loss leaders or tie-ins to the sale of other services.[14] In particular, if patients' decisions to initiate a visit to a doctor are much more sensitive to the price of a visit than to the price of subsequent tests and procedures, then physicians may set their office visit fees such that marginal cost exceeds marginal revenue. More formally this can be modeled by assuming that the demand for visits depends on the out-of-pocket cost of a visit, while the demand for tests depends on both the out-of-pocket costs of tests and the cost of an office visit. Under the simplest profit-maximizing assumption, the physician produces office visits beyond the point where marginal cost equals marginal revenue of the office visit alone since an extra office visit generates additional marginal revenue from tests as well as from the office visit itself. If the average revenue function lies above the marginal revenue function, however, then the fee may still exceed average cost, although it is less than it would be under strict adherence to the rule that marginal revenue should equal marginal cost.

There is little empirical evidence on the existence of loss-leader pricing of office visits. One implication of this model may be that physicians who either own testing equipment or bill for tests may charge less for office visits than other physicians. Danzon and colleagues, using data from a 1975 physician survey, found that when Medicare- and Medicaid-allowed fees were lower, the charge for a complete blood count tended to be higher, by forty to fifty cents, for each dollar reduction in the office visit fee.[15] Furthermore the coefficient of variation for office visit fees was lower than the coefficient of variation for a complete blood count fee, 0.37 compared with 0.59 for all specialties combined.

The aggregate importance of loss-leader pricing is unknown. The key issue for the RBRVS, however, is whether the market for loss-leader services is perfectly competitive. Although research cited above suggests that the market for primary care services has competitive elements, there are no definitive tests for the existence of perfect competition. Thus there is no firm evidence that office visits are priced below cost as opposed to below a profit-maximizing level in a world without loss-leader services.

Indirect evidence on entry into various specialties, however, as measured by the growth between 1974 and 1988 in the number of residents by specialty, does not suggest that primary care specialties are having significant problems attracting practitioners (table 5–2). Family practice and internal medicine had above average growth, while pediatrics was below average. But general surgery and major surgical subspecialties were all below average. (Ophthalmology and pathology were actually negative.) Other pieces of indirect evidence are the facts that the proportion of Medicare claims accepted on assignment is at an all-time high between 70 and 75 percent and that between 1987 and 1988 balance-billing liability declined from about $83 per beneficiary to $72.[16] These facts also suggest that Medicare payments, which are about 30 percent less than physicians' charges, are not too low and therefore that physicians' charges are probably not below cost.

Economic Theory of Cost. There is extensive economic literature on the specification and estimation of cost functions, a literature that the Harvard study appears to have ignored. One of the fundamental

TABLE 5–2
NUMBERS OF RESIDENTS BY SPECIALTIES, 1974–1988

Specialty	1974	1988	Percentage Change, 1974–88
Anesthesiology	2,044	4,480	119.2
Family practice	2,669	7,175	168.8
Internal medicine	11,024	18,074	64.0
Neurology	1,045	1,326	26.9
Obstetrics and gynecology	3,421	4,426	29.4
Ophthalmology	1,568	1,479	−5.7
Orthopedic surgery	2,375	2,758	16.1
Otolaryngology	994	1,036	4.2
Pathology	2,835	2,054	−27.5
Pediatrics	4,784	6,321	32.1
Psychiatry	4,370	5,097	16.6
Radiology (diagnostic)	2,068	3,322	60.6
Surgery	7,354	7,739	5.2
Urology	1,117	972	−13.0
All specialties[a]	52,499	81,093	54.5

a. "All specialties" category includes some specialties not listed.
SOURCES: Liaison Committee on Graduate Medicinal Education, *Directory of Accredited Residencies 1975–1976* (Chicago: American Medical Association, 1976), p. 8; *Journal of the American Medical Association* (August 25, 1989), p. 1030.

propositions of the economic theory of the firm is that the firm's production technology can be represented by a cost function that relates the total cost of production to the levels of all of the firm's outputs and the prices of all of its inputs. This theory has had extensive application in the area of hospital costs but surprisingly little in the area of the cost of physicians' services.[17] Physicians, like hospitals, produce a wide array of services and treat many different types of patients, although for most physicians the range of both services and patient types is small relative to an average hospital. Unlike hospitals, physicians do not pay for all of the inputs they use in producing services. Since the cost of inputs not hired by the physician are usually billed separately, for example, hospital operating room charges or independent laboratory or radiology services, this may not be a severe problem, however.

In principle, then, estimating a multiproduct cost function for physician firms may be a feasible task. Necessary data include counts of the different services the physician firm provides over some accounting period; the total cost of the practice over the same period, including payments made to physicians, the prices of the inputs employed, for example, hourly or weekly incomes of the physicians, nurses, secretaries, and other office help, supply prices, equipment and office rental rates and interest payments, if any; and descriptive information about the patients, for example, age, sex, and race distributions, and possibly insurance coverage as well.

Since cost depends on the volume of output, if the market is noncompetitive and physicians can set their own fees and thus affect output levels, cost itself depends on fees and all the factors, specifically insurance coverage, that affect fees. This notion should be most evident in the estimation of opportunity costs, which depend on physicians' incomes. Physicians' incomes are higher the greater their ability to set fees and manipulate volume. Thus the fact that the cost function does not explicitly include fees does not mean that costs are independent of fee levels.

The literature provides extensive guidance about both the functional form and estimation problems and methods. While the concept of a statistical cost function may be mysterious to physicians and policy makers, at least it is not arbitrary and has well-known properties. Furthermore these functions, if successfully estimated for different specialties, can be used to calculate marginal costs and average costs under current levels of output, minimum average cost, and average costs at different assumptions about physician compensation. If some specialists earn "too much" because their services are overpriced, then the cost function can be used to calculate average cost

115

under different assumptions about physician remuneration, for example, an equal rate of return to specialty training across specialties. Finally, all of the estimates of marginal and average costs could be denominated in a well-known unit of measure, dollars. Thus cross-specialty comparisons of marginal or minimum average costs could be straightforward and theoretically valid.

Are the data needed to estimate statistical cost functions currently available? No, but in principle they are not hard to obtain. Should estimating statistical cost functions to construct resource-based relative values be advocated? The chapter's last section shows why not.

Harvard RBRVS and Economic Theory of Cost. As noted at the outset of this chapter, the goal of the Harvard study is to "develop a resource *cost-based* relative value scale by investigating the resource *input costs* of physicians' services and developing methods to measure them." In particular, for each service, the resource-based relative value is

$$RBRV = (TW) \times (1 + RPC) \times (1 + AST)$$

where TW is the total work input of the physician for that service, RPC is an index of relative nonphysician practice costs across specialties, and AST is an index of the amortized value of the opportunity cost of additional training across specialties.

How well does the Harvard RBRVS adhere to the economic theory of costs? Not very well, for three major reasons. First, although the goal of the Harvard RBRVS is to base relative values on input costs or resource costs, the actual formula used is keyed to an index of physician work effort, not the cost of the effort. Second, nonphysician practice costs and opportunity costs are allocated to specific services in proportion to the relative work for that service since those two components of the formula vary only by specialty and not by service. Third, the formula itself is arbitrary and inconsistent with the cost function derived from economic theory.

The Harvard RBRVS is not based on input costs since it does not include the cost of physician work. It follows then that the relative scarcity of physicians who perform various services is not a part of the Harvard RBRVS. If practice costs and opportunity costs are the same, a service that requires twice the work effort of another has a relative value twice as large regardless of whether many or few physicians perform that service.

To some, this may not be troublesome. It clearly violates, however, a basic assumption underlying the cost function derived from economic theory, namely, that the cost of all of the inputs is included in calculating the average cost of a service. The repair of an inguinal hernia by a general surgeon, for example, has an RBRV of 476, more than four times the RBRV of an initial history done by an internist.[18] But if there were 80,000 general surgeons in practice instead of the nearly 40,000 currently active, would the cost of the required work stay the same? Would consumers need to pay the same fee to get general surgeons to perform the operation? If the answers to these questions are yes, then in effect one must believe that the cost of an input is independent of its supply or availability.

For another example, suppose that the Japanese developed a process for manufacturing lithotripters at half the cost of the current machines. Suppose that they flooded the U.S. market with these machines at half the price of current models. The new machines are identical to the old; that is, they do exactly the same work. Nevertheless the RBRVs of the services associated with those machines would be expected to fall precisely because the cost of a major input falls.

How does the Harvard study allocate nonphysician practice costs among services? Basically a service that takes twice as much work as another has twice the relative practice costs assigned to it regardless of whether it requires twice the equipment, is done in the office or the hospital (where presumably the physician incurs minimal practice costs), or needs twice the support to run the equipment and to prepare the patient for the service.

A thirty-minute office visit may require much more physician work than interpretation of test results, for example. But the equipment, staff, and space required to perform the test may have much higher nonphysician input costs than the half-hour office visit. Nevertheless the office visit has a bigger share of nonphysician costs implicitly assigned to it if it involves more physician work.

This type of misallocation may be one of the reasons RBRVs for office visits are so high relative to charges; that is, too much of the practice's nonphysician costs are assigned to visits. Malpractice insurance premium costs are implicitly assigned to specific services in the same way although it is well known, for example, that not performing a relatively easy service, delivering a baby, can have a profound effect on the malpractice premiums of gynecologists and family and general practitioners. Thus services that are performed primarily in settings other than the office, that is, in settings where physicians bear little of the cost of other inputs, or services that take a lot of physician time but not much equipment or ancillary help, such as a complete medical history, are overvalued relative to nonphysician practice costs.

The Harvard study's paper on practice costs summarizes the situation fairly well. "Without detailed information on the actual practice costs of providing each service, it is difficult to evaluate what distortion, if any, is caused by the impact of incorporating practice costs on the basis of total work."[19] In other words, the nonphysician costs of providing individual services is simply unknown.

In addition to the strong assumption that practice and opportunity costs are allocated in proportion to total work, the formula itself is arbitrary and inconsistent with the economic theory of cost. First, the cost of producing a service depends on the volume of that service in relation to the volume of other services produced by the physician firm. Second, the cost depends on the prices of all the inputs, including the physician. There is no such thing as a fixed and invariant cost of producing a service. Rather cost depends on the circumstances of production. Thus, to produce consistent resource-based relative values, one needs to evaluate costs under a consistent set of assumptions about volume and input prices.

Ignoring the multiproduct aspect of a physician's practice may be another reason the RBRVs for office visits appear to be so high relative to charges. Many of the physician's inputs, including time, are "hired" to produce a wide range of services. Since the inputs are there to produce other outputs, not just office visits, the marginal cost of an office visit may in fact be quite low. A recent study of hospital costs using the multiproduct cost function approach found that the marginal cost of a hospital outpatient visit (excluding outpatient surgery) was only $27, well below the usual cost-accounting estimates.[20] Using an arbitrary formula, even one that appears simple, reasonable, and understandable, can lead to wrong estimates, however.

Although the Harvard RBRVS is not a true cost-based relative value scale, the study has nevertheless made three significant contributions. First, it demonstrates that panels of physicians can be used to reach consensus about the relationships among services. Unfortunately they were asked the wrong questions.

Second, the study demonstrates the feasibility and acceptability to physicians of creating families of services and using a small number of services for which an RV is explicitly developed in each family as the basis for extrapolating relative values to the other services in that family.[21] The creation of these families was no small task and can be used in future relative value studies.

Third, the study developed a useful method for linking relative values across specialties.[22] If relative values are not expressed in monetary terms, then some way to calibrate specialty-specific relative values to a common scale must be found. The approach developed by the Harvard study can be used in future relative value studies.

Alternatives to RBRVS

Estimates of the cost of producing a service should obviously be a factor in constructing both relative values and relative fees.[23] Cost, however, should not be the sole determinant of relative values precisely because cost does not take value into account. Rather than focusing on the relationship of fees to costs, payers should worry about the relationship between fees and outputs. To say that the fee for an office visit is too low relative to that for an electrocardiogram or a colonoscopy or a hernia repair should be interpreted to mean that patients are either not getting enough office visits or getting too many cardiograms, colonoscopies, or hernia repairs. Will paying more for office visits and less for cardiograms result in more office visits and fewer cardiograms? Will a higher fee for an office visit result in longer or better visits? Is this a better mix of services? Will more or better office visits lead to better outcomes? Can patients get the same quantity and quality of care at a lower fee? Viewing the problem as how to get value for money implies that Medicare should concentrate on what it gets as a result of a fee schedule, not on how physicians combine inputs to produce services.

The debate over how much to pay for evaluation-management services relative to procedural services provides an excellent example of these points.[24] The primary issue seems to be the difference between fees and costs. One side argues that EM services are undervalued relative to procedural services because the implicit rate of return per unit of physician effort appears to be so much lower for EM services than for procedural services. The other side argues that these calculations do not properly take into account differences in skill, complexity, training, risk, and the like, required to perform a procedural service relative to an EM.

It can be argued that EM services are undervalued simply because the payment per hour of physician effort is low relative to payment per hour for procedural services. Most other occupations, such as ballet dancers, teachers, and gas station attendants, have no opportunity to perform procedural services; they receive a low payment per hour of work. But this fact would hardly justify paying more for ballet tickets, school budgets, or gasoline. Nor would paying more for these other services, to eliminate the apparent inequity in providers' payment per hour, make procedural services any less lucrative.

The same point can be made by looking at the other extreme of hourly remuneration. Some professions, such as lawyers, stockbrokers, and corporate executives, earn high rates of return per hour from EM activities. Yet the resource cost per hour of their time may be even lower than that of physicians. The key to this paradox is that resource cost or payment per hour is not the sole, or necessarily even the primary, determinant of payment rates. Value to the user or patient also plays an important role.

Relative fees for EM and procedural services may be out of line. But this judgment should be based on assessments of the benefits of those services and whether people are getting too many or too few of one or the other kind of services. Again, making these assessments is not easy. It requires gauging whether people have trouble obtaining EM services, whether more EM services would improve outcomes (medically and fiscally), whether raising fees for EM services would increase their volume, and whether too many procedural services of marginal or no benefit are being performed. Answers to these questions, not comparisons of rates of return per hour of physicians' time or estimates of how much work is needed for a service should signal how relative fees ought to be adjusted.

To some extent, this perspective on the physician payment issue begs the question since it does not solve the problem of what are the right quantity and quality of services. But there are two important differences between trying to evaluate quantities and qualities of services and trying to identify the true cost of production. First, focusing on access and quality shines the light in the right place. Second, quantities of services, unlike production costs, physicians' time, and input prices, can be easily and inexpensively measured. Through the use of uniform and detailed procedure coding terminologies, which are already widely in place, information on quantities for specific services can be generated as a byproduct of the claims payment process in a fee-for-service system.

Relative fees could be changed by increasing the fees for office visits. Do beneficiaries receive more office visits? Do physicians actually spend more time with patients per visit? Does it make any difference to outcomes, subsequent service use, or the total cost of care? Do patients get fewer diagnostic and surgical procedures? If the quantities of some procedures are thought to be too high, then those fees could be lowered. Ultimately both relative and absolute fees could be manipulated to produce volumes of care consistent with both budgetary constraints and good medical care.

Access indicators can also be generated from claims data. In the Medicare program, for example, changes in the proportion of claims for which physicians accept assignment signal the beneficiaries' degree of access. Another signal is the distribution of Medicare part B services across physicians' practices. If physicians begin to find the Medicare fee schedule unacceptably low, then Medicare patients will probably become increasingly concentrated in low-cost practices since only those practices will find that Medicare fees cover their costs. Another indication of access is the magnitude of balance billing. The all-time high rate of assignment in Medicare hardly suggests that current fees are too low relative to other payers' fees or to current physician supply.

Defining the quality of care and measuring how it and the quantity of services change in response to fee changes are elusive and difficult tasks. But to avoid them because they are difficult brings to mind the man, allegedly an economist, who searched for his lost key under the lamppost, although it had dropped into the shrubs by the dark house. Searching may be easier where there is light, but having light guarantees neither relevance nor success. And in the case of trying to measure service-specific resource costs, the light is both low wattage and flickering.

The primary implication of this discussion is that the right price from Medicare's point of view need not bear any direct relationship to underlying costs. If providers are willing to supply as many services of a given quality and convenience as Medicare wants at the price it is offering to pay, then the price is right.

Perhaps Medicare should take costs into consideration in establishing fees, especially to guard against paying too much for a service. Having information on costs may be one way of identifying where large profits exist. For some services, especially those involving new technologies or rapidly changing technologies, charge and quantity data may not be reliable indicators of whether the fee is too high or too low. Charges may not adjust rapidly to changing costs, and quantities may be influenced by the new technological and clinical capabilities of a procedure, as well as by its profitability. Under these circumstances, cost data can provide useful additional information for deciding how much to pay for a service. Recent efforts to identify services whose fees are inherently unreasonable are precisely in this vein and can easily continue without any resort to a resource-based relative value scale.

While a relative value scale based on judgments about access, volume, and quality could be developed de novo, charge data are a readily available and practical starting point. According to prior research on relative value scales, those built from charge data are largely invariant with respect to the charge data used and appear to be reasonably constant over a five-year period, although absolute fee levels grow dramatically.[25]

Starting with a charge-based scale need not implicitly ratify possible distortions contained within existing charges. If the group responsible for developing relative values believes that some services are provided too often and some too infrequently, or that technological change has lowered the cost of a procedure well below its going fee, then that information should be used to diverge relative values from existing relative fees, as in the case of services with inherently unreasonable fees.

This approach does not purport to be a purely objective, politically free method. Many of the factors to be considered in valuing a service are inherently subjective. Consequently the goal of the process is not to seek the objectively true relative value scale or fee schedule. There is no such thing.

Rather the process should try to identify directions of change from existing relative charges. Furthermore, since this is a grope in the dark for a lost key, changes from existing relative charges should be implemented gradually. The ultimate extent and pace of implementation should depend primarily on how physicians and patients respond in quantities of services, access, and quality.

Although this process for determining relative values is inherently judgmental and political, structured methods are available; these use informed opinions as a substitute for precise information to reach consensus on directions for changing relative charges. The Harvard RBRVS study has admirably demonstrated how to tap physicians' knowledge of the process of delivering services. Similar procedures could be used to garner physicians' views on the effectiveness and profitability of various services. Instead of asking physicians about how much skill, effort, and the like, are required to provide a service, they should be asked which services are big money makers, which are provided too often in marginal situations, and which, if any, are not provided often enough. Physicians will not have the final word, but they can and should be part of the process.

As a practical matter, it may not be desirable to implement immediately a fee schedule that departs too radically from existing average charges. For one thing, major changes are likely to create substantial political opposition from physicians who would be financial losers and from patient groups who might fear disruptions in access and reductions in quality of care. For another, there is little actual experience in constructing a relative value scale from other than charge data, converting that scale into a fee schedule for achieving specified objectives in addition to paying for services, and knowing precisely how physicians will respond.

To increase political acceptability and to minimize the costs of making mistakes in calculating fees, Medicare may wish to constrain changes to no more than 5 or 10 percent greater or smaller than existing average or prevailing charges. It might also be desirable to start with a relatively small number of procedures including those responsible for a high proportion of expenditures or those thought to be seriously over- or underprovided. If major problems or unexpected effects did not surface over the first year of the fee schedule, then fees could be adjusted another 5 or 10 percent on a periodic basis until the transition to the desired fee schedule is completed.

The case for gradual implementation of a fee schedule is all the stronger because no administrative or structured process, including the one outlined above, can precisely identify true relative values. A subjective process informed by available data may be able to identify procedures thought to be substantially under- or overvalued. But these evaluations should be taken as recommendations to increase or decrease relative fees. How much to change them ultimately depends on how quantity, quality, and access respond to each round of changes in both relative and absolute fees.

However these processes are ultimately resolved, it is critical that insurers set up systems to monitor the quantities of services provided, to assess changes in the quality of those services, and to evaluate beneficiaries' ease or difficulty in obtaining services at the fee schedule prices. This information is essential to identifying both the impact of changes made in the fee schedule and the needs for future changes. Changes in political objectives and changes in budgetary constraints also influence annual modifications to the fee schedule.

Recalibration of the underlying relative value scale probably needs to be done less frequently, perhaps every five years. Changes in costs due to changes in technologies and changes in the prices of inputs, especially the cost of malpractice insurance and of time for physicians, nurses, and other labor, could be incorporated into the scale revision process. New procedures could be incorporated into the scale as they become clinically acceptable, although reexamination of their costs and efficacy might occur more frequently than every five years until they become standard or routine services. Various studies of cost, efficacy, and quality could be performed on an ongoing basis for selected procedures to build a larger and better data base for future considerations of changes in scale values.

To the extent that the modern fee schedule is no more than the ancient just price, will market forces make fee schedules anachronistic? Can regulatory fee schedules incorporate or take advantage of market-generated pressures?

One approach, which is in keeping with existing Medicare practice, to incorporating market forces is to permit physicians to bill patients for charges exceeding the fee schedule amount. Unlike the current system, Medicare could also permit rebates for charges below the fee schedule amount. In this way patients would not be denied access to quality care when demand is high or physicians are in short supply. Nor would they have to pay more than the going rate when demand is soft and physicians are engaging in widespread fee discounting.

Another, perhaps equally, important reason for maintaining a dual system of fee schedule amounts and physicians' charges (above or below the fee schedule) is that average charges can serve as a continuous monitor of how closely the fee schedule reflects market conditions.[26] Thus they could also provide a mechanism for making adjustments to relative values and relative fees. Not all changes in market conditions affect all services uniformly. Comparing relative and absolute charges to relative and absolute fee schedule amounts may provide good information about how to change the fee schedule.

Permitting physicians to bill patients for amounts different from the fee schedule may be desirable for other reasons as well. Despite the large number of procedures and the precision with which a procedure coding terminology defines them, variation is inevitable in the quality, convenience, and amenities people wish to purchase and providers are willing to provide. A uniform fee schedule that applies to all physicians and to all patients discourages these variations. To the extent that high-quality (as opposed to average-quality) care is more expensive to provide, physicians are reluctant to offer it. To the extent that patients want high-quality care, they have difficulty finding it. These types of conflicts are likely to arise especially when specialists and generalists provide services identified by the same procedure codes.

The choice between equity and uniformity, on the one hand, and freedom of choice and diversity, on the other, is essentially political. Generally the American way seems to favor the latter. If this choice is made, then separate means of ensuring low-income people adequate access to care of acceptable quality should also be an objective of the health care financing, payment, and delivery systems.

The approach outlined for constructing a relative value scale may frustrate those who seek to determine truth, just as economic realities frustrated the ancient theologians who sought the just price. Even with the right data, whoever is paying must decide what is desired so that fees are set correctly. No objective truth exists for an issue like this. Instead insurers should concentrate on evaluating what they get for their payments rather than the relationship between payments and resource costs.

Similarly policy makers should be cautious about jumping aboard the RBRVS train. The RBRVS could create far greater distortions, and thus disruptions, than currently exist. Its apparent political popularity as a mechanism for creating a fee schedule should not outweigh the harm that a wrong fee schedule could create. If anything, the RBRVS's lack of strong intellectual underpinnings should strengthen the case for creating a fee schedule from existing charge data and then modifying relative fees as experience and research direct.

Beyond Payment Reforms

A Commentary by Charles E. Phelps

These comments center on three main areas: (1) further clarification of the nature of input costs, factor substitution, and final product costs; (2) the role of administrative fee schedules in determining the quality of care; and (3) the role of information in medical care, which may have more profound effects on health care and health outcomes than price or fee mechanisms.

Input Costs, Output Costs, and Condition of Entry. The chapter discusses, although incompletely, the distinction between input costs and final product costs, and it does not draw into the discussion possible distortions in factor markets that could possibly account for some of the observed patterns in the relative pricing of physician services. In entirely competitive markets, as Hadley has discussed well, the minimum average cost AC_j of the provision of service j would constitute the appropriate reimbursement for Medicare or any other regulatory insurance plan. This average cost would come from combining the costs of inputs, combined intelligently according to cost-minimizing rules and the production function.

Unfortunately Hadley stopped short in his discussion of the costs of physician labor as an input to the firm. In concept the labor input of physicians in a physician's firm could be considered separately from those of the physician as owner, manager, and entrepreneur. Indeed in some firms physicians are separately hired with no management or ownership role. How are such services priced? This necessarily depends on the conditions of supply and how the factor markets are organized and perform, even if the final product market is perfectly competitive. Two examples can be considered. First, if the supply curve of physician labor is perfectly elastic, then the cost of that physician time enters directly into the cost of the final product, and the cost of that input does not vary with the aggregate demand either for the input or for the final product. Second, if the input is

126

supplied with zero elasticity (fixed supply), then its market price varies with the intensity of final product demand, and the supply curve of the final product also incorporates some inelasticity. Indeed, under the extreme case of zero elasticity of substitution between this fixed supply input and other inputs, the final product also has a completely inelastic supply curve, even in competitive markets. In the intermediate case, if the input supply has some price responsiveness, then the competitive supply curve also has finite supply elasticity, except when perfect substitution with other inputs is possible. In a competitive final product market, if an input market behaves noncompetitively, with monopoly pricing an extreme case, then the output price of the firm reflects that higher input cost.

A separate consideration in the production process is the role of factor substitution. As a crude generalization, those services commonly classified as procedure-based (that is, surgery) apparently have relatively little opportunity for substitution of less costly labor for physician labor. One would not expect internists to perform neurosurgery, let alone nurses. In cognitive services such as diagnosis, however, much of the information gathering can be, and often is, performed by persons other than the principal physician in charge of the patient's case. Nurses and physician assistants often take the primary history and some of the physical examination of some patients. Without understanding the roles of substitution in production, one cannot meaningfully talk about the appropriateness of the cost-based RBRVS proposed by Harvard's project. This is particularly true since the Harvard approach, as this chapter clearly discusses, tacitly assumes that physician labor and all other factors, combined, are used in fixed proportions.

These same considerations broadly hold in final product markets that are monopolistically competitive. If a specific input has a restricted or fixed supply, then its shadow price rises, and the apparent costs of the firm rise. Hadley's discussions of the opportunity costs of physician time hint at this issue but do not directly discuss it. This approach raises the possibility that some of the differences in apparent (inferred) average billings per hour for physician time correspond to different conditions of entry for physicians and surgeons into the relevant specialty, or different opportunities for substitution in production.

Hadley's table 5–2 suggests that conditions of entry into various specialties may not be the same. With an overall 62 percent increase in medical and surgical residents (all specialties) between 1974 and 1988, most of the surgical specialties (those emphasizing procedure-based compensation) showed much smaller increases in supply than did many of the cognitive specialties, most notably family and general practice and internal medicine. In Hadley's table 5–1, every CPT-4 procedure code with a charge/RBRV ratio exceeding 1 came within the domain of surgeons, and every procedure with a ratio less than 1 came within the general category of cognitive services. This table is not unrepresentative of the findings of Hsiao and his colleagues. If entry into surgical specialties were more restricted than for cognitive specialties for whatever reason, then this sort of result would naturally appear.[1] Comparison of the internal rates of return within various medical specialties corresponds with this notion, at least approximately. In 1980, for example, the internal rate of return for specialty training in internal medicine was estimated by Marder and Willke, chapter 13, at 9.8 percent, versus 13.8 percent for general surgeons and 14.8 percent for obstetrician-gynecologists.[2]

If some market distortions in the input market exist, then even the cost function methods discussed by Hadley provide distorted pictures of the true competitive costs of provision of one procedure versus another. Precisely for this reason Hsiao and his colleagues adopted the adjusted work effort scale. In effect they attempted to derive a measure of the value of physicians' time that would emerge in a fully competitive market with equal returns to time in every activity.[3] This issue sits at the heart of Hadley's criticism that the Harvard group ignored the cost of physician services. He states that the cost of physician services varies with the relative scarcity of the input. He does not address why such differences in the supply cost exist and persist across specialties, or if it would be desirable to peg a reimbursement system in such a way as to alter these relative scarcities in the long run.

Neither the Harvard analysis nor subsequent discussions have focused on the likely long-run market response to a fee index based on relative cost, whether that proposed by Harvard or any comparable system. Surely, if the Harvard approach (or any near cousin) were implemented, the returns to various specialties would shift greatly. This would provide some important evidence on two issues: (1) the ability of physicians to induce demand and (2) the nature of supply into various medical specialties. It would be astonishing if one of the responses did not include a major shift away from surgery and into medical specialties. The political debate is already shaping up, since some specialists would have a windfall decline in the value of their specialty training, and others a windfall gain. Thus the implementation of these ideas depends more on political than economic issues.

The Role of Fee Schedules in Determining Quality. Hadley's chapter and the Harvard project's work generally ignore the issue of quality of the service provided. Quality can vary along many dimensions, including the diagnostic acumen of the doctor who treats the patient; the amount of time the doctor, nurse, or other professionals spend with the patient; and the ambience of the medical office. In general, patients' willingness to pay for a given quantity of care rises with the quality. Thus a family of demand curves and cost curves generally exists from which a physicians' services firm might choose one or more for its particular style. Some firms choose more quality, others more quantity. Setting a specific fee for a particular service (à la the Harvard cost-based RBRVS) may have as its primary determinant the setting of quality in the market, more than anything else.

A central question in such matters is whether the physicians' services firm would be permitted to charge in excess of the fee schedule limit and to bill the patient directly for the balance (so-called balance billing). Without balance billing, higher-quality producers who have prices above the fee schedule limit would surely reduce their quality. Any analysis of the welfare effects of a fee schedule must include the status of balance billing. The Harvard study does not discuss this question in general, nor does Hadley in general. Zuckerman and Holahan, in chapter 6, provide some useful discussion of these and other issues.

The Role of Information in Physician Services. A third, and perhaps most important, issue remains: much of Hadley's discussion, following the standards of economics, assumes that if the right price is offered for medical services, the market supplies the right quantity. Insurance distorts those decisions, but the mainline idea remains intact: correct pricing is all that is needed to get the market performing as well as desired. Demand inducement may also alter market performance, but that question is set aside as well. Hadley suggests that a useful approach to physician fee regulation would be based at least in part on better-informed buyers, for example, with well-grounded cost estimates. That is valid. A more fundamental problem exists in the market, however: physicians, in their crucial role as advisers and agents for patients, disagree wildly about the marginal productivity of various types of medical care. Thus setting the right prices alone does not give all the gains in health care markets that might be achieved. In addition the diffusion of information problem in medicine should be approached more directly. The new Agency for Health Care Policy and Research programs to study medical care use and health outcomes reflect a growing, and sorely needed, addition to the agenda of health care economics.[4]

The statement about disagreement among physicians regarding the marginal productivity of medical care arises from the repeated and well-documented evidence on the variability of use of specific medical services for apparently similar populations. This work, developed extensively over the last decade by Wennberg and various colleagues at Dartmouth and elsewhere, Roos and colleagues in Manitoba, Chassin and colleagues at Rand, and McPherson and colleagues in Britain, among others,[5] has established the following:

1. Variations are reproducible and systematic. Procedures with relatively high variations appear similarly in all studies, for example, tonsillectomy and back surgery. Low-variability procedures remain so in all studies (for example, hip fracture surgery).

2. Variations are not caused by random chance. Several approaches have established that most of the observed variations are systematic, not random.

3. Variations are not caused by price differences, at least in the main. The most compelling evidence for this is the occurrence of the same patterns of variations in the British national health system and in Canada, although price is the same to all patients, and providers (especially in the BNHS) are compensated by salary. Separately the degree of variability in some procedures is wholly inconsistent with known price responsiveness of consumers. In the Rand Health Insurance Study, for example, fully insured persons used hospital care about half again more than persons with relatively little insurance (large deductible plans).[6] Thus the largest difference in use across regions that might be expected because of price differences confronting patients would be on the order of 50 percent or so, even if one region had full insurance and the other stingy insurance. Yet, with much smaller variations in actual coverage, the observed differences in the rates of use of many surgical interventions often exceeds an order of magnitude across regions.

4. Variations are not caused by patient decisions or patient characteristics. They seem to be primarily related to physicians, not patients.

5. Variations do not arise because of the lack of medical training. Wennberg's study of different rates of hospitalization for patients living in New Haven and Boston (where almost all hospitalizations take place through doctors affiliated with medical schools) demonstrates that the disagreements persist even across some of the nation's finest medical schools.[7]

6. Variations occur for both surgical and nonsurgical procedures. Variations now appear more important for nonsurgical than surgical hospitalizations.

7. Variations are not caused by classic inducement. The BNHS example serves to refute this idea in part. In addition several studies have shown that informing doctors about the presence of variations suffices to cause the variation to collapse, usually with the high-rate doctors reducing their rates of application of surgical techniques.

All of these aspects of variations imply that something is taking place outside of the price system in the use of medical care. This is a problem in the economics of information, rather than in the economics of medical care per se. Little is known about the causes of these variations or their sustained presence. While the emphasis on payment schemes remains valid, one should not lose track of what may prove to be a more important problem in medical care, namely, the apparently large disagreements among physicians about the marginal productivity of medical care. If this problem is as large as it appears to some, it suggests that the institution of payment reforms alone will not achieve the goals of fully rational and appropriate medical care.

The Art of Paying Physicians

A Commentary by Clark C. Havighurst

One hears again and again from doctors that practicing medicine is an art as well as a science. According to Jack Hadley, paying a doctor is also not entirely a scientific matter. A lot of art is involved as well. Apparently, however, the state of this art remains quite primitive. Indeed, it is amazing how little is known about how to approach the fundamental task of paying physicians for patient care rendered at the expense of a third-party payer, either government or a private insurer. One wonders why the art of paying physicians was not perfected long ago. Medical insurance has been around for over fifty years, and Medicare has been paying doctors for nearly half that time. Yet physician reimbursement is still a mystery. It is important to ask why this problem remains unsolved.

One clue lies in the expression "physician reimbursement." It is notable that, even though the term "reimbursement" had been in general use for many years, Congress set up a Physician *Payment* Review Commission, not a Physician Reimbursement Review Commission. Despite its general use, "reimbursement" is clearly a misnomer for what is going on in compensating physicians for their services to beneficiaries of public or private health insurance programs. Reimbursement implies that the payer is making someone whole, simply compensating him for outlays made or specific costs incurred. The term is not at all accurate as a description of what today's insurers do when they pay doctors.

It was long the common practice for most payers to reimburse hospitals directly for costs actually incurred, and one might think that the term "reimbursement" was simply carried over unthinkingly to the physician context. But there was more to it than that. One reason why the term was employed, I suspect, was that it successfully avoided any implication that a third party's payment to a physician was in fact a purchase price. Indeed, certain interests found it advantageous to delude the public into thinking that they were

132

looking at something other than a commercial transaction. Ever since medical insurance began, there has been a concerted effort by the medical profession, without resistance from the health insurance industry, to prevent people from thinking of payers or consumers simply as buyers of personal services and of physicians simply as sellers. Partly as a result of that effort, the public went along with the nonmarket paradigm of medical care for many years, during which there was a systematic neglect of the art of buying physician services—what is now called prudent purchasing.

Some of the reasons why payers approached doctors in such a gingerly fashion for so long are familiar. The doctors set up the first important medical insurance plans, the Blue Shield plans, and designed them as noncommercial prepayment schemes. As joint selling agencies rather than independent middlemen, these plans could be counted upon to be allies of their sponsoring providers rather than agents of their subscribers. Physicians used these early plans to set an example for commercial insurers, which were allowed into the market only if they did business in ways that physicians approved. As Goldberg and Greenberg have shown in a classic article,[1] there were occasional boycotts, and always a threat of boycott, against plans that adopted an adversarial stance toward physicians and attempted to act as bargainers on behalf of the consumer. As a result of the profession's activities, the commercial health insurers generally fell into line and allowed themselves, as a cartel might do, to be policed by physicians. They thereby avoided the necessity for competitive innovation in the control of moral hazard and in the prudent purchasing of insured services. When all that is added up, there were a lot of years of physician "reimbursement" and no private experimentation with prudent purchasing.

As Lee Benham has noted, regulation of various kinds strongly inhibited commercial activity by corporate intermediaries in the health care field. The corporate practice of medicine was prohibited, or at least was legally suspect, for many years, and its status is still not fully clarified. In addition, free choice of physician was exalted as a firm tenet of all insurance plans, largely because physicians made it a prime criterion of a plan's acceptability. Although freedom of choice sounds like a good thing, "guild free choice," as Charles Weller has called it in distinguishing it from "market free choice,"[2] had the effect of limiting the ability of insurers to reward with more patients any practitioner who would reduce fees. Under the free-choice principle, payers had to let the patient choose the physician, whose fees could then be set without confronting a bulk purchaser. Because patients would be reimbursed by their insurers and lacked good information, they did not drive hard bargains.

When the Medicare program came along, its design essentially imitated the reimbursement practices that had emerged in the private sector. Congress adopted the Blue Shield approach to paying practitioners, including the free-choice principle. The idea that a payer should not interfere in the sacred doctor-patient relationship was enshrined in federal law. Precluded from practicing selectivity, government was foreclosed from using its bargaining power in dealing with individual physicians.

Another feature of the era during which it was bad form to speak of insurers *buying* physician services was the tendency to treat physician reimbursement as if it were a purely technical problem, to be addressed scientifically through a formula designed into the system. Thus, insurers developed the system of referring to "usual, customary, and reasonable" (UCR) fees to determine the maximum fees that they would pay or reimburse. That idea originated with the physician-dominated Blue Shield plans and was adopted by Medicare. Essentially it embodied the assumption that the appropriate fee to pay a doctor is what other doctors are charging for the same service. On the face of it, that method of paying physicians sounds like using the competitive price to determine appropriate compensation. But with widespread health insurance and its attendant moral hazard and with ignorant consumers facing huge search costs and a market where they could not shop effectively on the basis of price, the prevailing market price was hardly a perfectly competitive one. Furthermore the market price that emerged under these conditions was not external to the Medicare program and other third-party payers, whose reimbursement practices strongly influenced it in an upward direction.

On the face of it, UCR fees looked competitively and objectively determined and thus seemed to have scientific legitimacy. In reality, however, the UCR approach reflected the incredible premise that the majority of physicians, as ethical practitioners, would not abuse their discretion or market power in setting their fees. In effect, payers treated professional norms as if they were just as useful in evaluating the level of professional fees as they were in evaluating the quality or appropriateness of care. Although it is also a mistake to regard the latter issues as purely technical ones, they are certainly more so than are professional fees.

Relative value scales (RVSs) were another part of the effort to treat payment issues as a technical rather than an economic matter. Physician organizations produced RVSs in large numbers in the 1950s

134

and 1960s. The idea was to resolve fairness issues by careful scientific study rather than by letting relative values "float." Schedules were developed only for each specialty, however, and not for the profession as a whole. Political conflicts within the profession apparently prevented it from providing a scale that related surgical procedures, for example, to the activities of internists and other specialists. Nevertheless, within each specialty the profession produced quite detailed RVSs that aided in the effort to make the payment formula seem fair and technically sound, thereby keeping payers from initiating their own methods of buying professional services.

Phillip Kissam and I wrote an article in 1979 in which we discussed profession-sponsored RVSs from an antitrust perspective.[3] The main point of that article, in addition to observing the value and occasional use of RVSs as formulas to facilitate price fixing, was that RVSs were instrumental in the medical profession's larger campaign to keep insurers from becoming active purchasers of medical services. Evidence that we found in the medical literature revealed the profession's overriding fear that innovation in paying physicians might occur on the purchasers' side of the market. But as long as the profession could supply credible payment tools, payers would not be tempted or forced to invent new ones independently.

It took payers, both public and private ones, until the 1980s even to begin to study the art of physician payment. The learning process and innovation have only begun, however, and have much farther to go. The public would have been much better off today if the innovation that began tentatively when medical insurance itself began in the 1930s had been allowed to continue instead of being snuffed out by the efforts of organized medicine, as poignantly recounted by Goldberg and Greenberg. Indeed, one must grudgingly admire the success that the medical profession had in preventing health insurers from discovering for over a generation how to buy medical services effectively in a competitive market.

It is now probably time finally to jettison the myth that how to pay physicians is a scientific question, a technical matter than can be resolved by a magic formula developed by experts sitting around a table. If, though, the magic-formula chimera is still pursued, it would be an improvement if the work on any such formula were done by doctors and other experts who are not sponsored by medical interests. Although Jack Hadley praises the Hsiao study for involving doctors, the cooperation of organized medicine with that study suggests that the profession still hopes that a formula approach can keep physician payment out of the competitive marketplace.

Now that it has finally begun, innovation in paying physicians is

135

likely to proceed faster and more creatively and effectively in the private sector than previously seemed possible. In the private sector, politics will not get in the way of implementing new ideas, and competing health plans can try out a variety of methods, including fee schedules and formulas, in different circumstances. The market now seems to be free enough of the old constraints and inhibitions that real innovation can occur. Thus the public can now expect some real progress where so little was made for so many years. Innovation under market constraints and without fear of retaliation by organized medicine should soon allow payers finally to master the art of compensating physicians.

These observations strongly suggest the desirability of some kind of capitation in the Medicare program. That approach would leave the problem of how to pay physicians largely in private hands, sparing government the task of fashioning a global solution. A decentralized approach would also allow the private sector to work on solving the problem that Charles Phelps has stressed—that is, how to curb inappropriate spending on marginally beneficial health services. Decentralization of decision making on such issues as how to pay physicians and precisely what to pay them to do seems much more promising than trying to solve these problems by official, ostensibly scientific formulas, regulations, and protocols dictating medical practice. One can only hope that physician payment reform under Medicare will not freeze the art of paying physicians in its current, still primitive state.

Physician Markets

A Discussion

HENRY AARON: Jack Hadley is saying that the resource-based relative value scale is a rather primitive instrument and that total cost is a function of quality, inputs, and substitution possibilities. The correct analysis is far more complicated than the RBRVS estimation. From the standpoint of policy analysis, however, this is not helpful. People do not understand production costs right now. There is no good device for measuring health services. As several people pointed out, one cannot measure quality. There is no good measure of what the medical profession does. To apply the theoretically correct procedures, one would have to wait a long time.

One should step back and ask oneself to suppose that the exact marginal social benefit and marginal social cost of each and every medical procedure are known. Now, if that price were put into place in a world of insurance and uncertainty, would the right, socially ideal, benefit-maximizing quantities of each service result? They would not.

Conversely, if one asked the price that would elicit the social benefit maximizing quantity, it would not emerge from cost analysis carried out to perfection with complete information along the lines that Jack Hadley suggested.

To defend the RBRVS approach, one should reduce, not fully correct, the anomalies in existence between resource costs and perceptions of these marginal social benefits. It is theoretically not sophisticated, it is not exactly right, it is also not the last word.

Even if Hsiao's plan is modified by the various criticisms, few people think it is the last word. It is the part of the political process to generate the kinds of information that Havighurst called for. One should not criticize it as an exercise in microeconomics. Rather it is a step in political economy.

JACK HADLEY: I agree with everything that Henry Aaron said except the suggestion that I call for estimation of statistical cost functions. That would be a bad idea for exactly the same reasons that he cited.

137

This is a very political process. While we might well want to seek out excess profits and to try to drive those profits out through a fee mechanism, a technical statistical approach is not the way to do that. In fact I agree with some of the other comments that this process requires judgment about how markets respond to fee changes. We need to do a lot more in trying to measure quality, responses, and so forth.

RITA RICARDO CAMPBELL: I am amazed that a conference is being held on what I call the comparable worth theory of physicians' payments. The literature on how women should be paid in the state of Washington reads the same way as the RBRVS: resource values, skills to be evaluated, and so on. I suggest reading that literature.

Since business firms through coalitions to a degree led changes in national policy in the 1980s, I am disappointed that this conference does not include speakers from business firms to discuss utilization reviews. As a member of the board of a company that has plants in Van Nuys, California, and in Waco, Texas, I wonder why a coronary bypass is one-third more in California. The quality is much the same.

WILLIAM C. HSIAO: I would like to bring out three aspects of Jack Hadley's presentation. Do economists have a valid model for physicians' market pay? Or are we trying to borrow the neoclassical economic theory and the models that already exist and force them on a marketplace where behavior is perhaps different from what we have hypothesized about how consumer and suppliers behave?

In that context Jack believes the market behaves like monopolistic competition. I would like to ask, Is that model valid? Then we can judge whether Jack's conclusions are valid.

Second, Jack laid out the first-best solution and then looked at the RBRVS to ask, "How close does the RBRVS come to that first-best solution?" If we cannot find a first-best solution, is the RBRVS closer to that first-best solution or is some other alternative or is the status quo? Let us not compare this work to perfection.

And last, this is not a seminar on pure economics but rather a seminar on political economy. To what extent do the people who are most affected by it, both the consumer and the providers, think this is a good thing? At least one group has spoken: organized medicine. They by and large say no. This is imprudent from their perspective.

MARK A. SATTERTHWAITE: First, certainly some try to push physician pricing into economic models. Monopolistic competition is quite different from perfect competition, and it does seem to fit the facts. To explain fees by a noneconomic model, one has to ask the question, Why are fees so low? and not, Why are they so high?

138

Physicians seem to have a lot of unexploited economic power. Why are pediatricians willing to settle for lower incomes than surgeons? My working hypothesis about people is that none of us is greedy but that we just need 15 percent more.

Second, there is a lot of support for something like a resource-based relative value scale. As pointed out by Rita Ricardo Campbell, it is really an argument about comparable worth. And if we try to impose that without understanding why those discrepancies in income across specialties came about, we may just transfer a lot of income in the short run from one specialty to another, and then have an expensive long-run adjustment to return to those same old income disparities, toward which underlying economic forces may be driving us. That would be a great shame. We do not know the source of these disparities, and so there is a certain amount of danger in changing fees across specialties.

Third, it is a political process. We are not going to jump the whole way, so we probably will not do a great deal of damage if we move a bit of the direction of the RBRVS.

PETER ZWEIFEL: Going forth and back on income disparities would occur if you change to relative value-based payment.

German and Swiss fee schedules look just alike. Some countries have forty, fifty, sixty years of experience of working with those scales. The outcome is just about the same. Through the political process of negotiating, those physicians have had the upper hand, and the economists have the feeling that they are lagging behind, ten years at least, with technological development. But the power of those medical associations is enhanced because they are the negotiators, and the single physician is rather tied to them.

JOEL IRA FRANCK: I am a physician. Does the panel think there should be an Economist Payment Review Commission, instead of the PPRC? The theme of many of the talks here is that somehow doctors have incredible market power in gouging the public. There has been no net increase in real income for physicians in the United States in two decades, after accounting for inflation. Further, net income for doctors in the United States accounts for less than 10 percent of the medical bills of this country. There is no statistical evidence that this market has somehow changed or has always been noncompetitive.

Now people have been claiming that somehow there is a lack of consumer information, that doctors have life and death power over their consumers, the patients. When I bring my Chevrolet to Louis Chevrolet in Lewiston, Maine, I am putting my life in their hands. When I go to my lawyer to set up my Keogh plan, I am putting my life in his hands, and I have little knowledge of what is going on. Americans put their wealth in the hands of the stockbrokers. In October 1987, on Black Tuesday, 15 percent of the capital wealth of this country disappeared in six hours. There is no difference between medical care and any other personal service in this economy. Should we socialize all of these personal services? Should there be national price and allocation control of all of these essentially personal services?

LEE BENHAM: The argument is well stated. If you were going back to the eighteenth century and you could take only a few items, what would you take? Most individuals would take medical information or medicines.

Technological innovation has been enormous in medicine. No one would deny that. There are some major problems, however. The Washington University Medical School has sales revenue of $1 or $2 billion a year. If one speaks to individuals there about the outcomes associated with their practices, they have little information to give. Very little money goes into that.

Birds Eye spends proportionately more money for systematic quality control than the Washington University Medical School does. This is not to denigrate the people who work hard there. There are no proper incentives to get the research done so that people can understand the real outcomes. A deal could be struck in this regard. Go to the state legislatures and say, "We will cut liability to physicians to a modest level. In exchange, some of the significant resources that have been going into insurance would be applied to producing systematic information, which links actual consequences of medical practices to the actual inputs."

I congratulate the physicians on their hard work. At the same time other groups of specialists, perhaps not economists, need to present relevant information here.

CHARLES E. PHELPS: We could halve or double the resources going into the pockets or bank accounts of physicians and not make a large dent in what is going on in our health care resource use. The important thing about physicians is not how much we pay them. But they are running the controls of a large vessel, and that vessel consumes a lot more resources than go to the physicians individually.

I have become concerned about the information we have to guide that vessel. The front page of the second section of the *Wall Street Journal* today has a long discussion about physician variation. Rita Ricardo Campbell is worried about a 30 percent difference in how much the coronary bypass surgery was costing her firm. But the

140

difference between having one or not in Utica, New York, and in Manhattan is a 2:1 ratio: not 30 percent but 100 percent. For pregnant women, the chances of a Caesarean section in Oneida, New York, are almost 40 percent; they are 18.5 percent in Rochester.

Some of those people are not making the right decisions. Perhaps all of them are wrong. We do not know. But to get some more money into the evaluation of the outcomes into these variations is terribly important. The HCFA outcome studies and the National Center for Health Service and Research Outcome studies that are under way are enormously more important than tinkering around with the way we pay physicians.

Paying physicians is not the question here as much as helping them understand what to do and then giving them incentives to use the information.

WARREN GREENBERG: Except perhaps for the physicians' comments, we have been talking about a static system. Yet we have had a tremendous number of technological changes. Suppose we set a price today. What happens tomorrow with technological change? Are we going to be here at AEI the next year with the same discussion?

After all this is said and done, I agree with Clark Havighurst. We should go the capitation route and pay physicians that way. But how about the dynamic aspect of this? What happens in 1991, 1992?

FRANK A. SLOAN: You cannot focus on 10,000 procedures. You cannot monitor technological change. But if we were able to identify high-volume, high-cost procedures, we could perhaps monitor those. The obvious example of a tremendous change in cost is cataract surgery. Medicare spends about $3 billion per year on cataracts. That is a substantial amount of money. We could spend some amount to figure a reasonable fee for that procedure.

On the issue of prediction, economists have done a much better job of predicting GNP and similar variables than physicians have at predicting outcomes of common diagnoses. And it is easier. We can do a great job there relative to knowing the outcome of medical care. The public believes that medicine is an exact science; private payers do. But it is not.

MR. FRANCK: I agree with Frank Sloan about the lack of precision in medicine. That is an important point because the attempt to apply the model as if it were well-defined is wrong. Medicine is not cut and dried. It involves tremendous subjective evaluation.

I am not a defender of the status quo. The problem with the status quo, however, is not a lack of regulation of doctors through

Medicare and such. There has been too much regulation of doctors, insurance companies, hospitals, and so on. This regulatory apparatus has removed the incentives of the market.

I present a challenge to economists. Instead of studying this relatively trivial part of the total economic bill for medicine, that is, the 10 percent physicians take home—if you cut it 50 percent, you cut the health bill only 5 percent—you should study the effect of the regulatory apparatus that evolved in the past twenty-five years. Regulation is crushing this country with a burdensome medical bill that perhaps would not be there in a true market in medicine.

Doctors would accept more competition—not the AMA perhaps but rank-and-file doctors—if they were also told that along with the slings and arrows of competition, they would get the benefits of competition.

MR. HADLEY: I agree with Bill Hsiao that the Harvard study has taken us a step in the right direction. But we should be careful about accepting it as is and about accepting the notion that cost is the correct peg on which to base fees.

In response to Dr. Franck, no one on this panel wants to regulate doctors' incomes or say how much every doctor should earn. Fees are signals, and Medicare and other insurers have some interest in what those signals convey to practitioners. How we change those signals, that is, how we change those fees, depends on suggestions regarding average assessments of efficacy, of quality, of what collectively we think works and does not. Many things like balance billing are an important part of some ultimate system that stops well short of socialized medicine with government determining everything.

6
The Role of Balance Billing in Medicare Physician Payment Reform

Stephen Zuckerman and John Holahan

In the fall of 1989, the Congress enacted a major change in the way physicians are reimbursed for services provided to Medicare patients. The cornerstone of the reform package was the enactment of a fee schedule, based on the Harvard resource-based relative value scale,[1] that will reduce payment rates for many high-cost services, while raising them for others. Because of concerns that lower payment rates could result in lower assignment rates and an increased financial burden on beneficiaries, Congress also limited the actual fee that physicians could charge. These limits on physicians' charges increase financial incentives to accept assignment by reducing the difference between the billed and allowed amount. In a real sense, this new policy moves Medicare away from its historical commitment to case-by-case flexibility in assignment and toward mandatory assignment.

The theoretical arguments and empirical evidence for and against a policy of mandatory assignment are the subject of this discussion. In general, we find that mandatory assignment may in fact reduce the financial burden for many beneficiaries, but that it is also likely to reduce access to some segment of the physician population and to increase program costs. We argue that it is unnecessary to incur these risks in order to protect beneficiaries from large financial burdens while simultaneously controlling program costs.

From the beginning of the Medicare program until October 1983, physicians were permitted to assign claims on a case-by-case basis. Those choosing to accept assignment were reimbursed directly by the

The authors are grateful for comments provided by H. E. Frech, Jack Hadley, Jesse Hixson, and Margaret Sulvetta. Opinions expressed are those of the authors and do not represent the views of the Urban Institute or its sponsors.

program for an amount equal to the Medicare allowed charge less the patient's deductible and coinsurance liabilities, which they had to collect from the patient directly. They could not bill the patient for any charges in excess of the Medicare allowed amount. Physicians who did not accept assignment had to bill the patient directly. On nonassigned claims, physicians could charge beneficiaries more than the Medicare allowed charge. Patients could collect from the program the Medicare allowed charge less the deductible and coinsurance. By not assigning, a physician was able to charge more than the allowed amount and balance bill for the difference; but he or she had to collect the entire amount from the patient and bear the cost of collection and the risk of bad debts.

The problem with this policy was that assignment rates were relatively low (for example, approximately 50 percent in 1983), efforts to control costs by lowering allowed amounts pushed the financial burdens onto the patient, and the burden of balance billing was distributed unevenly among patients. Thus, the following corrective measures were included in the 1983 Deficit Reduction Act (DEFRA): physicians had to choose either to participate or not to participate in the program; participating physicians had to accept Medicare fees as payment in full on all claims; and nonparticipating physicians could accept assignment on a case-by-case basis, as in the past. Participants were to have their fee screens updated after fifteen months (by January 1, 1986). Other providers were not to have their screens updated and were not permitted to increase actual billed charges to patients. These last two measures provided the principal incentive to participate.

Subsequently, Congress extended the freeze on Medicare physician payments and on nonparticipating physician charges until January 1, 1987, but the 1986 Consolidated Budget Reconciliation Act provided for an increase of 4.15 percent in the allowed charges for participating physicians. These changes created further incentives for physicians to participate, since both the actual and allowed charges of nonparticipating physicians remained frozen.

The Omnibus Budget Reconciliation Act of 1986 then eliminated the freeze on actual charges by nonparticipating physicians, but it placed limits on their balance billing and formally established a differential in prevailing charges favoring participants over nonparticipants. This legislation also included a provision limiting the maximum allowable actual charge (MAAC) and thereby the extent to which nonparticipating physicians could increase their rates. Physicians whose actual charges exceeded 115 percent of the national average prevailing charge for the procedure, that is, the MAAC, could only increase charges by 1 percent. Those whose fees were less than 115 percent of the national average could increase by up to 25 percent as long as they did not exceed the maximum allowable charge. In addition, the statute established a 4 percent differential between prevailing charges of participating and nonparticipating physicians. This differential was increased to 4.5 percent in 1988 and to 5 percent in 1989.

The DEFRA physician participation policy appears to have been extremely successful. Between 1983 and 1985 assignment rates grew substantially in every state and, with a few exceptions, grew again between 1985 and 1987 (table 6-1). Rates vary greatly across states, however. In total, the assignment rate grew from 51 percent in 1983 to 67 percent in 1985, to 74 percent in 1987. The ratio of billed to allowed charges on nonassigned services, a measure of balance billing burden, increased slightly from 1.31 in 1983 to 1.38 in 1985, but then fell to 1.32 in 1987. Assignment rates increased in each specialty and for each type and place of service (table 6-2). Similarly, the ratio of billed to allowed charges changed for each specialty, place, and type of service.

Although policy makers find the increase in assignment rates encouraging, there are three reasons to view it with some caution. First, rapidly accelerating Medicare expenditures ensure even greater constraints on physician fees in the future. If, as several research efforts have shown, the decision to assign claims depends in part on the ratio of billed to allowed charges, assignment rates could eventually decline.[2] More recent evidence indicates that physicians' willingness to participate in the program increases with the level of Medicare fees, holding constant private charges and other factors.[3]

Second, a relative value scale that reduces fees for surgery and other high-charge services could discourage assignment in such cases and lead to significant increases in balance billing. Reductions in Medicare fees in high-charging areas would produce the same result. Although assignment rates could go up for medical care services and in low-fee geographic areas, it is the potential for increases in balance billing that worries policy makers. It is for these reasons that the recent payment reform legislation included further limits on the extent of balance billing in the future.

Third, assignment rates are still low in many areas of the country. In 1987, assignment rates topped 80 percent in twelve states and 90 percent in five, but were below 50 percent in five others and below 60 percent in another ten. Assignment rates also vary according to specialty and type and place of service. For some types of services in some parts of the country, they are very low, with substantial

TABLE 6-1
ASSIGNMENT RATES AND BALANCE BILLING, BY STATE, 1983, 1985, AND 1987

State	Assignment Rate			Ratio of Billed to Allowed Charges		
	1983	1985	1987	1983	1985	1987
U.S. total	0.51	0.67	0.74	1.31	1.38	1.32
Alabama	0.56	0.76	0.85	1.35	1.43	1.31
Alaska	0.46	0.57	0.70	1.33	1.35	1.36
Arizona	0.34	0.55	0.64	1.30	1.35	1.27
Arkansas	0.58	0.84	0.85	1.32	1.37	1.29
California	0.53	0.70	0.78	1.28	1.36	1.24
Colorado	0.42	0.57	0.61	1.37	1.45	1.42
Connecticut	0.44	0.64	0.79	1.31	1.48	1.37
Delaware	0.75	0.83	0.87	1.28	1.37	1.33
District of Columbia	0.76	0.85	0.83	1.33	1.41	1.33
Florida	0.34	0.66	0.71	1.29	1.34	1.22
Georgia	0.55	0.66	0.73	1.30	1.38	1.30
Hawaii	0.42	0.64	0.76	1.34	1.40	1.40
Idaho	0.22	0.34	0.28	1.32	1.37	1.32
Illinois	0.36	0.55	0.63	1.29	1.36	1.32
Indiana	0.28	0.50	0.63	1.33	1.36	1.29
Iowa	0.33	0.50	0.60	1.34	1.38	1.31
Kansas	0.48	0.74	0.84	1.30	1.34	1.33
Kentucky	0.39	0.55	0.71	1.29	1.32	1.26
Louisiana	0.37	0.65	0.73	1.37	1.40	1.35
Maine	0.73	0.82	0.89	1.28	1.34	1.27
Maryland	0.72	0.84	0.92	1.30	1.38	1.31
Massachusetts	0.85	0.95	0.99	1.28	1.38	1.18
Michigan[a]	0.79	0.78	0.74	1.32	1.53	1.30
Minnesota	0.27	0.49	0.68	1.30	1.34	1.39
Mississippi	0.58	0.67	0.68	1.37	1.41	1.39
Missouri	0.44	0.64	0.73	1.28	1.32	1.28
Montana	0.19	0.42	0.48	1.27	1.31	1.29
Nebraska	0.19	0.34	0.51	1.28	1.37	1.26
Nevada	0.61	0.79	0.89	1.30	1.38	1.35
New Hampshire	0.51	0.66	0.65	1.32	1.42	1.39
New Jersey	0.58	0.65	0.69	1.34	1.43	1.38
New Mexico	0.41	0.61	0.65	1.34	1.38	1.33
New York	0.62	0.73	0.77	1.37	1.47	1.47
North Carolina	0.49	0.65	0.74	1.31	1.39	1.34
North Dakota	0.29	0.33	0.42	1.27	1.33	1.28
Ohio	0.34	0.52	0.65	1.32	1.38	1.28
Oklahoma	0.30	0.45	0.56	1.37	1.40	1.38

TABLE 6-1 (continued)

Oregon	0.25	0.43	0.52	1.28	1.30	1.28
Pennsylvania	0.76	0.89	0.92	1.28	1.36	1.30
Rhode Island	0.90	0.92	0.95	1.39	1.43	1.41
South Carolina	0.57	0.80	0.79	1.32	1.43	1.42
South Dakota	0.18	0.25	0.32	1.29	1.33	1.31
Tennessee	0.46	0.58	0.72	1.34	1.38	1.33
Texas	0.53	0.63	0.72	1.37	1.43	1.35
Utah	0.45	0.64	0.75	1.27	1.31	1.32
Vermont	0.58	0.64	0.91	1.31	1.40	1.33
Virginia	0.56	0.69	0.75	1.31	1.36	1.41
Washington	0.30	0.44	0.53	1.27	1.33	1.27
West Virginia	0.51	0.69	0.80	1.39	1.48	1.34
Wisconsin	0.32	0.55	0.57	1.25	1.30	1.27
Wyoming	0.26	0.42	0.33	1.32	1.40	1.39

NOTE: Assignment rates are based on the ratio of assigned allowed charges to total allowed charges for all physician specialties. Nonphysician practitioners are excluded. The ratio of billed to allowed charges is based on the same practitioners.
a. We are aware that the assignment status of claims from Michigan beneficiaries may have been improperly coded in the BMAD data. There was no way to pinpoint the precise coding problems and correct them, however, and so the 1985 statistics for Michigan should be treated with caution.
SOURCE: 1983 Bill Summary Record and 1985 and 1987 BMAD Beneficiary Files.

amounts of balance billing. In 1987 assignment rates for orthopedic surgeons, for example, were 63 percent and the ratio of billed to allowed charges was 1.36; thus, almost 40 percent of elderly Americans needing the services of an orthopedic surgeon could have faced balance billing of rather large amounts. As data that follow show, this burden is not spread evenly across the beneficiary population. Rather, it falls on a very small number of people.

In this paper, we first employ economic theory to analyze how a policy of mandatory assignment might affect the physician service market. We then draw on empirical evidence from the Medicaid program, which has had a policy of mandatory assignment throughout its history, and from Medicare, which has not. We also examine the evidence on physician volume responses to fee changes, which offers some insight into how physicians would respond to fee reductions in a world of mandatory assignment. Some readers may wish to skip the rather technical discussion on the economic theory of assignment behavior and the findings presented in the literature and move directly to the results and policy section, where we explain an alternative proposal—one that would protect beneficiaries against

TABLE 6-2
ASSIGNMENT RATES AND BALANCE BILLING, BY SPECIALTY, TYPE, AND
PLACE OF SERVICE, 1983, 1985, AND 1987

	Assignment Rate			Ratio of Billed to Allowed Charges		
	1983	1985	1987	1983	1985	1987
U.S. total	0.51	0.67	0.74	1.31	1.38	1.32
Specialty						
General practice	0.47	0.62	0.69	1.30	1.36	1.27
General surgery	0.53	0.66	0.72	1.32	1.39	1.36
Cardiology	0.56	0.69	0.76	1.28	1.33	1.24
Internal medicine	0.50	0.65	0.71	1.28	1.34	1.24
Ophthalmology	0.44	0.68	0.79	1.23	1.28	1.26
Orthopedic surgery	0.44	0.57	0.63	1.35	1.41	1.36
Radiology	0.58	0.71	0.76	1.27	1.33	1.25
Other	0.54	0.70	0.75	1.37	1.45	1.40
Type of Service						
Medical care	0.51	0.66	0.72	1.29	1.34	1.26
Surgery	0.49	0.65	0.72	1.30	1.37	1.33
Consultation	0.62	0.73	0.78	1.26	1.31	1.25
Diagnostic X ray	0.57	0.70	0.74	1.26	1.32	1.24
Diagnostic lab	0.55	0.76	0.87	1.30	1.44	1.30
Radiation therapy	0.60	0.68	0.75	1.28	1.36	1.27
Other	0.46	0.66	0.68	1.53	1.62	1.58
Place of service						
Office	0.40	0.59	0.69	1.26	1.32	1.24
Inpatient hospital	0.54	0.67	0.72	1.34	1.42	1.36
Outpatient hospital	0.61	0.73	0.77	1.30	1.36	1.33
Independent lab	0.69	0.97	0.97	1.38	1.44	1.48
Other	0.76	0.90	0.91	1.34	1.41	1.38

NOTE: Assignment rates are based on the ratio of assigned allowed charges to total allowed charges for all physician specialties. Nonphysician practitioners are excluded. The ratio of billed to allowed charges is based on the same practitioners.
SOURCE: 1983 Bill Summary Record and 1985 and 1987 BMAD Beneficiary Files.

large financial burdens while allowing Medicare to control program costs and preserve access to a wide range of physicians.

Theory of Assignment Behavior

The basic theory of physician behavior regarding the decision to accept assignment in Medicare has been presented in a number of studies.[4] This theory can be adapted to consider what might occur if Medicare placed further constraints on balance billing, by mandating assignment so that patients seeing physicians who were unwilling to assign claims would be essentially ineligible for Medicare benefits. Although this policy option is far more extreme than those considered in earlier studies, the theory remains applicable.

The physician is assumed to be a profit-maximizing monopolistic competitor facing some downward-sloping demand.[5] In general, physicians provide services to five classes of patients: private nonelderly, Medicare nonassigned, Medicare assigned, Medicare-Medicaid dual eligibles (for which assignment is already mandatory), and nonelderly Medicaid. The cost of providing services to each of these groups is assumed to be the same. For simplicity, we do not explicitly consider Medicaid patients—aged or nonaged—in the graphic analysis that follows.

Figure 6–1 shows the various demand curves facing an individual physician. Private nonelderly demand is represented by linear demand curve D_p. Demand by elderly patients is shown as D_e. This curve is drawn under the assumption that these individuals are covered by Medicare. Were Medicare not available to the elderly, D_e would be shifted down by an amount equal to the Medicare payment, 80 percent of the reasonable charge (0.8^*R). The horizontal summation of the D_p and D_e equals the *total* nonassigned demand (Medicare and private) available to the physician, represented as D_{pe}. Notice that D_{at} kinks at the price at which elderly patients begin to demand some positive quantity of services. This kink produces a discontinuity in the associated marginal revenue curve (MR_{pe} drawn as a solid line). In the market represented by D_{pe}, the physician is assumed to be a price setter.

The physician also has a price-taking market to which Medicare assigned services can be supplied. The price available in this market is administratively determined and is shown as R, the reasonable charge, in figure 6–1. Assigned demand is perfectly elastic at R, the marginal and average revenue of assigned services, but is not infinite. The maximum volume of assigned services that the physician could provide is limited by the fact that beneficiaries incur a copayment on

149

FIGURE 6–1
A Basic Model of Behavior under Mandatory Assignment

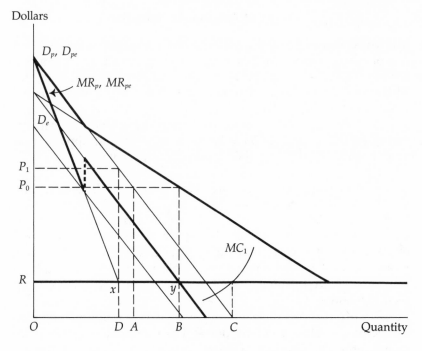

Dollars

all physician services; that is, assigned services are not "free" to the beneficiary.

The physician's output and pricing decisions will be determined by the intersection of the marginal cost and marginal revenue functions. Suppose a physician's marginal cost is given by MC_1. This physician will participate in both the price-taking and price-setting markets. As long as the discontinuity in MR_{pe} occurs above R, a physician with this cost structure will supply some nonassigned Medicare services. Reading from the graph, we see that this physician would like to supply OC total services, of which BC would be Medicare assigned, AB would be Medicare nonassigned, and OA would be private. The price charged in these last two markets will be P_0.

If the length of the horizontal assigned demand curve extends beyond point y (as in figure 6–1), then there is excess demand in the assigned market and BC assigned services will be provided. If available assigned demand is less than BC, however, there will be excess

150

supply in this market and both total output and assigned output will be less than the physician desires. Although not pictured, when there is excess supply in the Medicare assigned market, physicians can turn to the Medicaid market where services are typically provided as lower marginal and average revenues.[6]

When there is excess demand in the assignment market, the physician will necessarily need to engage in some form of nonprice rationing. The physician has the opportunity to treat certain patients and to not treat others. Although one might hope that these treatment decisions would be driven by medical necessity, there is no guarantee that this would be the case. Patients may be chosen on the basis of the physician's interest in a particular case, or the length and regularity of the relationship with the physician.

What would happen if assignment became mandatory for all Medicare services? The physician would incur a net loss in revenues since his ability to price-discriminate among Medicare patients would be lost. Mandatory assignment would mean that the downward-sloping portion of D_e above R would no longer be a relevant part of the demand structure for any physician. If a physician chose to become ineligible for Medicare benefits—that is, opt out—then the shift in demand would be even more radical. We address this situation below. First, let us consider what responses would be observed among physicians choosing to participate under mandatory assignment.

The downward-sloping demand curve would no longer be kinked, and MR would simply be given by MR_p to the left of its intersection with R (point x) and by R to the right of this intersection. The physician represented by MC_1 would not alter the total volume of desired services. This would continue to be equal to OC. Since the attractiveness of the price-setting market has been reduced with the prohibition of balance billing, the physician would want to expand Medicare assigned services. The types of changes in the Medicare market will depend, however, on the existence of excess supply or excess demand in the assignment market prior to mandatory assignment. If there was a state of excess demand, total Medicare volume would be expanded from AC to DC because beneficiaries willing and able to pay for services at R would no longer be "crowded out" of the market by beneficiaries willing to pay in excess of R. The potential for some type of nonprice rationing in this market would grow. Private volume would be reduced to OD and a new private fee would move in a direction related to the elasticities of D_p and D_e.[7]

When the initial position is characterized by excess supply, the size of the Medicare volume response to mandatory assignment is

151

indeterminate, but Medicare output can still be expected to rise. The reasons for this are twofold. The first is that, as above, AD units of Medicare output are added to potential assigned demand via a reduction in "crowding out." The second is that the length of the horizontal segment will increase as some of the patient resources spent on balance billing become available to purchase additional services; that is, the copayments required for more services can be met when balance billing is removed. Another way to think of this is that, given income, previously nonassigned patients can buy more services at the lower assigned price.

From the standpoint of the Medicare program, the potential for output to grow is probably the most important result of this model. Whether there is excess demand or excess supply of assigned services at R prior to mandatory assignment, Medicare faces the possibility of increasing its outlays by banning balance billing. Medicare output could expand without any shift in the underlying demand and without inducement. Although the program runs the risk of increased payments, the financial burden of the beneficiary is on average lower when services are provided by a participant.

If Medicare agreed to increase R in order to encourage physicians to accept mandatory assignment, Medicare volume and program outlays would be expanded further. Of course, a higher R would increase beneficiary copayments and would serve to reduce the length of the horizontal demand curve. A higher R might not affect volume if there was initially an excess of demand in the market. Mandatory assignment could be viewed as a policy that protects beneficiaries while R is reduced to cope with budget deficits. A lower R would reduce outlays in this model because physicians would respond by providing fewer Medicare services. With R reduced, the Medicare demand curve would lengthen (as a result of the lower copayment) and there would be less excess supply or a greater degree of excess demand and the potential for nonprice rationing.

Private sector patients would also be affected by changes in Medicare's reasonable fee. If budget pressures do lead to cuts in the price Medicare pays, then the attractiveness of Medicare relative to private patients will be reduced. The profit-maximizing physicians will then choose to supply more services to private patients. In order to sell these services, private prices will have to be cut. This process would work in reverse if Medicare decided to increase R.

For the physician depicted in figure 6–1, the results of a movement to participation with mandatory assignment are fairly straightforward. If R remains unchanged, Medicare volume increases, program outlays rise, beneficiary cost sharing (copayments plus balance

FIGURE 6–2
A Basic Model of Behavior If Physicians "Opt Out" of Medicare

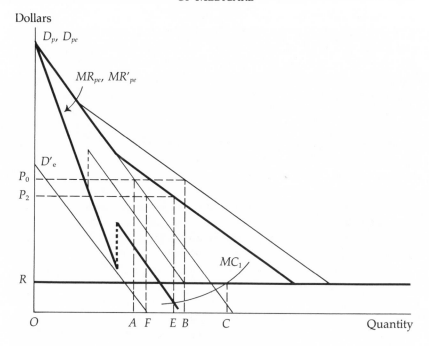

billing) falls, and private output contracts. All but one of these results would be stronger if R was increased at the same time that mandatory assignment was adopted. Beneficiary savings would not be as great since higher reasonable fees translate into higher copayments. If R was reduced, however, then a reorientation of the practice toward the private sector and away from Medicare would be likely. In this case, any monetary savings to the program or beneficiaries could be offset through nonprice rationing or informal black markets.

Figure 6–2 depicts the circumstances if a physician chooses not to participate when forced to assign all claims. The initial demand, marginal revenue, and marginal cost curves are the same as those in figure 6–1. The initial output, its division between Medicare assigned, nonassigned, and private patients, as well as the nonassigned price, are also identical to those shown above. Opting out will mean that D_e will shift downward toward the origin. If this physician's elderly patients do not purchase private insurance or in some other way compensate for the loss of Medicare benefits, the vertical shift in D_e

153

will be equal to $0.8*R$.[8] The new elderly demand curve, D'_e, will imply a new associated MR'_{pe} curve (the dashed line). The reasonable charge is included in this graph for reference but does not affect the marginal revenue curve for opted-out physicians.

The physician now finds that profits are maximized at output OE and price P_2, both at lower levels than in the initial price-setting market. The volume of services the physician wants to provide to the elderly has fallen from AC to EF, while private patients receive more care (OF as opposed to OA) at a lower price P_2. EF is the quantity of services the elderly will demand at P_2 given D'_e, their demand curve after the loss of Medicare insurance. By opting out, the physician sacrifices all program revenue from assigned claims ($BC*R$) and non-assigned claims ($AB*R$). A total loss in revenues in the price-setting market results from providing fewer services to the elderly at a lower price. Since firms with monopoly power will only provide services along the elastic portion of a demand curve, there will be some increase in revenues from private patients as a result of the drop in the private price. The growth in private revenues does not, however, offset the loss in revenues from the elderly.

Ignoring noneconomic considerations, physicians will choose to opt out or accept mandatory assignment, depending on the net loss (revenues minus costs) of each option. They will choose the situation with the smaller net loss. Although formal conditions for when this will occur are not derived, a number of informal results are apparent. Physicians will be more likely to opt out if they anticipate equating MR with MC at a quantity that can be provided totally in the private market, under either participation option. Physicians with MC curves that are well above MC_1 or those who face relatively little demand by elderly patients prior to mandatory assignment would be less likely to continue to see elderly patients. It is possible that even those physicians who treat significant numbers of Medicare patients could choose to opt out if the remaining demand for their services is strong.

One result that seems both apparent and intuitive is that physicians who see virtually none, if any, of their Medicare patients on an assigned basis will probably form the universe of potential nonparticipants. The relative changes in elderly demand would suggest that opting out would not be widespread in terms of pure numbers. If nonparticipation is concentrated in certain areas or among certain specialties, however, some elderly patients could face severe financial barriers to receiving care. Recall that under mandatory assignment patients of nonparticipants would not be receiving 80 percent of the reasonable charge as a subsidy to their costs.

Suppose that most physicians choose to participate, if for no

FIGURE 6–3
IMPACT OF ALTERNATIVE COST STRUCTURES ON BEHAVIOR UNDER
MANDATORY ASSIGNMENT

Dollars

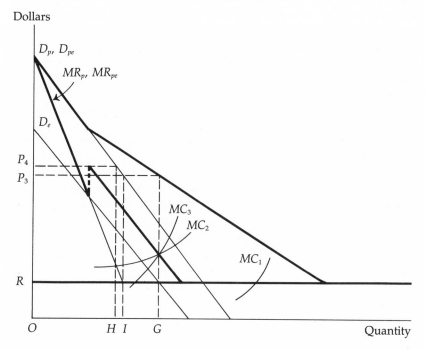

other reason than to keep open the possibility of assigning some Medicare services. Should we then assume that Medicare output would expand, as suggested in figure 6–1, and that Medicare beneficiaries need not be concerned about access problems or financial burdens? Clearly, the answer is no. Figure 6–1 depicts a market outcome based on a single type of cost structure. Other marginal cost curves, yielding alternative outcomes, are equally plausible. Two potentially important scenarios are considered in figure 6–3.

The demand and marginal revenue curves are the same as those drawn in figure 6–1. Consider physicians with marginal cost curve MC_2. Before mandatory assignment, these physicians produced OG units of total output; OI of these were to private patients, and IG were to Medicare nonassigned patients. The price charged in both markets was P_3. These physicians provide no care on an assigned basis. After they agree to participate, total output falls to OH. As in figure 6-1, the private price effects shown depend on the relative elasticities of

D_p and D_e. Now, however, they do not provide any services to Medicare patients. As marginal cost becomes steeper, say, moving toward MC_3, the chances that those who provided no assigned services initially will continue to see Medicare patients (or even expand Medicare output) grows. Given reasonably shaped marginal cost curves, it is not implausible to suggest that a new participant who did not previously assign services will curtail the volume of Medicare services.

Are there many physicians for whom an initial position such as that shown in figure 6–3 is relevant? In an absolute sense, probably only a few treat some Medicare patients yet assign zero services, whereas many may provide a token number of assigned services, perhaps to fulfill some charitable objectives in the practice of medicine. In 1978, more than 40 percent of California physicians assigned claims for fewer than 5 percent of their Medicare services (excluding Medicaid-Medicare dual eligibles).[9] Of course, this was at a time when assignment rates were well below their current levels. Minimal but nonzero program involvement has certainly been identified in Medicaid as well.[10] Mandatory assignment may have little impact on these services, since they are not being provided for profit-maximizing motives. If this type of physician is important in certain Medicare submarkets, however, then the supply of these Medicare services could be reduced.

Figure 6–3 also raises the clear potential for a "black market" in Medicare services. Some Medicare beneficiaries interested in seeing a physician with cost curve MC_2 are willing to pay a fee greater than the required 20 percent copayment. Although legislatively banned, such transactions may be difficult to prevent in light of the fact that balance billing has been permitted since the inception of Medicare. A black market would imply that, given MC_2, output would be greater than OH and that Medicare beneficiaries would receive some services from these physicians. The black market is possible because, by participating, these physicians have maintained Medicare eligibility for their patients. If these types of transactions were numerous, one could conclude that mandatory assignment was by and large ineffective and that current levels of balance billing were not excessive—at least, not excessive enough to encourage a change in physicians.

Literature Review

The model described in the preceding section suggests that physicians are more likely to participate under a regime of mandatory assignment if private demand for their services is relatively weak, if their costs of practice (for example, the costs of their own time or other inputs) are low, and if Medicare rates are relatively high. The model also suggests that the same factors will influence the number of Medicare patients and the amount of care that participating physicians will be willing to provide. We now examine evidence from Medicaid and Medicare programs on the responses of physicians to reimbursement rates to search for further clues to likely physician behavior under mandatory assignment policy.

As mentioned at the outset, Medicaid has had a system of mandatory assignment throughout its history. Physicians are required to make an implicit choice of participation and, perhaps more important, must decide how much service to provide if they participate. At first glance, the evidence from this program does not seem applicable to the Medicare situation. Medicaid finances care for an extremely poor population, reimbursement rates have historically been low in most states, and physicians are subject to a variety of controls (for example, prior authorization, extensive utilization review, and delays in payment), all of which affect physician willingness to participate. Moreover, the Medicaid population is a relatively small one. Many Medicaid recipients are not high users of services. Many others use primarily specialized services, such as care in nursing homes and in institutions for the mentally retarded. As a result, many physicians can simply decide not to participate in Medicaid without a significant income loss. The same statement is clearly not true for most physicians in Medicare. Nonetheless, some physicians may be in a position to not participate at all in Medicare or to reduce the extent of participation if the program becomes sufficiently unattractive. For these physicians, the Medicaid evidence may be quite applicable.

There is a substantial body of literature on the factors affecting physician participation in Medicaid, notably reimbursement rates. Such studies have usually included measures of physician costs, physician supply, Medicaid eligibility, and private market demand, but their data sets and methodology have varied. Even so, they have consistently found that Medicaid reimbursement rates are directly and positively related to the decision to participate and the number of patients seen by participating physicians.

There are eight major studies of physician participation that have appeared in the literature and one important unpublished paper. The first such study was based on a survey of more than 2,000 private-practice, fee-for-service physicians that was carried out by the National Opinion Research Center (NORC).[11] Data from the same survey were used to analyze participation by obstetricians/gynecologists, pediatricians, and general surgeons in 1977 and 1978,[12] and participation by nine other medical and surgery specialists.[13]

Another set of studies was based on claims data from California for 1972 through 1978. The first examined a large sample of general practitioners, general surgeons, and internists who were in practice in California continually from 1972 through 1975.[14] Another examined trends in claims data on more than 290,000 services provided by general practitioners, internists, obstetricians/gynecologists, pediatricians, general surgeons, orthopedic surgeons, and ophthalmologists for each year from 1974 to 1978.[15] Further work on the same period focused on the decision to participate and the number of patients seen per participating physician by both primary physicians and surgeons.[16] This period was of great interest because the state had adopted a fee schedule that on average increased fees for maternity care services by 30 percent, primary care services by 20 percent, anesthesia services by 65 percent, and all other services by 9.5 percent.

Two other studies examined participation in Medicaid by pediatricians. Both used data on participation and Medicaid caseloads from a survey conducted by NORC for the American Academy of Pediatrics in 1978 and 1983. The first investigated the decision to participate and the amount of care provided;[17] the second looked at the reported decision to participate fully (that is, to take on all available Medicaid patients) versus limiting participation.[18] Still another study focused on the effect of a 30 percent reduction in Medicaid payment on tonsilectomies/adenoidectomies and seven other surgery procedures in Massachusetts.[19] Massachusetts reduced primary care fees at the same time, but this reduction was short-lived. The result was essentially a substantial reduction in surgery fees relative to primary care.

As noted above, these studies consistently showed a positive and significant relation between Medicaid rates and the decision to participate. The higher the Medicaid rates, the more physicians participated. There was some evidence that the responsiveness to Medicaid rates is sensitive to the definition of participation. In one study, a large number of physicians (the exact percentage depending on the specialty) participated in Medicaid if the definition was one or more patients per calendar quarter.[20] If the definition was changed to ten or more or twenty or more patients, however, about one-third fewer physicians qualified as participants; moreover, the decision to participate became much more sensitive to Medicaid reimbursement rates. This suggested a high degree of "casual" participation in which physicians either see patients on a charitable basis or see a long-standing patient who has temporarily entered the Medicaid program.

Past research also suggests that the level of Medicaid rates strongly affects the number of patients that participating physicians are willing to treat. The elasticities of participation and number of patients seen per participating physician tend to vary, but appear to be somewhat higher when claims data are used rather than survey data. There is also some variation in whether the decision to participate or the number of patients per participating physician is more sensitive to Medicaid rates. For example, Hadley and Held and Holahan found both to be important,[21] whereas Mitchell found that the decision to participate was sensitive to Medicaid rates but that the number of patients per participating physician was not.[22] Perloff and her colleagues found that the ratio of Medicaid reimbursement to usual fees was significantly related to the decision to be full participants in Medicaid, that is, to accept all available Medicaid patients (as defined by the physician).[23] The higher the ratio of Medicaid reimbursement to usual fees, the more likely physicians were to be full participants in both years, 1978 and 1983, that were studied.

Three studies looked at the impact of changing relative fees in ways somewhat similar to that proposed by the Harvard resource-based relative value study. When primary care fees were increased relative to surgery fees, the number of patients per physician increased noticeably for the primary care physicians, who were the main beneficiaries of the fee schedule increases.[24] In the year following the fee schedule, Medicaid patients per physician increased by 37.5 percent for pediatricians, 36.4 percent for obstetricians/gynecologists, 23.4 percent for internists, and 23.2 percent for general practitioners. Medicaid eligibility increased by 12.8 percent during this period and went up even higher for the medically needy and disabled. Thus, not all of the increases in patients can be attributed to the increase in fees. These increases, however, were larger than that observed in the two earlier years, when there were also substantial increases in eligibility. For physicians who benefited less from the fee schedule increase, there were much smaller increases in patients per physician. Thus the California increase in physician fees coupled with the twisting of relative fees in favor of primary care appeared to have the desired results.

An econometric analysis of the same data confirmed that both primary care physicians and surgeons were sensitive to changes in fee levels.[25] The elasticities of the participation rate and the number of patients per participating physician with respect to the Medicaid price were roughly twice as large for the surgical specialties as for primary care physicians.

The impact of the reduced surgery fee was assessed by comparing the mean level of surgery volume before and after the fee cut.[26] No effort was made to control for other factors that could have caused changes during this period. The principal finding was that tonsilectomy/adenoidectomy was the only procedure in which there was a strong indication of a decline in the level of surgery following the fee cut. There was a statistically significant decline at the .05 level in three of the four professional standards review organizations (PSRO) areas (of 25 percent or more). The results for the other procedures showed little consistent pattern, which is not surprising given the relatively small amount of data available on other procedures.

The econometric studies also identified other factors behind participation decisions, after controlling for the level of private demand by including a variable to capture private prices. Although the definition of this variable varied to some degree, findings were consistent: the higher the level of private demand, the less participation in Medicaid and the fewer patients per participating physician. Second, the variables that capture the costs of physician practices were found to be significant. For example, variables that might capture the practice opportunity costs of physicians (for example, employee wage rates, board certification, foreign medical graduate, and being a member of a subspecialty such as cardiology or dermatology) were all found to be statistically significant in one or more studies.

Thus, the evidence clearly indicates that increases (decreases) in Medicaid reimbursement rates lead to increases (decreases) in the willingness of physicians to participate and the number of patients they will see. At the same time, increases (decreases) in private prices reflecting increases (decreases) in demand from private patients, all else held constant, reduce (or increase) physicians' willingness to participate in Medicaid and the number of patients they will see. A change in relative fees also appears to affect physician behavior. The two studies that address this issue suggest that increases in primary care fees relative to surgery would lead to an increase in the willingness of primary care physicians to see Medicaid patients. The evidence from California also suggests that, holding private fees and other factors constant, surgeons are more responsive to Medicaid fees than primary care physicians. Similarly, surgeons appear to have responded to the reduction in surgery rates in Massachusetts.

Empirical Evidence from Medicare

Although Medicare has had a much more liberal policy toward assignment and balance billing than Medicaid, physicians' willingness to accept assignment under different Medicare arrangements over the years may be currently relevant if only because the same beneficiaries are involved. Five recent studies on the decision of physicians to accept assignment and one on physicians' willingness to participate in Medicare under the Physician Participation Program enacted in October 1983 are of particular interest. The results from Medicare are remarkably consistent across these studies.

One study based on the 1976 NORC survey of 711 general practitioners, general surgeons, and internists found that Medicare reasonable charges were positively related to Medicare assignment rates but that billed charges were not significant.[27] Another study using claims data from physicians in northern California also revealed a positive relationship between assignment and reasonable charges, but physicians' billed charges were negatively related.[28] Elasticity estimates were extremely large in this study (the elasticities on the reasonable charge and billed charge variables were approximately 2.0 and −1.4, respectively), but it was argued that billed charges were not truly independent of reasonable charges since the net effect of changes in reasonable charges was substantially smaller than implied by the initial elasticity estimates. A third analysis using the 1978 AMA Periodic Survey of Physicians revealed the same positive and negative relationship for reasonable charges and billed charges, respectively.[29] A cross-sectional analysis of 1979 data on all Colorado physicians along with a survey of Medicare beneficiaries showed that the ratio of billed to reasonable charges was positively related to assignment rates.[30] The elasticity on the ratio variable was .05. In a fifth study using time-series data, Medicare reasonable charges were found to be positively related to changes in assignment rates for medical care, laboratory, and radiology services.[31] In a sixth, more recent study, the participation rate of physicians was positively related to the level of Medicare allowed charges.[32] The level of Blue Shield fees was not related to the decision to participate.

Several other variables have been included in these studies. Four found area income to be negatively related to assignment rates or, in one case, to the decision to participate. This variable is interpreted as a measure of private demand. Thus, the greater the private demand, the lower the assignment rates (or participation rates). Three studies found that foreign medical graduates had higher assignment rates. One study found board-certified physicians were less likely to accept assignment. Others did not confirm this effect. Another found that assignment rates declined with age up to a point and then began to increase again for older physicians, and still another found age to be negatively related to assignment rates. Almost no studies found

161

physician input cost to be related to the decision to accept assignment. One did find malpractice rates negatively related to participation rates.

Thus, the evidence on Medicare seems reasonably consistent with that from Medicaid. In all of the studies we examined, Medicare reasonable charges were positively related to assignment rates or to the decision to participate. The evidence on private charges was generally negative, but was sometimes insignificant. Decisions to accept assignment or, in more recent years to join the Medicare participation program, are also negatively related to the strength of private demand and to physicians' opportunity costs.

Physician Responses to Price Changes

One drawback of using the theory of physician assignment behavior or empirical evidence from Medicaid or Medicare is that neither may be entirely appropriate for predicting responses to Medicare mandatory assignment. This theory has already been used to predict that physicians faced with an "all or none" assignment option would choose the "none" option in most cases.[33] Although it has been shown that two-thirds would in fact choose "none," a substantial minority of physicians violated the general rule. The point is that it may be fruitful to explore a range of theoretical and statistical avenues in order to forecast responses to mandatory assignment.

In light of the fact that Medicare fees are likely to be altered in tandem with a change in assignment policy, physicians' responses to price changes are of particular interest. The theoretical debate has centered on whether the physician has the ability to "induce" demand[34] or is subject to competitive pressures in a more traditional neoclassical fashion.[35] The intent here is not to assess this debate, but note that two of the numerous empirical studies on this issue merit attention.

One study examined physician response to changing relative fees in Colorado.[36] In 1976 the Medicare program adopted a statewide fee schedule in Colorado. The net effect was an increase in fees in all areas other than Denver by about 20 percent, whereas Denver physicians experienced an increase of about 5 percent. The increases varied considerably among physicians because of differences in their initial customary charges. It seems that most services increased in response to declining fes: specifically, service intensity (complexity) of medical services and surgery increased, with elasticities of .61 and .27, respectively. The volume of surgery and laboratory services also increased, with elasticities of .15 and .52, respectively. The volume of medical services and radiology was unaffected. The increases were attributed to a supply or inducement response because (1) the demand for services could not have increased sufficiently to explain the volume growth in view of the widespread presence of supplementary insurance and Medicaid before and after the fee change; and (2) reduced fees would increase balance billing, thus offsetting any demand effect associated with lower amounts of coinsurance. As such, a volume increase occurring when fees fell would be a supply response because the balance billing growth would be so much greater than the coinsurance cuts that it would be implausible to attribute the volume increase to a demand response.

The argument in the second study was that the responses of volume to price levels can be interpreted as either a demand or supply response and that the true effect is hard to determine.[37] The authors estimated regression equations using 1983 and 1985 data from 350 geographic areas in the United States for medical care, surgery, radiology, and consultation volume. They controlled for demographic characteristics, incomes of the elderly, supplementary insurance, assignment rates (that is, a proxy for balance billing), physician supply, malpractice premiums, and hospital admission rates and lengths of stay. The authors found negative and significant relationships between prevailing charges and the amount of surgery and radiology, using a weighted quantity measure that encompasses both volume and intensity. The volume of medical care services was not significantly related to price. Consultations were positively and significantly related to the prevailing charge index. The short-run elasticities in the surgery and radiology equations were $-.14$ and $-.32$, respectively; the elasticity in the consultation equation was a positive .20. The elasticity of total volume with respect to price was less than -0.1.

These results suggest that the response to fee policy within a regime of mandatory assignment may be somewhat different from that observed in Medicaid. That is, physicians who choose to participate may be likely to increase their supply of services in response to a decline in fees. Similarly, they may reduce services in response to an increase in fees. In support of physicians' desires to provide more services in response to fee reductions, coinsurance and deductible payments by beneficiaries would also decline as fees are reduced.

Without doubt, physician responses to a regime of mandatory assignment are extremely difficult to predict. It is likely that many physicians, presumably those not highly dependent on the Medicare program, would behave as physicians do under Medicaid and reduce the extent of participation in response to lower Medicare fees. The evidence clearly indicates that the extent of participation is highly sensitive to private demand, the opportunity costs of a physician's time, and the level of other practice costs. These same factors are likely to affect physicians' willingness to participate in Medicare.

Results and Policy

The evidence cited above suggests that balance billing has given some beneficiaries access to physicians who would be unwilling to supply Medicare services at allowed charge levels. The costs of maintaining access have been borne by beneficiaries, who may face copayments well in excess of 20 percent. In addition, by imposing a higher implicit rate of cost sharing on nonassigned services, balance billing has in all likelihood reduced volume and lowered program outlays.

Physicians have gained from balance billing by being able to price-discriminate among Medicare patients and earn monopoly profits on some Medicare services. Also, since they are allowed to receive different prices from different Medicare patients, physicians have generally accepted the fact that Medicare rates do not explicitly incorporate legitimate factors that may affect prices, such as costs, service quality, and training. As assignment rates grow, however, the concern is that Medicare allowed amounts should be, in a broad sense, reasonable.

Prohibiting balance billing—for example, through mandatory assignment—would represent a departure from Medicare's flexible approach to assignment decisions. Recall that under the current approach assignment rates have risen to 74 percent. Those opposed to balance billing argue that a ban would reduce the beneficiary's financial burden at little or no cost to the public sector. Even if the policy were "successful" and every Medicare provider became a participant with no increase in allowed amounts, however, public sector costs could rise.

Theory predicts that as monopoly profits are redistributed from physicians to Medicare beneficiaries the total quantity of Medicare services could grow. This occurs because physicians who provided both assigned and nonassigned care are now willing to provide more services at the allowed amount; the allowed amount becomes relatively more attractive because the more profitable nonassigned market is no longer available. Since the program pays only 80 percent of the allowed amount (with or without balance billing), an increase in volume will increase outlays. This tendency to see volume grow under mandatory assignment would be somewhat offset by physicians who choose to curtail Medicare output. Some of their patients may seek care from physicians trying to increase output. Although the magnitude of these countervailing forces is unknown, it is evident a priori that prohibiting balance billing is likely to increase Medicare costs. A policy that provides incentives to expand volume at a time when volume increases are seen as the primary forces behind Medicare expenditure growth seems particularly ill-advised.

Perhaps the most widespread concern about a ban on balance billing is that some physicians would not participate and might simply stop treating Medicare patients altogether. Access could be threatened if these physicians were concentrated in certain areas or within particular specialties or were the most experienced, knowledgeable, and skillful ones available. At a minimum, patients being cared for by nonparticipants would face substantial increases in out-of-pocket costs unless they changed physicians. Our theoretical analysis suggests that the costs to the physician of this choice could be high and, therefore, this response would not be widespread. This does not mean that this choice would never occur, however.

A less dramatic, but potentially more prevalent, response would be for physicians to participate but to cut back on their volume of Medicare services. This behavior would no doubt be associated with some forms of nonprice rationing on the part of physicians. Although physicians might adopt a triaging scheme so that those patients with the greatest medical need received care, this may not always occur. Even under current policy this is an issue for physicians facing excess demand in the assignment market.

The empirical studies of Medicaid participation and Medicare assignment provide more consistent evidence than does the economic theory as to the types of physicians who might opt out or, at least, curtail access. A broad range of studies show that physicians with high practice costs or in markets with strong private demand see fewer Medicaid patients, assign fewer Medicare claims, and are less likely to choose formal Medicare participant status. Public program involvement is also lower among more experienced physicians, those educated at U.S. medical schools, and board-certified physicians.

Further limits on balance billing would mean that Medicare's allowed amount would in practice come to represent the full (and sole) price physicians received for Medicare services. Although current allowed amounts would be altered by the adoption of a fee schedule, they would not necessarily reflect all or most factors that contribute to price variations among physicians. These include practice costs, product quality, physician experience, and demand conditions in the local market. Without balance billing, it becomes important to account for these factors by new allowed prices, but the adjustments needed to convince physicians the policy was equitable could be extremely complex.

Concerns about program costs, access, and the complexity of the fee schedule suggest that a shift toward mandatory assignment might only be desirable if current policy imposes severe financial hardship on the elderly. Table 6–3 presents data on the volume and distribution of balance billing by physicians in 1987. For each beneficiary, we compute the amount of balance billing as the difference between billed and allowed charges. In all likelihood, this approach provides an upper bound on the amount of balance billing. First, because some Medigap policies cover fees above the Medicare allowed charge, part of what we count as balance billing will be covered by Medigap. (Some of these savings are offset because these types of Medigap policies require higher premiums.) Second, some physicians may not try to collect all or part of the balance bill on unassigned claims. Little information is available on this second point.

In 1987, Medicare beneficiaries faced approximately $2.3 billion in balance billing. Furthermore, the distribution of balance billing was quite skewed. Almost 42 percent of beneficiaries receiving services had all of their claims assigned and, therefore, were not subject to any balance billing; 92.6 percent of beneficiaries incurring some balance billing were liable for less than $500 for all of 1987; however, 2.9 percent of beneficiaries with at least one nonassigned claim in 1987 faced more than $1,000 in balance billing (this group accounted for 35.7 percent of all balance billing in the system).

Two conclusions can be immediately drawn from these data. First, balance billing is likely to impose little, if any, financial burden on the vast majority of Medicare beneficiaries. Of course, even small amounts of balance billing could be a hardship if incomes are inadequate. Second, there exists a small group for whom balance billing is quite high. To the extent that balance billing is a mechanism to ensure access for most beneficiaries, it may be inequitable to have so few beneficiaries bear such a disproportionate share of the costs. The issue of equity, however, depends not only on the distribution of incomes and relative access to participating physicians. If policy makers wish to protect financially vulnerable beneficiaries and to encourage more physicians to select participant status, mandatory assignment may not be a prudent policy at this time.

An Incentive Strategy

An alternative strategy would be to increase the incentives to participate while exempting beneficiaries with low incomes or poor health

TABLE 6-3
CHARACTERISTICS OF MEDICARE BALANCE BILLING, 1987

Level of Balance Billing ($ per year)	Beneficiaries[a] (millions)	Total Amount (millions of dollars)	Amount per Beneficiary	Percent Distribution		
				Beneficiaries	Beneficiaries with some balance billing	Total balance billing
Zero	10.7	0.0	0.0	41.8	N.A.	N.A.
1–200	12.3	549.1	44.72	48.1	82.6	23.8
201–500	1.5	469.3	315.70	5.8	10.0	20.4
501–1000	0.7	463.7	697.30	2.6	4.5	20.1
1,001–2,000	0.3	437.5	1,371.10	1.3	2.1	19.0
2,001 or more	0.1	384.8	3,154.39	0.5	0.8	16.7
All categories	25.6	2,304.4	154.96[b]	100.0	100.0	100.0

N.A. = not applicable.
a. Only Medicare enrollees with at least one allowed claim were included in these computations. If all of the approximately 32 million enrollees had been included, the numbers not exposed to balance billing would have been greater.
b. This average is based only on those beneficiaries with some balance billing.
SOURCE: 1987 BMAD Beneficiary File.

from balance billing.[38] The incentives to participate would come from paying less than allowed charges to nonparticipants, but the full allowed charge, less cost sharing, to participants. The present 5 percent differential between participant and nonparticipant allowed charges might be increased until participation rates reached some desired level. Under this approach, patients would not lose Medicare benefits when seeing a nonparticipating physician, as they would in mandatory assignment. They would, however, have strong incentives to be treated by a participant. If Medicare reimbursed the patient choosing a nonparticipating physician at an allowed charge, say, 20 percent below that of participants, out-of-pocket costs would rise considerably.

As patients began to see the financial benefit in using participants, some would change physicians. At the same time, nonparticipating physicians who continued to attract patients could balance bill. (Some form of the MAAC limits might be retained, although the data from table 6–3 suggest they might not be needed as financial protection.) This would ease the pressure on the system to compensate higher-cost physicians, while reducing the current subsidy available to patients who wished to exercise this choice.

Program costs would be reduced by paying, say, only 80 percent of the allowed fee to nonparticipants. Medicare would also probably have greater control over fee increases because physicians could opt for nonparticipant status if fees were perceived as being too low. With mandatory assignment, the level and rate of growth in fees are of paramount importance. As long as balance billing remains an option, but with reduced public subsidy, greater control can be exercised over payment rates.

Beneficiaries could be exempted from balance billing on the basis of income or health status. Currently, physicians must accept assignment on Medicaid patients, regardless of their decisions on other patients. The Medicare Catastrophic Coverage Act of 1988 extended Medicaid eligibility to all elderly below the poverty line as of January 1992; subsequent legislation made these new Medicaid eligibles exempt from balance billing. A broader group of beneficiaries could be exempted from balance billing on a patient-by-patient basis.[39] For example, Medicare could exempt all beneficiaries who would have reached the new Medicare catastrophic threshold, had the law not been repealed. Together, these exemptions should protect most potentially vulnerable groups.

Physicians treating those exempted from balance billing would be paid full Medicare allowed charges, independent of their participant status. Patients would generally be responsible for deductibles

168

and coinsurance (unless covered by Medicaid). These provisions would ensure that the incentive strategy did not impose financial burdens on the poor and very sick patients.

Furthermore, most physicians would be available because non-participation and balance billing would be permitted, though not generously underwritten. At the same time, this policy would eliminate financial burdens on those least able to afford them, while allowing others to avoid them by enabling them to select from a large pool of participating physicians. Medicare would find less resistance to efforts to constrain rate increases and program costs because nonparticipating physicians could compensate for low allowed rates by increasing charges to most of their patients. Interphysician compensation differences would be permitted for those physicians able to retain a sufficient number of Medicare patients able to pay balance billing charges.

The goal of Medicare has always been to provide the elderly access to mainstream medicine. This can best be done by keeping the relationship between physicians and patients flexible. Mandatory assignment would move the program away from this historical commitment and could push program costs up if access became a problem. Our proposed incentive strategy is an extension of the successful DEFRA policy in that it permits voluntary participation and assignment as well as balance billing (for nonparticipants). It goes beyond DEFRA in that it would impose greater costs for nonparticipation while exempting the most potentially hard-hit segments of the Medicare population from balance billing.

Maintaining Market Discipline

A Commentary by Jesse S. Hixson

Holahan and Zuckerman argue that allowing physicians to charge patients in excess of Medicare indemnity rates will serve a number of desirable public policy objectives of the Medicare program. Their one reservation is that unrestricted balance billing might cause the poor or high users of Medicare services undue financial hardship. Therefore, they recommend exempting this class of beneficiary from balance billing.

In 1978, Frech and Ginsburg came to the same conclusion—that balance billing would produce a number of desirable results if incorporated into a system of public health insurance.[1] Otherwise, they concluded, there would be nonprice rationing, and the production and distribution of medical care would cease to reflect consumer preferences. Not only would rationing to individuals be distorted, but the specialty and geographic distributions of physicians could be profoundly affected. Frech and Ginsburg offered other alternatives to deal with the financial hardship problem: cover only the poor and needy; vary cost sharing with income; or set very high levels of reimbursement.

It seems that most analysts who consider the theoretical pros and cons of balance billing from time to time arrive at the same general conclusion—that it is a desirable and even necessary adjunct to a physician fee-for-service insurance system. There are also numerous empirical demonstrations of the perverse effects of prohibiting prices from performing a market-clearing function, which are much the same as the effects of prohibiting balance billing: The results of mandatory assignment in the Medicaid program and of rent controls across the country are examples. Given the logic and the evidence, why has there been a steady movement to restrict or prohibit balance billing in the Medicare program?

A clue can be found in the testimony of Philip R. Lee, chairman of the Physician Payment Review Commission, before the U.S. Senate

Finance Committee on March 17, 1989: "The market for physicians' services does not function well enough to preclude the need for financial protection for Medicare beneficiaries. Without limitations on balance billing, beneficiary financial protection would suffer." The objection of those opposed to balance billing is based on the absence of price competition among physicians. Without price competition, they believe nothing will prevent physicians from charging excessive prices. Therefore, it seems necessary to propose a system of payment that combines balance billing with the market discipline of price competition.

A necessary condition for price competition is that suppliers realize an adequate demand response to changes in price. This in turn requires that consumers both perceive and respond to price differentials. The incentive to respond to a price differential is the reward for choosing a lower-priced good or service over a higher-priced substitute. Thus, it is essential that consumers be confronted by opportunity costs of adequate magnitude to induce choice among alternatives that in turn presents suppliers with a worthwhile demand response to changes in price.

The main barrier to price competition in the traditional fee-for-service market is the proportional copayment by which the consumer pays, after reaching the deductible limit, a constant percentage of the charge submitted to the payer. Copayment substantially reduces the price or opportunity cost perceived by the consumer of choosing among differentially priced alternatives, thus diluting incentives contained in price differentials. To present the consumer with a certain price reduction, a supplier must lower his price many times more than the reduction perceived by the consumer. Under copayment of 20 percent, which is the case under Part B for physician service, physicians must lower their price by $5 to present the consumer with a price reduction of $1. Thus, within the range of possible price variation for most services, there may be practically no demand response to price cuts by fee-for-service physicians, and hence no incentive for price competition.

Many consider the consumer sacrifice in this regard to be in direct conflict with the goal of financial protection for the elderly Medicare beneficiary. Yet, the program does require a considerable financial sacrifice. In 1985, beneficiaries paid, on average, one-half of the total Medicare Part B allowed charges out-of-pocket through premiums, deductibles, coinsurance, and balance bills.[2] One could ask, therefore, if it is possible to *restructure* this financial burden so that the sacrifice is the same or even smaller but more effective in providing the incentive for price competition among fee-for-service physicians.

One approach is to replace the current Part B premium, deductible, and copayment with balance billing, which would then be the vehicle for price competition. To protect the poor and near-poor elderly, a minimum benefit package or a minimum degree of access to free care could be made available to everyone; balance billing would be applicable to those services not included in the minimum benefit package or not covered by the access criteria. In this way, the necessary consumer sacrifice would be concentrated to minimize the burden on those elderly in need of financial protection while maximizing its usefulness as an incentive for price consciousness.

Such a system could be designed in several ways, but it would specify a minimum standard of benefits that Medicare would purchase for every beneficiary and thus would guarantee some level of adequate care for their needs. The Medicare benefit package could be augmented by open-market purchases of additional services or services of higher quality than those provided for in the standard package. The financial burden on the poor or needy elderly would thus be minimized or eliminated, while beneficiaries with greater financial means or tastes for additional services could buy them, and physicians could freely compete for their business.

If the services sought were of higher quality than those the program furnished at no charge, physicians would be free to balance-bill the patient for the difference. The cost to the patient would be 100 percent of this difference. *Thus, the patient would face, on the margin of choice between the standard level of quality and the higher level of quality, the full opportunity cost of this decision, which would maximize the demand responsiveness to a change in the physician's price.*

Although it might be too difficult or impractical to define the particular exclusions and inclusions of a minimum benefit package, a minimum level of access to care could be provided by offering enrollment in prepaid health plans (for example, HMOs). The negotiated levels of benefits could be provided at no charge to beneficiaries. Beneficiaries who wanted more lavish benefits could pay the marginal cost of a more expansive plan. For the fee-for-service market, government-administered fee schedules could be adjusted to guarantee a minimum level of access; this could be accomplished by adjusting indemnity rates to achieve target participation rates or assignment rates among physicians in *each local market*. Participating physicians would agree to accept the Medicare indemnity rate as payment in full, as would be the case for assigned claims in general.

The needy beneficiary can be protected in a number of ways that do not tax the physicians who choose to provide them care. Singling out a group of beneficiaries and requiring private suppliers of services to provide them special discounts is certainly a unique, and almost bizarre, approach to financing public programs. Beneficiaries evidently also object to being identified for differential treatment under the program.

A straightforward approach to subsidizing the elderly population's consumption of medical services that strengthens and exploits the traditional function of prices is within easy reach. Effectively functioning prices produce the desirable results: The government will not spend any more than necessary to buy the services that it does, consumers will not pay any more than necessary, and the desired degree of access to care can be ensured. To achieve these desirable results, however, the approach must be designed to overcome the skepticism concerning the market's ability to function effectively.

7
Paralyzing Medicare's Demand-Side Policies

Thomas G. McGuire

Recently enacted legislation offering Medicare beneficiaries coverage for "catastrophic" expenses renews interest in the issue of the role of privately purchased insurance policies designed to supplement Medicare coverage. This chapter reconsiders the trade-off between the risk-protection benefits of those policies and the expenditure-inducing costs in the light of catastrophic coverage and Medicare's interest in promoting beneficiary choice of alternative delivery systems such as health maintenance organizations (HMOs). The central question here is whether Medicare should discourage purchase of supplemental policies. I argue that what was once a difficult policy call has now become clear-cut. Even if (1) the elderly accurately foresee the expected benefits from purchase of such insurance, (2) are highly risk-averse, and (3) supplemental policies have a small impact on total utilization, supplemental policies appear to do more harm than good.

Before catastrophic coverage legislation, Part A of Medicare, covering hospital costs, required payment of deductibles, copayments, and full costs for days above covered limits. The deductible, set at $560 in 1989, applies to a benefit period or "spell of illness." Copayments were one-fourth of the deductible amount per day for days sixty-one through ninety during a hospital stay. The beneficiary could apply sixty "lifetime reserve" days (which themselves have a copayment) to days after ninety, but when these were exhausted the beneficiary was responsible for all costs. Under provisions of catastrophic coverage, the beneficiary is only responsible for the deductible. Optional Part B has a $75 annual deductible, with Medicare then paying 80 percent of the "reasonable charge." The beneficiary pays

I am grateful to Randy Ellis, Cindy Gallup, Marion Gornick, Chris Tompkins, and Ted Frech for helpful comments on an earlier draft. This chapter was written before repeal of Medicare's catastrophic coverage.

20 percent and may be subject to balance billing if the physician does not accept the Medicare reasonable charge as full payment. Under catastrophic coverage, the beneficiary's obligations are limited to $1,370 of cost sharing for Medicare-approved charges per year. Beneficiaries are still responsible for any charges above Medicare-approved rates.

Elderly beneficiaries have supplemented Medicare's coverage by purchasing insurance in many forms, including hospital indemnity and "dread-disease" policies. The majority of these are known as Medigap policies and are designed to supplement Medicare by paying some or all of the cost-sharing requirements in Medicare. In 1984, premiums for Medigap policies were $4.9 billion ($3.7 billion for BC/BS plans and $1.2 billion for commercial carriers), amounting to almost 10 percent of Medicare's $60 billion outlays in that year.[1]

Amy Taylor and her colleagues recently asked whether Medigap policies are a "friend or foe" to cost containment in Medicare, pointing out that while Medigap dilutes demand-side cost sharing and thereby interferes with cost-containment goals, it also protects beneficiaries against risk of health expenditures, reducing the pressure for expansion of Medicare benefits.[2] Other economists have labeled Medigap a "foe," stressing the classic overinsurance argument that by being able to purchase the supplemental policy for a premium reflecting only the costs covered by the supplemental policy and not the costs of induced services paid for by Medicare, Medigap policies are underpriced and overpurchased.

Forceful criticisms of Medigap have been made using the overinsurance argument since at least 1982, with no apparent effect on public policy.[3] The overinsurance position may have carried little weight in part because analysts have underestimated the risk-protection benefits of Medigap policies to the elderly. It is certainly true that supplemental policies are underpriced in that enrollees are not asked to pay the social marginal cost of additional coverage. Medigap may not have been overpurchased in relation to the socially efficient coverage of the elderly, however, if Medicare left an inefficiently high amount of financial risk with the elderly in the first place. The elderly are probably more risk-averse than the average younger person, and face higher expected health care expenditures and a much higher variance in those expenditures. Nonetheless, before the recent catastrophic legislation, the basic coverage in Medicare Parts A and B had significant coinsurance and no stop loss, and was generally inferior to policies elected by working populations in (admittedly tax-subsidized) private markets. It is possible that the elderly were "underinsured" with basic Medicare coverage, and Medigap may have served to redress this inefficient level of public insurance.

A test of this contention would be whether fully informed Medicare beneficiaries were willing to purchase Medigap if it were priced efficiently. Other authors have argued that efficiency would require a premium tax of 25–100 percent. I estimate that the efficient tax might be on the order of 50 percent. This tax corresponds to a loss ratio of 66 percent for a policy priced at actuarial cost. The elderly are evidently willing to pay "taxes" of this magnitude over actuarial value in the form of marketing/administrative costs and profits. The weighted average loss ratio for all Medigap policies is about 65.8 percent.[4] Unfortunately, the market behavior of the elderly may not be a convincing piece of evidence for this test because the elderly consistently overestimate the insurance coverage of both Medicare and supplemental policies they purchase.[5]

Recent events in Medicare, however, make a debatable issue much more clear-cut. The first of these changes is the persistent escalation of Part B costs. Medicare has been generally successful in containing Part A costs through its prospective payment system (PPS), holding incurred hospital payments to a 5.5 percent increase, for example, in the second year of the PPS.[6] Meanwhile, in spite of limits on the growth of fees for physician and other services, Medicare's Part B obligations are growing rapidly. In the two years between 1987 and 1989, the Part B premium charged to beneficiaries, calculated as a fixed fraction of projected Part B costs, rose 56 percent.[7] The savings to Medicare of any pricing reform for Part B would be hard-pressed to match the savings from a straightforward reinstitution of demand-side cost sharing for Part B following elimination or restriction of Medigap coverage.

Second, Medicare's policy initiatives involving alternative delivery systems, such as health maintenance organizations (HMOs), are foundering. Medicare began paying HMOs and qualified prepaid health plans on an at-risk basis for Medicare beneficiaries in 1985. Enrollment in risk contracts was 813,712 in December 1986, amounting to about 3 percent of beneficiaries.[8] By September 1988, enrollment in risk contracts had grown to only 1,040,966. The reasons for this policy failure are complex, but one fundamental problem is that in the eyes of the beneficiary any alternative delivery system must compete with the Medigap policy. A beneficiary can obtain nearly full insurance with full choice of providers at a subsidized premium through Medigap. The competing HMO or other plan must either offer enrollment at a lower premium or with increased benefits to attract beneficiaries. Pursuing either strategy costs money and decreases the attractiveness of Medicare participation. Without a revised policy toward Medigap, Medicare will continue to face a difficult task inducing beneficiaries to give up free choice of provider in the conventional fee-for-service medical system.

Third, Medicare's new catastrophic health insurance coverage beginning to take effect in 1989 significantly limits the risks beneficiaries face from acute care expenses.[9] Beneficiaries are responsible only for the $560 annual deductible on Part A expenses. Beginning in 1990, Medicare will pay 100 percent of covered charges for physician and other Part B bills once the beneficiary's cost sharing has reached $1,370. In 1991, Medicare will cover part of outpatient prescription drug costs. Medicare will also modestly increase its share of the costs of long-term care. Publicly provided catastrophic coverage erodes the risk-protection rationale for Medigap coverage.

Medigap as Overinsurance

The danger of overinsurance when more than one insurance policy may be purchased to cover the expenses, either in whole or in part, for the same event has been well-recognized in the insurance literature. Pauly articulated the issue in the health insurance context: "The premium for supplemental coverage . . . reflects only the claims on the supplemental coverage. It does not reflect additional claims on the 'basic' coverage, and so tends to underprice supplemental or shallow coverage."[10] Although Pauly did not mention Medigap insurance explicitly, he clearly had such an application in mind when he concluded that, with regard to the question of purchasing supplemental coverage to fill in around a public insurance program, "supplementary coverage should be taxed to reflect the additional use of the basic public insurance benefit." This tax remedy to correct the underpricing of Medigap has been repeated by a number of authors.

Christensen and others argue that "the prevalence of medigap insurance . . . eliminates the constraints on unnecessary use intended to result from Medicare's cost-sharing provisions. As a result, use of Medicare-covered services is higher than it otherwise would be, and most of the costs of the additional services used are paid by Medicare rather than by medigap insurers."[11] They estimate that the increase in the use of Medicare-covered services because of Medigap amounts to about $8.1 billion in 1987, or $440 per enrollee. Because the $440 is about the same as the average Medigap premium, the tax would have to be about 100 percent to ensure that beneficiaries paid the full cost of the supplemental coverage.

Ginsburg was one of the first to recommend restricting Medigap

FIGURE 7-1
MEDIGAP AND INDUCED EXPENDITURES FOR MEDICARE

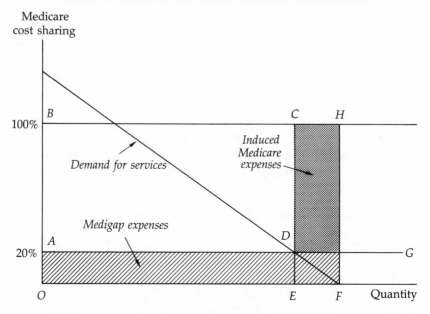

purchase.[12] He recently restated his argument: "Medigap insurance is implicitly subsidized by Medicare through the former's impact on use of services. . . . Since the costs that Medicare pays will not be reflected in the premium for the supplemental plan, the latter will be underpriced and too many people will purchase it."[13] Ginsburg proposes a tax of 35 percent on Medigap premiums to eliminate this distortion. Frech has made the same point, concluding after reviewing the empirical work of Taylor and others[14] that the tax required to achieve efficient pricing exceeded 100 percent.

Figure 7-1 shows why Medigap insurance is underpriced. If we assume for the sake of simplicity that Medicare requires a uniform 20 percent cost sharing for beneficiaries, demand for services is OE, Medicare payments are $ABCD$, and out-of-pocket payments are $OADE$. A Medigap policy that eliminates cost sharing altogether increases demand to OF, requires premiums to cover Medigap expenses of $OAGF$, and induces new Medicare expenses $DCHG$. The authors just mentioned have argued that Medigap should be taxed so

178

that premiums to the beneficiary cover all the extra covered charges due to the policy, the explicit Medigap expenses as well as the induced expenses for Medicare.

As figure 7–1 makes clear, the magnitude of induced expenses to Medicare and the efficiency tax on Medigap premiums depend on the volume of extra service use caused by Medigap. The nature of Medigap coverage and the effect of coverage on service use has been the subject of a number of investigations.

The degree of coverage among Medigap policies varies, although because of state and federal regulation most policies adhere to minimum coverage standards, and coverage features vary less than was true in the past. Using data from the 1977 National Medical Care Expenditure Survey (NMCES), before federal regulations took effect, Taylor and others report that 66 percent of the elderly had both Medicare and Medigap coverage.[15] Another 11 percent had Medicare and Medicaid. Of those with some Medigap coverage, two-thirds purchased coverage as individuals, and one-third had coverage through a group related to their former employment. Combining NMCES with a follow-up survey, the Health Insurance/Employer Survey, Cartwright and others categorized beneficiaries with some private Medigap coverage into "high," "medium," and "low" coverage groups.[16] A high-coverage policy, according to this classification, was complete coverage for A and B, cost sharing or complete coverage for A, and partial for B. Low coverage included partial A or partial B only. Medium coverage was all other combinations. According to this classification, 26 percent of all beneficiaries with Medigap were in the high, 56 percent in the medium, and 18 percent in the low-coverage categories.

Rice and McCall surveyed a random sample of beneficiaries in six states in 1982, the year federal regulation took effect.[17] Seventy percent or more of beneficiaries owned some policy in all six states. Most of these were Medicare supplemental policies but ownership included a significant number of other types of policies, such as hospital indemnity and major medical. Even though the Baucus legislation would not have had an effect, the Medicare supplemental policies conformed to the Baucus standards. A more recent GAO report also found widespread compliance with required coverage features.[18]

Empirical research on the impact of Medigap coverage on service use has been plagued by many of the same difficulties faced by nonexperimental research on the effect of insurance on health care demand among working-age populations. First, the key independent variable, insurance coverage, is observed imperfectly. In published

179

empirical research, it is simply entered as a "yes" or "no," when in reality, the degree of coverages studied can vary substantially.

Second, the observed set of other factors determining health care expenditures is quite limited in studies to date. The absence of a comprehensive set of controls in a nonexperimental study makes it more likely that the presence of Medigap insurance is correlated with some other unobserved determinant of utilization.

A very serious problem is that the presence of Medigap insurance must be regarded as endogenous in a model explaining health care expenditures. The majority of Medigap policies are individual purchases, not benefits automatically available through (former) employment. This is the opposite situation from health insurance for the working population, making the self-selection issue potentially much more troubling for empirical study of the elderly than for younger groups. No study of which I am aware does a satisfactory job of dealing with the selectivity issue. Authors generally recognize the problem, but inadequate data (particularly instruments for insurance purchase) preclude effective use of simultaneous equation methods.

Christensen and others use data from the 1984 Health Interview Survey (HIS) with usable information on 7,799 full-year Medicare enrollees.[19] A strong point of this survey is the detail on independent variables such as activity limitations and self-assessed health status. The Medigap variable can only be entered as a yes or no, and no attempt is made to address selectivity issues. They find a strong impact of Medigap on use compared with the Medicare-only group. Medigap apparently increases the probability of some hospital use by 27 percent (but no estimated effect on level of service), the probability of any physician visit by 12 percent, and the number of visits conditional on some visits by 11 percent. In general, the total annual use per enrollee is estimated to increase 24 percent for both hospital and physician office-based care.

Taylor and others used the 1977 NMCES data to estimate the effect of Medigap on hospital and physician use among the elderly by means of ordinary least squares.[20] They argued on the basis of a specification test that they could not reject the hypothesis of independence in the error terms of the equation determining insurance purchase and the equation determining expenditures. The presence of group-purchased Medigap increased the expenditures on hospital care about 30 percent, although no significant effect was detected for persons with nongroup or Medicaid coverage. The authors found very large effects on office-visit demand. Both group and nongroup Medigap plans increased the probability of making a doctor visit by greater than 10 percent, and conditional on seeing a doctor during the year, increased physician expenditures from 26 to 39 percent. According to their estimates, the impact of having any Medigap policy (with varying degrees of Part B coverage) increases demand for physician office visits by 40–50 percent.

The NMCES data have also been used in a two-part model of health care demand.[21] Applying a specification test, Hu and others could not reject the independence of the error terms in an equation determining Medigap purchase and an equation determining use. In comparison with the Medicare-only beneficiaries, those with Medigap were significantly more likely to use some medical care during a year, and given some use, Medigap was estimated to increase the extent of use by about 10 percent. The authors did not report the average estimated percentage increase in probability of the use given Medigap coverage, so it is difficult to compare the estimated impacts with other studies.

Using market-level data, Holahan and others studied growth in physician expenditures in Medicare for metropolitan areas and non-metropolitan areas of states between 1983 and 1985.[22] In a partial adjustment model including many determinants of the demand and supply for physician services, a higher percentage of beneficiaries with supplemental insurance had no clear impact on physician expenditures. Scheffler estimated a two-stage least squares regression model treating a measure of Blue Cross Medigap coverage at the area level as an endogenous variable in a model explaining Medicare expenditures.[23] He found a positive and significant relation between the number of covered individuals and area average expenditure.

In the light of the results from studies of younger populations, it would be very surprising if the elderly increased their demand for health care by 20 percent after elimination of a deductible for hospital care and the small deductible and 20 percent copayment of covered charges for Part B services.[24] There is no question that Medigap coverage would increase demand by the elderly by some amount, but the findings discussed above do not separate moral hazard from selection effects associated with Medigap purchase. In the next section, the effect of Medigap on use is assumed to range from 5 to 15 percent, with 10 percent chosen as the most likely value.

A Model for Evaluating the Efficiency Effects of Medigap

Medigap insurance can increase efficiency by protecting beneficiaries against risk. It can also have the opposite effect by inducing inefficient levels of health care expenditures. It will certainly have distributional effects because those electing the supplemental coverage do not pay for all of the costs associated with the policies. This section presents a simulation model that evaluates the magnitudes of the likely effects of Medigap coverage. The general purpose of the model is to describe the risk protection/cost trade-off presented by Medigap with and without catastrophic insurance in Medicare.

A stylized version of Medicare, Medigap, and catastrophic insurance are incorporated into the model to represent the effect of these coverages on beneficiaries. The assumptions used in the model are described below.

Assumptions for Simulations. The average expenditures for a Medicare beneficiary without Medigap coverage are $3,000 per year.[25] This includes Medicare-covered charges as well as acute care costs paid for by the beneficiary. In order to represent the presence of financial risk and to model the effect of a catastrophic plan offering protection against out-of-pocket costs after a deductible, it is necessary to be concerned with the distribution of expenditures as well as the mean. Assumptions about the distribution are contained in table 7–1. The population is divided into fourteen groups. There is a probability that a beneficiary will fall in each group, and there will be an "expenditure factor" for each group in terms of the overall mean of users. The distribution is skewed, representing the fact that a small percentage of the beneficiaries account for a large percentage of the costs each year. About 30 percent of the beneficiaries have no expenditures in any year. Christensen and others show that expenditures for the elderly are dominated by the question of hospitalization.[26] For the 20 percent of the elderly hospitalized during a year, expenses are much higher than the mean; for those not hospitalized, average expenses are much less. The distribution in table 7–1 is meant to capture this skewness. The distribution is also consistent with the anticipated effect of catastrophic coverage on average beneficiary cost sharing, as discussed below.

Medicare is assumed to cover a flat 80 percent of all acute care expenses. Christensen and others report that Medicare pays 72 percent of acute care costs for the elderly.[27] The 80 percent assumption overstates the coverage for physician services because of the Part B deductible and balance billing, and understates the coverage for most hospital care beyond a very short duration, since the main hospital out-of-pocket expense is the Part A deductible.

Medigap insurance is assumed to pay 80 percent of the beneficiaries' out-of-pocket costs. This assumption is meant to reflect the characteristics of a model Medigap plan, not the average plan, which pays less. Presence of Medigap induces some extra utilization in the

TABLE 7–1
DISTRIBUTION OF ANNUAL MEDICARE EXPENDITURES

Group	Percent of Population	Expenditure Factor
0	30.0	0
1	7.0	0.2
2	7.0	0.3
3	7.0	0.45
4	7.0	0.6
5	7.0	0.75
6	7.0	0.9
7	7.0	1.0
8	7.0	1.2
9	7.0	1.5
10	2.8	2.0
11	2.1	3.0
12	1.4	4.0
13	0.7	6.0
Total	100.0	

NOTE: The mean expenditure is $3,000. The mean conditional upon some use is $3,000 × (1/0.7) = $4,285.71. The expenditure for each group is the expenditure factor times the mean expenditure conditional on some use. Thus, group 1 is 7 percent of the population making an expenditure of 0.2 × $4,285.71 = $857.
SOURCE: Author.

population covered. The moral hazard effect of Medigap is alternatively assumed to be a 5, 10, or 15 percent increase in utilization. These demand impact assumptions are small in relation to some of the findings in the literature discussed above. Figures in the low range are chosen for three reasons. First, unsatisfactory controls for selection effects probably bias estimated coefficients upward in models estimated so far. Second, these lower figures accord with findings from the Rand Health Insurance Study on the difference in use between plans in which families paid 25 percent and 0 percent of expenditures.[28] Third, these assumptions are favorable to Medigap.

Medigap premiums are set such that the loss ratio is 70 percent. No selection effects are considered in the model. Beneficiaries with Medigap are assumed to have the same expected expenditures as those without, except for the supplemental insurance.

If beneficiaries desire to maximize the expected utility of income available for nonmedical expenses, the cost of risk is approximately proportional to the variance of the out-of-pocket expenses. The factor of proportionality is the coefficient of absolute risk aversion (the ratio of the second and first derivative of the income utility function) divided by two, so alternative assumptions about risk preferences and the cost of risk can be cast in terms of the coefficient of absolute risk aversion. In this discussion, it is assumed that the coefficient of absolute risk aversion may take on values of .0020, .0015, or .0010. These values correspond to a generally high level of risk aversion, as will be seen in the simulation where the cost of risk is quantified. The values were chosen in order to represent a high degree of risk aversion among the elderly, and again, to be favorable to the case for Medigap.[29]

Catastrophic coverage will take a simple form of paying all out-of-pocket costs of the beneficiary after $2,000. The actual legislation contains separate limits for Part A ($560) and Part B ($1,370),[30] summing to about $2,000. Assumptions in the model are summarized in table 7–2.

The Impact of Medigap—No Catastrophic. The workings of the simulation model embodying the above assumptions are illustrated in table 7–3, which compares the situation for Medicare and the beneficiary with and without Medigap, prior to catastrophic insurance. Initially, without Medigap, the $3,000 of mean annual expen-

---

TABLE 7–2

SUMMARY OF MODEL ASSUMPTIONS

Expenditures
  Mean expenditure of $3,000 per beneficiary per year
  Distributed as shown in table 7–1
  80 percent covered by Medicare; 20 percent out-of-pocket
Medigap
  Covers 80 percent of out-of-pocket obligations
  Increases total expenditure by (.05, .10, .15)
  No selection effects
  Premiums set to meet 70 percent loss ratio
Risk
  Cost of risk is approximated by the variance of income times the
    coefficient of absolute risk aversion divided by two
Catastrophic coverage
  Medicare pays all out-of-pocket costs after $2,000 per year
  No effect on total charges

SOURCE: Author.

THOMAS G. McGUIRE

TABLE 7–3
MEDICARE AND BENEFICIARY COSTS WITH AND WITHOUT MEDIGAP
(dollars)

	No Medigap	Medigap	Difference
Medicare	2,400	2,640	240
Beneficiary			
Out-of-pocket costs	600	132	−468
Medigap premiums	0	754	754
Cost of risk	419	20	−399
Total beneficiary	1,019	907	−112
Medicare + beneficiary	3,419	3,546	127

NOTE: No catastrophic insurance, moderate risk aversion, and moderate moral hazard assumed. Total annual expenditure without Medigap is $3,000. Moderate risk aversion means a coefficient of constant absolute risk aversion of .0015. Moderate moral hazard means a demand impact of Medigap of 10 percent.
SOURCE: Author.

ditures are paid 80 percent by Medicare and 20 percent by the beneficiary. The beneficiary bears considerable financial risk, valued at $419. In other words, the beneficiary would be willing to pay $419 above the actuarial value of the risk in order to avoid the risk altogether. The total cost borne by the beneficiary is the expected out-of-pocket cost of $600, plus the risk cost, for a total of $1,019. The total social cost of the program is the sum of Medicare and beneficiary cost, or $3,419.

Medigap affects all of the above costs. Medicare costs rise 10 percent (assuming a moderate moral hazard effect) because of the demand induced by Medigap. Out-of-pocket costs fall as the beneficiary pays a Medigap premium to cover 80 percent of out-of-pocket expenses. The cost of risk falls sharply. Total beneficiary costs, even accounting for the 70 percent loss ratio in Medigap and the higher total expenditures because of demand inducement, fall to $907, because of the fall in the cost of risk. The sum of Medicare and beneficiary costs rise to $3,546.

This example illustrates some key points about Medicare and Medigap. The first is that the cost of risk for the unprotected Medicare beneficiary can be quite large. A relatively inefficient Medigap policy, returning on average only 70 percent of premiums as payout, may still substantially improve the welfare of the average beneficiary. Second, this example shows the overinsurance problem. Medigap is a good buy for the beneficiary, but Medicare suffers a 10 percent cost

TABLE 7-4: COST IMPACT OF MEDIGAP WITHOUT CATASTROPHIC (dollars)

Moral hazard	High Risk Aversion[a]			Moderate Risk Aversion[a]			Low Risk Aversion[a]		
	H[b]	M[b]	L[b]	H[b]	M[b]	L[b]	H[b]	M[b]	L[b]
Without Medigap									
Medicare costs	2,400	2,400	2,400	2,400	2,400	2,400	2,400	2,400	2,400
Beneficiary									
O-O-P costs	600	600	600	600	600	600	600	600	600
Medigap premiums	0	0	0	0	0	0	0	0	0
Cost of risk	558	558	558	419	419	419	279	279	279
Total beneficiary	1,158	1,158	1,158	1,019	1,019	1,019	879	879	879
Medicare + beneficiary	3,558	3,558	3,558	3,419	3,419	3,419	3,279	3,279	3,279
With Medigap									
Medicare costs	2,760	2,640	2,520	2,760	2,640	2,520	2,760	2,640	2,520
Beneficiary									
O-O-P costs	138	132	126	138	132	126	138	132	126
Medigap premiums	789	754	720	789	754	720	789	754	720
Cost of risk	29	27	25	21	20	18	14	14	12
Total beneficiary	956	913	871	948	907	864	941	900	858
Medicare + beneficiary	3,716	3,553	3,390	3,708	3,546	3,384	3,701	3,540	3,378
Net Cost from Medigap									
Medicare costs	360	240	120	360	240	120	360	240	120
Beneficiary	-232	-245	-387	-71	-112	-155	62	21	-21
Medicare + beneficiary	158	-5	-168	289	127	-35	422	261	99

a. The risk aversion assumption is that the coefficient of absolute risk aversion is high (.0020), moderate (.0015), or low (.0010).
b. The moral hazard assumption is that Medigap increases total utilization by a high (.15), moderate (.10), or low (.05) amounts.
SOURCE: Author.

TABLE 7–5: COST IMPACT OF MEDIGAP WITH CATASTROPHIC (dollars)

Moral hazard	High[a]			Moderate[a]			Low[a]		
	H[b]	M[b]	L[b]	H[b]	M[b]	L[b]	H[b]	M[b]	L[b]
				Catastrophic alone					
Medicare costs	2,454	2,454	2,454	2,454	2,454	2,454	2,454	2,454	2,454
Beneficiary									
O-O-P costs	546	546	546	546	546	546	546	546	546
Medigap premiums	0	0	0	0	0	0	0	0	0
Cost of risk	300	300	300	225	225	225	150	150	150
Total beneficiary	846	846	846	771	771	771	696	696	696
Medicare + beneficiary	3,300	3,300	3,300	3,225	3,225	3,225	3,150	3,150	3,150
				Catastrophic + Medigap					
Medicare costs	2,814	2,694	2,574	2,814	2,694	2,574	2,814	2,694	2,574
Beneficiary									
O-O-P costs	126	120	115	126	120	115	126	120	115
Medigap premiums	718	686	655	718	686	655	718	686	655
Cost of risk	13	13	12	10	10	9	7	6	6
Total beneficiary	857	820	782	853	816	779	850	813	743
Medicare + beneficiary	3,670	3,513	3,356	3,667	3,510	3,353	3,664	3,507	3,209
Net cost from Medigap									
Medicare costs	360	240	120	360	240	120	360	240	120
Beneficiary	11	−26	−64	82	45	8	154	117	47
Medicare + beneficiary	370	213	56	442	285	128	514	357	159

a. Risk aversion assumption is that the coefficient of absolute risk aversion is high (.0020), moderate (.0015), or low (.0010).
b. Moral hazard assumption is that Medigap increases total utilization by a high (.15), moderate (.10), or low (.05) amounts.
SOURCE: Author.

187

increase. In general, costs to both parties go up slightly. On balance, in this example, Medigap results in higher costs than benefits.[31] This example also shows that although Medigap is inefficient with this combination of moral hazard and risk-aversion parameters, it is a reasonably close call. Medigap confers considerable benefits when beneficiaries are exposed to large out-of-pocket risks, and if demand inducement was lower or risk aversion higher, Medigap might be socially efficient.

Table 7–4 describes the results of the impact of Medigap in the absence of catastrophic coverage for the nine combinations of parameters for moral hazard and risk aversion. Medicare's costs are influenced only by the degree of moral hazard. Medicare's costs are 15 percent higher ($2,760) if Medigap increases demand 15 percent. Medicare costs rise 10 percent or 5 percent when the increase in demand is moderate and low.

Without Medigap, the beneficiary's cost of risk associated with expected out-of-pocket cost of $600 and a variance based on the distribution from table 7–1 is $558 when risk aversion is high, $419 when moderate, and $279 when low.

With Medigap, the beneficiary's costs of risk are small across all parameters. Demand response affects costs to the beneficiary as well as Medicare, increasing premiums and out-of-pocket payments. The beneficiary costs go up by a higher percentage than Medicare costs because the loss ratio for insurers is less than one. In the high moral hazard case, for example, when demand is increased by 15 percent by Medigap, nonrisk-expected costs to the beneficiary go from $600 to $138 out-of-pocket costs. With Medigap premiums of $789, the total is $927. Although this is a large increase in dollar costs, only in the case of low risk aversion does the beneficiary find the purchase of Medigap unattractive.

According to the calculations in table 7–4, Medigap ranges from very attractive to marginally attractive to beneficiaries, depending on the degree of risk aversion and demand response. For Medicare, Medigap is always associated with extra cost, directly in proportion to the assumed demand response.

When the costs to Medicare and the beneficiary are considered together in the final row of table 7–4, no clear conclusion about the efficiency of Medigap emerges. If beneficiaries are not very risk averse, even a small amount of moral hazard can increase total social costs of the program. But recognizing that the elderly may be more risk averse, a call for restricting Medigap on efficiency grounds is unpersuasive in the precatastrophic scenario presented here.

The Impact of Medigap with Catastrophic. Table 7–5 reports the same simulations as table 7–4 with the addition of catastrophic coverage. A $2,000 out-of-pocket limit has a relatively small effect on the expected out-of-pocket costs for beneficiaries, reducing these from $600 to $546 per year. This is a relatively conservative estimate of the impact of catastrophic coverage on beneficiary out-of-pocket costs. Initial estimates by the Reagan administration valued the benefit at about $60 per year, but this may have been an underestimate owing to the omission of projected costs of the expanded drug benefit.[32] By understating the value of catastrophic to the elderly, we again give Medigap the best chance to improve net welfare.

In table 7–5, Medicare expected costs have been raised to reflect the costs covered by the catastrophic provisions. Because these expenditures are the most risky from the beneficiary point of view, the gains from catastrophic are mainly in terms of the reduction in the cost of risk. The cost of risk has been almost cut in half in comparison with the cost to the beneficiary without catastrophic coverage.

Medigap affects the costs to Medicare in the presence of catastrophic coverage in the same manner as before, the percentage increase in Medicare costs being directly related to the percentage increase in demand induced by Medigap. The economics of Medigap for the beneficiary have been altered by catastrophic, however. For the beneficiary, Medigap is now a marginally attractive option if he or she is highly or moderately risk averse, and a poor option if the level of risk aversion is low. According to the calculations in table 7–5, only when risk aversion is high and moral hazard is moderate or low does the beneficiary come out ahead with Medigap.

From a social point of view, combining the costs to the beneficiary and to Medicare, Medigap always causes more costs than benefits.

Medigap and Choice of Alternative Delivery Systems. Alternative delivery systems (ADS), such as a health maintenance organization (HMO) or a preferred provider organization (PPO), are a potentially important part of a strategy to contain Medicare costs.[33] For the beneficiary, an ADS is an opportunity to avoid Medicare's cost sharing, and in this way, is an alternative to the purchase of Medigap. Medigap does two things in this context. First, it gives beneficiaries a subsidized means of avoiding out-of-pocket costs in the fee-for-service sector, decreasing the attractiveness of the ADS. Second, Medigap increases average Medicare payments in a locality, and thereby increases the premium Medicare will pay to an organization at risk for beneficiary costs. This second effect, if the organization could use the extra premiums to attract beneficiaries, would serve to increase the attractiveness of the ADS. Either effect could in principle dominate, but I suspect that the Medigap effect on ADS has on balance been an unfavorable one. Medigap eliminates the incentive to surrender the convenience and familiarity of the fee-for-service sector. The Medigap-caused increase in payment to an ADS is diluted, because not all beneficiaries elect Medigap and increase utilization. Furthermore, federal legislation regulates how an ADS may use premium payments from Medicare, limiting the way a plan can structure its competitive position.

Evidence is accumulating that enrollees take premiums and expected payouts into account in their choice of plans.[34] Marquis and Phelps studied families' hypothetical choice of supplemental insurance and found an elasticity of demand to insurance premiums of about −0.6.[35] Other studies, relying on price differences created by economies of group purchase, or marginal tax rate differences leading to different degrees of tax subsidy of insurance, have found responses ranging from nearly zero to much larger than −.6.[36]

Ellis found very strong evidence that employees select a health plan on the basis of expected benefits.[37] When a new "high option" plan was offered in the firm he studied, the employees choosing the better coverage at a slightly higher premium had health expenses in the prior year more than five times greater than those employees who chose the low option.

Friedlob and Hadley analyze the reasons Medicare beneficiaries join HMOs on the basis of the experience of four plans in the Minneapolis–St. Paul area.[38] Fifty-eight percent of the enrollees studied gave their main reason for joining an HMO as either better benefits or lower cost than the fee-for-service alternative. Garfinkel and others found the presence of Medigap coverage to have a significant negative effect on the probability of a beneficiary enrolling in an HMO.[39]

Quantifying the cost of Medigap to Medicare's ADS initiatives would be guesswork. If Medigap were eliminated, however, a substantial fraction of the 70 percent of beneficiaries with Medigap coverage could be expected to elect an ADS option covering most of their out-of-pocket expenses. At present, an ADS-based strategy is simply not a viable option for Medicare. Eliminating Medigap would give Medicare the ability to use reduction in demand-side cost sharing as an incentive to bring beneficiaries into delivery systems with more efficient patterns of care.

Discussion

Medicare is a leader in setting supply-side payment policy to control expenditures. A Medicare physician fee schedule may soon be added to the hospital prospective payment system as a prominent Medicare supply-side payment policy. In contrast, Medicare's demand-side policies, cost sharing in Parts A and B and initiatives using alternative delivery systems, are accomplishing little.

Following the lead of other researchers, I have argued that the effectiveness of Medicare's demand-side policies is seriously undermined by the widespread purchase of Medigap coverage. Medicare in effect subsidizes the purchase of supplemental insurance that has a paralyzing effect on its own demand-side payment policy. The demand-limiting effect of cost sharing is undone, and incentives to choose HMOs and other alternative delivery systems are weakened.

Although I have not stressed the consumer-protection argument, Rice and others have argued that the main rationale for regulating Medigap is that beneficiaries overestimate its value, particularly in regard to Medigap's coverage of long-term care expenses.[40] Expenses for long-term care represent the largest financial risk for the elderly. Eliminating or restricting the purchase of Medigap policies may redirect demand for insurance protection by the elderly into a more useful channel: buying protection against long-term care expenses.

Even though Medigap is a clear foe of Medicare cost-containment goals, it is not clear that, prior to catastrophic coverage legislation, Medigap did not serve a legitimate social purpose of financial protection for the underinsured Medicare beneficiary. The social role of Medigap in terms of risk protection is greatly diminished by the presence of catastrophic coverage, even in a model set up to be favorable to the case for Medigap.

The main implication of this analysis is that there is an opportunity for Medicare, as catastrophic coverage is phased in, to take steps to limit or eliminate Medigap coverage, which could lead to a Medicare program saving on the order of 5–10 percent of expenditures. No other viable public policy, on the demand or the supply side, can promise savings of this magnitude in a move that should *increase* the social efficiency of the Medicare program.

There are a number of options for Medicare to consider, which can only be mentioned briefly here. The first, as already proposed by numerous authors, is to tax Medigap policies, that is, impose a premium tax on Medigap insurance designed to compensate Medicare for the extra services induced by Medigap coverage. Medicare would save under this approach by the collection of the premium tax, and by the lower level of induced services because the beneficiaries would be discouraged from buying Medigap. The tax argument has much more appeal in the postcatastrophic world, because it is much more likely to represent an efficiency improvement as well as a means to reduce Medicare net program costs.

A possibly superior approach to the tax option is for Medicare itself to offer optional insurance through a self-financing mechanism, similar from the point of view of the elderly, to the way Medigap must be purchased. Because of lower administrative costs, Medicare should be able to charge about the same as the average Medigap premium, yet build in a tax of about 50 percent. In this way, Medicare could recover at least some of the extra costs induced by Medigap coverage without much extra financial burden on the beneficiary.

Medicare Part B coverage itself could be expanded to eliminate the need for the elderly to buy a Medigap policy at all. One strategy would be to eliminate all beneficiary cost sharing except for the Part B deductible. This Medicare benefit expansion could be financed in a fashion similar to the financing of catastrophic, a combination of premiums and taxes on the elderly. Because the loss ratio for most catastrophic insurance is so low, this form of balanced-budget finance could leave the elderly better off than with an administratively inefficient market for private insurance. It would represent a great simplification for insurance coverage for the elderly. By fully covering Part B, this policy would give Medicare more power in setting fees for physicians and other Part B services, and would work well with an aggressive Medicare physician fee schedule policy.

Issues in Medicare Benefits

A Discussion

STEPHEN ZUCKERMAN: Balance billing is indeed an important safety valve. The point is, there are some people representing beneficiary groups, and there may even be some people within the government, who feel that once you have gone to the trouble of spending millions of dollars to develop a relative value fee schedule, that should be it and balance billing is not necessary.

The quality issue, in terms of which physicians may choose not to participate, is something that people establishing the fees need to be sensitive to. The physicians currently with the highest fees are the ones most likely to be driven out of Medicare if balance billing is too restricted. They may be the better physicians, if they can attract those fees from the private market or from nonassigned Medicare patients.

As for the sole local provider, the issue is really not so much protecting beneficiaries—if they don't have enough income, or if their expenditures are high—but protecting beneficiaries where the market simply can't work because there are very few specialists in a particular area. That will be a problem.

Medicare catastrophic limits exclude balance billing, so that reaching the catastrophic limit may imply that a certain level of Medicare copayments has been reached, but expenditures could be far greater than that if the consumer paid balance bills. So the catastrophic limit may be an imperfect trigger mechanism for exempting people from balance billing, but we thought it might be fairly simple to administer.

THOMAS G. McGUIRE: It is true that there was no empirical basis for my calculations of the cost of risk. Very little work has been done on the cost of risk. There are some models around, and I tried to be extremely conservative by exaggerating risk aversion.

FREDERICK R. WARREN-BOULTON: My personal demand for medical

193

procedures is pretty inelastic. When I want my appendix out, I definitely want my appendix out. I wouldn't say, "Well, I think I will have you cure my cold instead."

The quality of the process is a different matter. I am likely to be very elastic with respect to how many days I spend in the hospital, how good the meals are, and things like that. My question is, can you argue that balance billing is much more important in handling moral hazard than coinsurance, because balance billing directly attacks the quality dimension? It shifts the extra cost of additional quality entirely to the consumer, whereas with coinsurance the consumer only pays 20 percent. So, could you say that balance billing is more efficient at handling the problem than coinsurance, because it operates on the quality margin more?

MR. ZUCKERMAN: Medicare is currently structured much like a complicated fee schedule. A physician can increase expenditures by increasing volume. But the beneficiary pays 100 percent of the extra cost of intensity, through the amount of balance billing. So, some of the good incentives of balance billing are in there now because the physician has to ask the beneficiary to pay for extra intensity.

COMMENT FROM THE AUDIENCE: For nonassigned claims, the average balance billing burden is greater than the coinsurance. The coinsurance is about 20 percent of the allowed charge, and the balance billing now is about 30–35 percent of the allowed charge. One of the issues about the relative scale is that balance billing will be directly affected, dollar for dollar, as the fees are charged, so it can be more important than coinsurance.

QUESTIONS: Mr. Hixson stated that under the current system, from the demand side—because of the 20 percent copayment—a $5 fee hike, for example, would only be reflected to the patient in a $1 cost, so there is a market distortion, but that is only true if the charge is within the allowed charge of Medicare. If balance billing is permitted, anything above that allowed charge is completely borne by the patient, and is a further incentive for a real market force. Can you explain a little more how, under your proposal, the patient would bear 100 percent of the marginal costs?

JESSE S. HIXSON: To deal with the problem of the burden on the low-income beneficiary, you could simply have a minimum benefit package for everyone, and then for any additional services—more, high-quality, or more extensive services—the patient would pay 100 percent of the additional cost.

For the preferred provider plan (PPO) and the health maintenance organization (HMO), it is easy to imagine how one would do that. For fee for service, if you define a level of assignment that you want to achieve, and adjust your fees to achieve that target and level of assignment, you can assume that you are achieving the desired level of access for the low-income patient.

That would be an indicator of the level of access in the local market. Then, for whatever reasons, if some patients did not want to go to a participating physician or to one who assigned Medicare claims, they could do so and pay whatever the difference in fees the physician charged.

QUESTION: Does Mr. Zuckerman have a sense of where you could go with these policies, even if you didn't know the magnitudes of the response? Should you have a little more or a little less coinsurance or balance billing?

MR. ZUCKERMAN: Many of the policies that are being discussed—from the relative value scale and fee schedule to banning Medigap, or even moving toward mandatory assignment—are quite different from past policies in the Medicare program. There won't be a lot of hard data about the response to these policy changes and people are going to have to make educated guesses. An example of this was the predicted sharp increase in hospital admissions under the Medicare prospective payment system. In fact, hospital admissions fell. So you have to be cautious, but should still try to systematically analyze it and make some predictions.

H. E. FRECH III: The thing that we are least ignorant about seems to be the response of consumers to copayments. The Rand study has nailed that down pretty well. An important finding of that study was that the response to the out-of-pocket price did not vary with age.

We can work through their examples and predict responses to changes in cost sharing better than anything else—say, a change in fees, resource-based fees, new kinds of utilization controls, or restrictions on balance billing. With the changes being proposed these days, we are really guessing.

Because of Medigap and also because some physicians waive deductibles and coinsurance (which is common, although illegal), we don't even know what copayment Medicare patients have now. We have a very poor idea of the baseline copayment. Further, existing statistics wildly overstate the amount of copayment in Medicare. They ignore Medigap coverage, the waiving of deductibles and coinsurance, and the waiving of balance bills when physicians do not take assignment.

JOEL IRA FRANCK: Do you think that the decision about physician participation in Medicare was a bad idea—that is, the decision to have a new class of participating doctor and thereby eliminate, on a case-by-case basis, physicians talking frankly with patients about what it may cost them? Do you think that has had an antimarket effect on physicians' fees and utilization of services? Would it be better to have no such thing as participation in any insurance program and always have copayment, even if there is Medigap insurance?

MR. ZUCKERMAN: To the extent that the participation program has encouraged higher assignment rates, there is some evidence that this has contributed to growth in volume over the last few years. It stands to reason that the higher assignment rates lower the price to the patient. You would expect that, without inducement, volume will be higher when prices are lower.

MR. FRANCK: But would it be beneficial, from a market point of view, to eliminate the concept of participation, so that on a case-by-case basis, a patient and physician would discuss whether the physician is going to accept assignment or not?

JOHN HOLAHAN: Even before 1983, there were many physicians who assigned virtually 100 percent of claims, so it wasn't a situation where every claim was being negotiated. The participating physician program probably didn't have much impact on individual, claim-by-claim negotiation.

COMMENT: There seems to be a viable insurance market to take care of the dollar cost of care. There is very little insurance you can buy to eliminate the pain and suffering aspect of medical care.

ROGER G. NOLL: The point of buying insurance is to shift income to where you value it higher. At best, insurance can equate the marginal utility of money or wealth. Usually, when I am in a great deal of pain the marginal utility of my money is probably even lower, so I probably would like to have a reverse insurance policy.

COMMENT: Most physicians contribute to the common good by taking care of certain parts of the population. Maybe physicians should show that they have a certain percentage of Medicaid patients on their list in order to be able to balance-bill. That way they would be forced into contributing something to the common public good.

MR. ZUCKERMAN: We would certainly favor reducing the subsidy to the physicians who are not willing to participate. That is the direction in which policy has moved and will probably continue moving. We would favor continuing down that road, but as for mandating that everyone take Medicaid patients, that is not going to work.

MR. WARREN-BOULTON: Earlier in the discussion, we were trying to settle on the right price, but now we are not sure that we can and so we want to keep balance billing. The consensus seems to be that the need for a safety valve through balance billing is probably still there. But there are also many people who believe that once you have the "just price" you don't need balance billing. That implies greater confidence in the ability to establish these prices for the 7,000–10,000 procedures and 450,000 physicians than makes sense.

The fact is, if you want to exercise monopoly power over physicians, you have to stop balance billing. That is the one thing that you have to do if you want to transfer significant amounts of income from doctors to someone else. It depends on what your goals are. If you simply want to set up a more efficient system, you allow balance billing. If you want to tax doctors, then you ban balance billing.

Perhaps a simpler and more efficient way to do it would be just to have a surcharge on your income tax: Anybody who is a doctor pays 30 percent extra.

MR. FRECH: There is a right distribution of prices, different prices for different physicians, different locations, and different towns. So even if you did the Hsiao-type exercise absolutely perfectly, it would be like finding the right price for a bottle of wine. The point is, there is going to be a big role for balance billing, even if it were possible to do the Hsiao project exactly right, which is a wild assumption in itself.

PART TWO

Alternatives for Setting and Adjusting Fee Schedules

8
Toward an Adjusted-Charge Relative Value Scale

Janet B. Mitchell, Jerry Cromwell, Margo L. Rosenbach, and William B. Stason

The principal criticism leveled against the usual, customary, and reasonable (UCR) method of physician payment used by Medicare and by many private payers is that it has no mechanism for readjusting physician reimbursement rates downward. The incentives are to increase, or at least maintain, existing fee levels. This is particularly a problem for new technologies. Fees are set high initially, and then remain high even when the costs of providing the service have fallen. Coronary artery bypass graft (CABG) and pacemaker surgery are two frequently cited examples. Better equipment, better surgical techniques, and just "learning by doing" have greatly reduced the time and effort involved, and probably the relative difficulty as well.[1] The historic insurance bias in favor of surgery undoubtedly has also served to widen the payment differential between surgical procedures and visits.

As a result of these concerns, Congress has already begun to reduce Medicare payment levels for selected surgical operations and to increase reimbursement for primary care services (as part of the Omnibus Reconciliation Act of 1987). Some policy makers, including the members of the Physician Payment Review Commission, believe that the payment system needs a more thorough overhaul and are considering a resource-based relative value scale (RBRVS) that would take into account the work effort involved, practice costs, and the opportunity costs of residency training.[2]

This research was supported by HHS Contract No. 100-86-0023 cosponsored by the Assistant Secretary for Planning and Evaluation (ASPE) and Health Care Financing Administration (HCFA) and by Cooperative Agreement No. 17-C-98999/1-02 from the Health Care Financing Administration. The views and opinions are those of the authors, and no endorsement by ASPE, HCFA, or Department of Health and Human Services is intended or should be inferred.

Those strongly in favor of such a scale assume that the current reimbursement system is irrevocably flawed. But are relative prices *so* distorted that we need to construct an entirely new price list? Could we get away with just some tinkering, at least in the short run? If charges are distorted only for some services and procedures, then a charge-based relative value scale, with corrections for those procedures that are egregiously mispriced, might be an equally valid basis for a fee schedule. Given the dramatic income redistributions implied by the RBRVS, a charge-based relative value scale might also serve as a transitional payment model.

In this chapter, we seek to test the relationship between physician effort and current Medicare charges. We use regression analysis to determine the association between Medicare fees and the time and complexity of selected medical and surgical procedures. Based on estimated fee-effort equations, outlier procedures are identified as potential candidates for higher or lower payment. We then compare our results with those obtained in the RBRVS study.

Methods

This analysis is based on the Physicians' Practice Follow-up Survey of 1987. Physicians participating in the 1983 Physicians' Practice Costs and Income Survey (PPCIS) were recontacted and questioned about the effort (time and complexity) involved in performing selected medical and surgical services.

Sample Description. The original sample for the PPCIS had been drawn from the physician master file maintained by the American Medical Association and included all active, nonfederal physicians practicing patient care at least twenty hours per week. A single-stage, stratified element-level, random sampling design was used, with oversampling in several small specialties. The PPCIS response rate was 67.6 percent for a total sample of 4,729 physicians.

In the follow-up survey, we contacted 3,368 eligible physicians in the following specialties who had responded to the 1983 survey: general practice, family practice, internal medicine, cardiology, dermatology, gastroenterology, neurology, general surgery, ophthalmology, orthopedic surgery, cardiovascular/thoracic surgery, plastic surgery, otolaryngology, neurosurgery, urology, obstetrics-gynecology, radiology, and anesthesiology. A total of 2,499 physicians (74.2 percent) responded. Anesthesiologists were excluded since all reported times had to be based on estimates by the physician personally performing each procedure. Medicare payment for anesthesiologists who perform the complete procedure differs from that for those who direct certified registered nurse anesthetists (CRNAs). Unfortunately, this distinction cannot be reliably determined from claims data.

Time and Complexity Estimates. Each physician was asked to assess time in ten to fifteen services performed by the specialty. The list of services varied by specialty.[3] Time was defined as the period required to perform the service for a typical patient in each physician's practice. Where applicable, this included separate estimates of preoperative and postoperative times (including follow-up after discharge from the hospital). Surgeons were also asked about their billing practices with respect to posthospital office visits. At least three out of four surgeons included *all* such visits in their global fee, and another 5 to 10 percent included *some* visits, depending on the specialty or procedure.[4] This reported behavior is confirmed by an analysis of Medicare claims data in ten states, which showed that surgeons rarely bill separately for pre- and postoperative and posthospital visits.[5]

Each physician was also asked to rank the list of services according to relative complexity independent of the time it takes to perform the procedure and to take into account the judgment, skill, effort (mental and physical), and stress involved in performing the procedure. First, physicians were asked to select the *most* complex procedure on the list and assign it a score of 100. Then, they were asked to select the least complex procedure and rank it on a score of 1 to 100 relative to the most complex procedure. Physicians were then asked to rank remaining procedures in relation to the least and most complex procedures. The final rankings were reviewed by the respondent to ensure the reliability and validity of their responses. Physicians were asked to rank all procedures regardless of whether or not they personally performed the procedure.

Average time and complexity scores were internally consistent and had face validity.[6] Initial office visits were rated as being longer and more complex than follow-up visits, for example, and original hip replacements were considered less time consuming and less complicated than procedures involving revisions of previous hip arthroplasty.

Furthermore, physicians were in close agreement in the time and complexity values they assigned to each procedure. Intraclass correlation coefficients for service and procedure time ranged from .42 to .91, and coefficients from thirteen of the seventeen specialties were greater than .60. Comparable correlation coefficients for complexity ranged from .43 to .83, with those for ten specialties at .60 or higher.

There was considerably more variability in self-reports of pre- and postoperative time, especially for ophthalmologists and orthopedic surgeons. This may have been due to practice pattern differences, especially in the location of care (for example, inpatient versus outpatient care).

Before performing cross-specialty analyses, we standardized complexity estimates across specialties using the interpretation and report of a chest X-ray, since this procedure was asked of each specialty and its content was believed to be more standard and familiar to physicians than an office or hospital visit or surgical procedure. Each complexity score for a specialty was divided by that specialty's chest X-ray score. The resulting scores thus rank complexity *relative to* that for chest X-ray interpretation within each specialty, and the complexity score for a chest X-ray is 1.0 for each specialty.

Surgeons typically rated a two-view chest X-ray as less complicated than medical specialists and general practitioners. On a scale of 1 to 100, surgeons ranked the X-ray between 15 and 25, whereas medical specialists' scores ranged from 25 to 45. A lower rating of the index procedure by surgeons will tend to raise the relative complexity of their complicated surgeries. This "decompresses" their scale relative to medical specialists and reflects the inherent complexity of their most difficult surgeries. One could argue, however, that surgeons still have not ranked an X-ray low enough, thereby understating complexity. We acknowledge that this method may result in the compression of complexity scales across specialties, although physicians had the opportunity to rate their most difficult procedure a hundred times more complex per minute than their simplest one. The multivariate analysis, discussed below, should detect such compression and empirically test the validity of the standardization technique.

By design, there was considerable overlap in the procedure lists for each specialty. Both general and thoracic surgeons were asked to report on pacemaker insertion, for example, and internists shared certain endoscopies in common with gastroenterologists. To perform the multivariate analysis (described below), we aggregated common procedures to produce one observation per procedure. Mean times and standardized complexity values were combined for these common procedures, weighted by the relative frequencies of performance by specialty (as reflected in the Medicare claims data base). Aggregation was not done for visits and consultations, however, because they represent fundamentally different services when performed by different specialties.

Fee Data. Physician fees were proxied by national average Medicare-allowed charges obtained from the 1985 Part B Medicare Data (BMAD) beneficiary file maintained by the Health Care Financing Administration. This file contains all claims submitted by a 5 percent random sample of Medicare beneficiaries for calendar year 1985. Mean allowed charges were calculated for each service and procedure included in the study, weighted by the relative frequencies of performance by specialty. Medicare allowed, rather than submitted, charges were used in view of the policy interest in justifying actual Medicare payments in terms of relative physician effort. Scales based on the two sets of relative charges were found to be correlated .99, so it makes little difference which is used. Moreover, because charges are aggregated to the national level, they reflect a national "relative value scale" devoid of geographic variation. This is appropriate for our purpose, which is to relate average fees to time and complexity and not to explain fee variation across areas.

Statistical Analysis. Time and complexity estimates derived from survey responses need to be combined in some fashion to produce a predicted fee. The original resource-based relative values had been developed with the aid of a simple multiplicative model, which implicitly assumes that effort doubles when *either* time or complexity doubles.[7] Actual physician charges may or may not follow such a rule, and a more general formulation would be

$$F_i = A \times T_i^\alpha \times C_i^\phi$$

where F_i = the average allowed charge for the ith procedure, T_i = average time, C_i = average complexity, and A = a base fee for a hypothetical procedure taking one minute at unit complexity. If the exponents α and ϕ were estimated to be less than 1.0, then fees would rise more slowly than under the simple model, which assumes one-for-one percentage increases. On the other hand, if physicians tend to compress the scale on which they report simple versus complex procedures, the ϕ complexity coefficient could exceed 1.0 and fees would rise faster percentagewise than reported complexity.[8] This adds a flexibility that compensates for systematic under- or overreporting of complexity which is missing from a simple model.

Two important modifications were made to the predicting equation. First, the sum of pre- and postoperative times was treated as a separate variable with its own exponent. If pre- and postoperative times are ignored, their effects will produce an upward bias in the estimated procedure time and complexity coefficients because all are positively correlated. On the other hand, if pre/post times are combined with procedure time, this implicitly assumes that they have the

205

same marginal value (in terms of fees) as procedure time. Although it is reasonable to expect physician fees to rise with more pre/post time, they should do so at a slower rate than the more "valuable," more "complex," procedure time.[9]

As a second modification, a multiplicative dummy variable was included to distinguish surgical from medical procedures. (The variable was set equal to 1 except for invasive diagnostic or therapeutic surgical procedures, where it was set to 2.) If no surgical adjustment is made, one implicitly assumes that all procedures fall on the same time and complexity curve, which could make a whole class of surgical procedures appear overpriced. Patients' perceptions of the value of surgery, reinforced by broader and deeper insurance coverage, could explain systematically higher fees for surgical procedures. Whether the effects of insurance coverage should be reflected in the fees is debatable, however, and we present the results with and without the adjustment.

The multiplicative model was estimated in double-log form using least-squares regression on 139 unique services and procedures.[10] Predicted values from the regression were compared with actual fees to identify over- and underpriced procedures. As predicted values from a logged equation will underpredict fees, depending on the explanatory power of the equation, all values were adjusted upward using a formula developed by the staff at the Rand Corporation.[11] A 95 percent confidence interval was constructed around each adjusted predicted fee that indicates the potential error in the predicted value.[12] Actual allowables falling within this band may not involve over- or underpayments if the true predicted value is at the low or high end of the interval. Without such a band, policy makers would not know how much confidence to place in an estimate and therefore how large a rollback or increase might be defensible. Clearly, a narrower 80 or 90 percent confidence interval may be equally appropriate and would produce more outliers. Note that any confidence band reflects the decision makers' perceptions of the true number of outliers once time, complexity, and possibly surgery are held constant.

Results

The results of our analysis are presented in the next three sections and then are compared with those of the RBRVS study.

Time and Complexity Estimates. Table 8–1 presents data for twenty-one services and procedures representing a range of physician activity and are identical to the ones included in the RBRVS study. Thus, services provided by certain specialties, like cardiology and neurology, have been omitted here. All services, of course, were included in the regression analysis.[13]

Three measures of time are shown for major surgical procedures: procedure (skin-to-skin) time; in-hospital preoperative time; and postoperative time, both in hospital and following discharge. We assume all three times are included in the global fee. For diagnostic surgery and for nonsurgical services, only the procedure time was collected. Table 8–1 also presents the mean standardized complexity score for each procedure and service, ignoring the complexity of the pre- and postoperative times.

Of the specific procedures, coronary artery bypass surgery (CABG) averaged 221 minutes (3.7 hours) in the operating room and another 272 minutes (4.5 hours) in postoperative follow-up. Three-graft CABGs had an average complexity score of 5.10, making them one of the most complicated surgeries per minute, exceeded only by modified radical mastectomies (5.28), aortic valve replacements (5.26), and one-stage lens procedures (6.87).[14] Cataract surgery is particularly noteworthy for its long pre- and postoperative times (176 minutes), in contrast to the operation itself, which takes less than an hour on average.

Direct comparisons of complexity can also be made from table 8–1. For example, the general surgeon rated an initial comprehensive hospital visit at 2.18 versus 2.57 for an internist, which is an 18 percent difference. The internist's visit was also 38 percent longer (58 versus 42 minutes), implying substantially greater total work effort for this one service. By extension, we can also infer that a transurethral resection of the prostate (TURP), say, is 29 percent more complex than an internist's initial comprehensive hospital visit (3.32 versus 2.57).

Fee Equations. Table 8–2 presents the estimated coefficients, first without, and then with, a surgical adjustment. To test the sensitivity of the model to time and complexity interactions, all variables were entered in stepwise fashion, beginning with procedure time alone. Each coefficient can be interpreted as the percentage effect on fees of a 1 percent increase in either time or complexity. For example, a 1 percent increase in procedure time results in a 1.53 percent increase in physician fees (column 1). The explanatory power of the model ranges from 66 to 91 percent, and all included variables are highly significant, both statistically and in their marginal effect on payments.

TABLE 8–1
Mean Time and Complexity Estimates for Various Medical Procedures and Services

Procedure or Service	Time (in minutes)				Standardized complexity[a]
	Procedure	Preoperative	Postoperative	Total	
Modified radical mastectomy	109	64	183	356	5.29
Total hip replacement	127	42	208	377	4.78
Operative laryngoscopy with biopsy	35	—	—	35	1.24
Permanent pacemaker insertion; ventricular	68	52	119	239	2.03
Aortic valve replacement	201	56	278	535	5.26
Coronary artery bypass; three grafts	221	63	272	556	5.10
Proctosigmoidoscopy	20	—	—	20	1.31
Cystourethroscopy with small bladder tumor resection	38	—	—	38	1.94
Transurethral resection of prostate (TURP)	68	43	159	270	3.32
Dilation and curettage (D&C)	20	—	—	20	1.42
One-stage lens procedure	56	32	144	232	6.87
Chest X-ray, two views; interpretation and report	5	—	—	5	1.00
Hip X-ray, two views; interpretation and report	5	—	—	5	0.73

Initial comprehensive office visit					
By family practitioner	41	—	—	41	2.13
By general surgeon	37	—	—	37	1.93
Follow-up intermediate office visit					
By internist	23	—	—	23	1.31
By family practitioner	19	—	—	19	1.12
Initial comprehensive hospital visit					
By internist	58	—	—	58	2.57
By general surgeon	42	—	—	42	2.18
Follow-up hospital visit					
By internist	21	—	—	21	1.48
Comprehensive consultation					
By family practitioner	45	—	—	45	2.13
By dermatologist	27	—	—	27	3.00

Empty cell = not applicable.

a. Raw complexity scores have been standardized across specialties by dividing each complexity score by that specialty's score for interpretation and report of a chest X-ray. See text for details.

SOURCE: 1987 Physicians' Practice Follow-up Survey.

TABLE 8-2

REGRESSION OF TIME AND COMPLEXITY ON 1985 (LOGGED) MEDICARE
ALLOWED CHARGES

	(1)	(2)	(3)	(4)
Logarithm of procedure time	1.53[a]	.91[a]	.56[a]	.55[a]
	(.09)	(.14)	(.11)	(.08)
Logarithm of pre/post time	—	—	.34[a]	.21[a]
			(.03)	(.03)
Logarithm of complexity	—	1.04[a]	.54[a]	.49[a]
		(.19)	(.15)	(.11)
Logarithm of surgery dummy (= 1 or 2)	—	—	—	1.50[a]
				(.15)
Intercept	−.64	.79[b]	1.95[a]	1.72[a]
	(.35)	(.40)	(.32)	(.24)
R^2 Adjusted	.66	.72	.85	.91
F	268[a]	179[a]	260[a]	362[a]

NOTE: Standard errors appear in parentheses. Coefficients for time and complexity can be interpreted as the percentage increase in charges associated with a 1 percent increase in time or complexity. Coefficients of the surgical dummy and the intercept can be evaluated as exponents of 2 or the base of the natural log, e, respectively. In equation (4), for example, a surgical procedure is $2^{1.50} = 2.8$ times more expensive than a medical service. The intercept coefficient in equation (4) implies that a medical service of complexity $= 1$ involving 1 minute of procedure and pre/post time would cost $e^{1.72} = \$5.58$.
a. $P \leq .01$.
b. $P \leq .05$.
SOURCE: 1987 Physicians' Practice Follow-up Survey.

This confirms the hypothesis that physician fees in general are strongly related to reported time and complexity.

When Medicare-allowed charges are regressed on procedure time alone, the time coefficient is almost twice as large as that obtained when complexity is controlled for. A doubling of procedure time results in a 153 percent increase in fees versus 91 percent after adjusting for complexity (columns 1 and 2). Complexity and time are positively correlated, which explains the significant drop in the procedure time coefficient once complexity is entered into the equation. Hence, longer procedures are paid more, in part because they are also more complex. The explanatory power of the model is also substantially increased by adding the average complexity score.

The statistical significance of the complexity coefficient is particularly noteworthy given the use of a single procedure (chest X-ray interpretation) as a cross-specialty link. If *true* relative ratings of X-ray complexity varied widely by specialty, the pooled complexity variable that assumes them all to be equal would contain too much "noise" to be statistically significant. Our results support the use of physician-reported complexity ratings in adjusting procedure times for work intensity, as well as the use of a single service as a numeraire, at least as a good first approximation.

When pre and post times are added to the model (columns 3 and 4), we obtain a statistically significant coefficient (p < .01) that is substantially smaller than the coefficient for procedure time. A pre/post time elasticity of 0.34 implies 3.4 percent higher fees for every 10 percent increase in such time, other things being equal. This effect is reduced to 0.21 once surgery is held constant, but it is still significant. Although substantial, the effect of pre/post times on fees is considerably less than that of the surgical time itself. This finding has two significant policy implications. First, it demonstrates the importance of measuring pre- and postoperative times for surgical procedures. Second, it suggests that patients and physicians differ in the values they assign to actual operating room and follow-up times, and that they also differ among themselves in this regard.

By accounting separately for pre- and postoperative time, we also substantially reduce the marginal effect of complexity on allowed fees. More complex procedures often require more pre- and postoperative time as well. If such time is included in the predictions, we need not weight complexity ratings nearly as heavily.

The surgical dummy enters with a positive coefficient of 1.50 and is highly significant, both statistically and in absolute impact. For surgical procedures, the multiplicative shift effect = $(2)^{1.5}$ = 2.8, implying that, other things being equal, surgical procedures are 2.8 times more expensive than nonsurgical procedures. Note, too, the improvement in R^2, from .85 to .91. The complexity coefficient falls slightly, reflecting a positive correlation between complexity and surgery, although surgical procedures are clearly being paid a premium over and above the time and complexity differences.

The pre/post time coefficient falls by nearly 50 percent. Controlling for surgery purges it of any extra premiums associated with surgery so that it now reflects more of a pure time elasticity. Such a large fall in the pre/post elasticity also warns against overvaluing pre/post time, as would be the case if the .34 coefficient was used. Indeed, as shown in the next section, predicted fees will be higher for some surgical procedures (that is, where no explicit surgical adjustment has been made). This happens precisely because these

211

procedures involve lengthy pre- and postoperative follow-up, which is valued much higher if surgery is not controlled for. A more complete analysis (col. 4) would allow a standard, across-the-board markup for surgery, but would greatly reduce the value of pre/post time. How much of the surgical markup itself is legitimate is still debatable, of course. If it was all the result of a surgical insurance bias, then the markup should have to be excluded from predicted payments.

Predicted Medicare Payments. Table 8–3 compares actual 1985 Medicare-allowed charges for physicians with predicted payments based on time and complexity alone (column 2). In column 3, this base is expanded to include the surgical adjustment. The 95 percent confidence limits are shown beneath each predicted payment. (The predicted payments do not lie precisely between the upper and lower confidence limits because of the log-normal distribution of the charge data.) Actual payments that are substantially above the predicted payment imply that this service or procedure is "overpaid" relative to the physician effort involved, particularly if it is also above the upper confidence limit. Where current reimbursement levels are below predicted payments (and below the lower confidence limit), we can infer that the service or procedure is likely to be "underpaid."

With a time and complexity adjustment alone (column 2), reimbursement for office and hospital visits would double or even triple, which is consistent with the relatively high time and complexity estimates assigned to these services (see table 8–1). Consider, for example, an initial office visit to a general surgeon and a cystourethroscopy with resection of a small bladder tumor. Both are reported to be of equal complexity and to take equal amounts of time to perform, yet Medicare currently pays 8½ times more for this surgical procedure than for the visit. On the basis of the physician effort involved, however, both services would be reimbursed about the same ($95–96).

Interestingly, it is not only the two types of visits that appear "underpaid." On the basis of relative time and complexity alone, predicted payments would be higher than current rates for a modified radical mastectomy and proctosigmoidoscopy as well as for some other common operations not shown here, such as a cholecystectomy or hysterectomy.

By contrast, three of the surgical procedures appear substantially "overpaid": operative laryngoscopy, pacemaker insertion, and cystourethroscopy with bladder tumor resection (see table 8–3). All of these are relatively uncomplicated procedures and (with the exception of pacemaker insertion) take relatively little time to perform.

What impact does the inclusion of the surgical adjustment make in these predicted payments? As expected, predicted payments for nonsurgical services fall, although visits still appear "underpaid" by 40–70 percent. Although predicted payments for relatively simple invasive procedures like endoscopies increase, those for longer operating room procedures (for example, CABGs) actually decline. This occurs because the predicting equation places a relatively lower weight on the surgeon's time, especially for pre- and postoperative care, after adjusting for the 2.8 across-the-board multiplier favoring surgical fees. At the same time, the 95 percent confidence limits associated with all the predicted payments narrow considerably. The net effect is to produce three *additional* "overpaid" surgical procedures: total hip replacement, CABG surgery, and one-stage lens procedures.

Inclusion of the surgical adjustment in the predicting equation thus has the counterintuitive result of identifying more outlier surgical procedures. In view of the more precise and more reliable estimates produced by this equation (as evidenced by the narrower confidence band), however, these results may be preferred.

Comparison of Adjusted-Charge and Resource-based Relative Values. The predicted payments shown in table 8–3 can be thought of as the basis for a charge-based relative value scale in which "outlier charges" have first been increased (or reduced) to make them consistent with the physician effort involved. How do our adjusted-charge relative values compare with those of the RBRVS study? In order to make such a comparison, we first need a numeraire, or index procedure. Since the results can be very sensitive to the choice of a numeraire, we sought a procedure that was appropriately paid on the basis of *both* our methodology and that of the RBRVS study. We selected the interpretation and report of a chest X-ray (two views) for two reasons: (1) it had the advantage of being neither a surgical procedure nor a visit; and (2) its average payment of $14 (as of 1985) seemed reasonable given the physician effort involved.[15]

Table 8–4 compares adjusted-charge and resource-based relative values, using the chest X-ray interpretation and report as the index procedure in each case. Column 1 simply presents relative Medicare-allowed charges; thus (in 1985), Medicare was paying 67 times more for a modified radical mastectomy than it was for chest X-ray interpretation. Column 2 presents adjusted-charge relative values (that is, values based on the predicted payments from table 8–3, column 3).

TABLE 8–3
ACTUAL AND PREDICTED MEDICARE ALLOWED CHARGES, 1985
(dollars)

Procedure or Service	Actual Allowed Charge	Predicted Amount without Surgical Adjustment[a]	Predicted Amount with Surgical Adjustment[b]
Modified radical mastectomy	951	1,905 (1,551–2,334)	1,642 (1,404–1,920)
Total hip replacement	2,252	1,976 (1,603–2,437)	1,707 (1,456–2,002)
Operative laryngoscopy with biopsy	295	72 (60–87)	137 (112–168)
Permanent pacemaker insertion; ventricular	1,058	759 (586–984)	728 (597–888)
Aortic valve replacement	2,895	2,968 (2,315–3,806)	2,447 (2,024–2,959)
Coronary artery bypass; three grafts	3,714	3,075 (2,366–3,997)	2,537 (2,077–3,098)
Proctosigmoidoscopy	36	54 (48–62)	103 (86–124)
Cystourethroscopy with small bladder tumor resection	322	96 (84–110)	178 (148–213)
Transurethral resection of prostate (TURP)	1,038	1,067 (869–1,309)	972 (832–1,136)
Dilation and curettage (D&C)	250	220 (168–289)	249 (202–308)
One-stage lens procedure	1,546	1,359 (1,023–1,806)	1,214 (977–1,507)

Chest X-ray, two views; interpretation and report	14	21 (15–29)	15 (11–19)
Hip X-ray, two views; interpretation and report	16	18 (13–25)	13 (10–16)
Initial comprehensive office visit			
By family practitioner	39	105 (91–121)	68 (60–77)
By general surgeon	38	95 (83–109)	62 (55–70)
Follow-up intermediate office visit			
By internist	25	58 (51–67)	39 (35–44)
By family practitioner	20	48 (41–56)	33 (29–37)
Initial comprehensive hospital visit			
By internist	59	141 (118–169)	91 (78–106)
By general surgeon	51	108 (93–124)	70 (62–79)
Follow-up intermediate hospital visit			
By internist	32	59 (52–67)	46 (42–52)
Comprehensive consultation			
By family practitioner	67	111 (95–129)	72 (63–82)
By dermatologist	67	102 (83–124)	65 (55–77)

NOTE: 95 percent confidence limits in parentheses.
a. Predictions based on regression model shown in table 8–2, column 3.
b. Predictions based on regression model shown in table 8–2, column 4.
SOURCE: 1985 Part B Medicare Data, Health Care Financing Administration; authors' calculations.

TABLE 8-4

COMPARISON OF ADJUSTED-CHARGE AND RESOURCE-BASED RELATIVE VALUES

Procedure or Service	Actual Allowed Charges (1)	ACRVS (2)	ACRVS Purged of Surgical Adjustment[a] (3)	RBRVS Work effort only (4)	RBRVS Full model (5)	PPRC Fee Schedule Payments[b] (6)
Modified radical mastectomy	67.0	112.1	40.0	57.5	63.8	53.8
Total hip replacement	158.6	116.6	41.6	98.5	134.4	116.8
Operative laryngoscopy with biopsy	20.8	9.4	3.4	18.7	22.0	16.5
Permanent pacemaker insertion; ventricular	71.2	49.8	17.8	26.8	28.8	42.1
Aortic valve replacement	203.9	167.2	59.7	122.8	132.2	162.8
Coronary artery bypass; three grafts	261.5	182.4	65.1	124.1	133.6	166.4
Proctosigmoidoscopy	2.5	7.1	2.5	4.9	5.3	3.1
Cystourethroscopy with small bladder tumor resection	22.7	12.1	4.3	34.3	39.2	24.2
Transurethral resection of prostate (TURP)	73.1	66.4	23.7	57.8	66.1	54.2
Dilation and curettage (D&C)	17.6	17.0	6.1	12.5	14.1	13.7
One-stage lens procedure	108.9	82.9	29.6	65.8	73.8	68.5

Hip X-ray, two views; interpretation and report

Initial comprehensive office visit						
By family practitioner	2.8	4.6	4.6	5.5	6.1	3.6
By general surgeon	2.7	4.2	4.2	5.5	6.1	3.4
Follow-up intermediate office visit						
By internist	1.7	2.7	2.7	3.1	3.4	2.1
By family practitioner	1.4	2.2	2.2	3.1	3.5	1.9
Initial comprehensive hospital visit						
By internist	4.2	6.2	6.2	9.3	10.1	5.9
By general surgeon	3.6	4.8	4.8	9.3	10.3	5.5
Follow-up intermediate hospital visit						
By internist	1.8	2.7	2.7	3.7	4.0	2.4
Comprehensive consultation						
By family practitioner	4.8	4.9	4.9	8.9	9.9	5.7
By dermatologist	4.7	4.5	4.5	8.9	9.4	6.5

NOTE: All values have been indexed to a chest X-ray (two-view) interpretation and report.

a. Predicted payments have been divided by the exponent of the coefficient associated with the surgical dummy (2.8).

b. These represent payments simulated by PPRC (as of April 25, 1989).

SOURCE: 1987 Physicians' Practice Follow-up Survey (ACRVS); National Study of Resource-based Relative Value Scales for Physician Services (RBRVS); unpublished PPRC simulations.

Thus, if we take into account the physician effort involved, the mastectomy should be paid 112 times more than the chest X-ray interpretation.

These adjusted-charge relative values, however, are based on the regression model that included the dummy surgical adjustment, the results of which suggest that surgical procedures *as a class* are 2.8 times more expensive than medical services of equivalent time and complexity. One reason for this may be an insurance bias in favor of surgery; if so, then this surgery payment premium may be neither efficient nor equitable. Column 3 presents relative values *purged* of this adjustment, that is, by dividing the values for surgical procedures by 2.8. The resulting relative values should be viewed as an absolute lower bound, however, as there may be other legitimate explanations for the premium, such as patient willingness to pay more for surgical intervention, longer training residencies, and higher nonphysician practice costs.[16]

Columns 4 and 5 present relative values calculated from the RBRVS. The relative values in column 4 are based on work effort alone, that is, without the other two factors (practice costs and opportunity costs of training). These values may be more directly comparable with our results, since our adjusted-charge relative value scale (ACRVS) is based on time and complexity alone and does not include these other factors. Column 5 presents relative values based on the full RBRVS model: total work multiplied by the practice cost and opportunity cost indices.

In column 6, relative values are calculated from the simulated fee schedule payments developed by the Physician Payment Review Commission (PPRC). These payments are based on the Hsiao estimates of work effort with an "additive" approach to specialty-specific practice costs (unlike the multiplicative approach used in the RBRVS).

In columns 2 and 4, we see that the RBRVS values of work effort only are consistently lower for surgical procedures and higher for visits and consultations, in comparison with our adjusted-charge values.[17] Whereas our ACRVS results suggest that total hip replacement should be paid 117 times more than chest X-ray interpretation, for example, the RBRVS results imply a differential of "only" ninety-nine to one. Similarly, whereas regression-based relative values suggest a follow-up hospital visit differential of 2.7, RBRVS values would reward that visit considerably more: 3.7 times higher than a chest X-ray interpretation.

How can we explain these differences between the two scales? Probably the main reason is the failure of the RBRVS to include postoperative time following discharge from the hospital. Surgeons consistently report spending considerable amounts of time providing follow-up care in their offices, and our regressions confirmed that pre/postoperative time is an important predictor of relative fee levels. By understating the "true" amount of work associated with operating room procedures, the RBRVS will bias values for surgery downward, particularly for operations that have long follow-up times relative to the procedure time itself, such as lens procedures. (Predicted payments based on regressions *without* pre- and postoperative time would be substantially lower for such operations than the payments shown in table 8-3, for example.) Furthermore, because of the way in which the cross-specialty linkage was performed in the RBRVS study, values for nonsurgical services will automatically be inflated.[18]

The effect of the full-model RBRVS is to increase the relative values for virtually all of the services shown in table 8–4. This happens because (1) the combined multiplier for the numeraire procedure is only 0.90 (the product of the practice cost and opportunity cost indices for radiologists); and (2) the multiplier for the nonradiology services ranges from 0.95 to 1.23, depending on specialty. The relative values for surgical procedures in the full-model RBRVS begin to approximate those in table 8–4, column 2, but in general remain lower. In the case of visits and consultations, however, the full model widens the difference between the RBRVS relative values and those of our study.

In general, the relative values of the PPRC fee schedule resemble those of the RBRVS based on work effort only. There are some exceptions, however. Notably, relative payments for the three cardiovascular procedures (pacemaker insertion, valve replacement, and bypass surgery) are more similar to those implied by the ACRVS.

Discussion

Our results suggest that there is some validity to the current relative fee structure. The variation in Medicare reimbursement can be explained in large part by the physician effort associated with providing different services. That is, the fact that surgeons are paid more for hip replacements than for TURPs, and more for both of these surgeries than for visits, can be justified by the longer times and greater complexity of the former in each case.

Nevertheless, charges for some services do appear distorted relative to others. Like the RBRVS study, our work shows that surgical procedures are relatively overpaid and visits underpaid. This is consistent with the widely held view that more generous insurance coverage for surgery has increased the demand for surgical services.

219

The two studies differ, however, in their estimate of the *magnitude* of the distortions. The RBRVS study implies that surgical reimbursement needs to be reduced greatly (by as much as 50 percent in the case of bypass graft operations) and that visit payments need to be doubled. Simulations performed by many researchers have shown that the resulting redistributions of Medicare revenues across specialties would be so profound that they might affect access to care.[19]

In contrast, changes introduced by our ACRVS would be more modest, and consequently more acceptable to physicians and beneficiaries alike. The predicted payments in table 8–3 imply "only" a 32 percent reduction in bypass surgery, for example. Rather than adopting an entirely new price list, policy makers could use the existing charge structure to make gradual changes in reimbursement for those services and procedures that are most egregiously mispriced. How might this be done? One way would be to calculate adjusted-charge relative values like those shown in column 2 of table 8–4. The problem, of course, is that these values include the full effect of the surgery dummy. To the extent that this dummy is capturing historic insurance bias, the values will be overstated for surgical procedures. If so, then policy makers might want to make across-the-board rollbacks in surgical payments *before* calculating the relative values.

If we attribute the entire surgery shift effect to insurance bias, on the other hand, the result is a draconian reduction in reimbursement (see table 8–4, column 3). Some amount of this surgery premium is undoubtedly due to other factors as well, such as patient preferences and greater training and practice costs.

We would propose a more modest across-the-board reduction in surgical payments—say, 10 percent—followed by construction of the adjusted-charge relative value scale. This would result in higher payments for visits and reductions for some surgical procedures. The actual size of those changes will depend on the conversion factor chosen: whether or not it is budget-neutral, for example, or whether it takes into account any factors not captured by the relative values themselves, such as geographic differences in practice costs.

How society (that is, Congress) defines the appropriate conversion factor will ultimately depend on its perception of a fair income, given the high costs of training physicians. Whatever relative value scale is chosen, the conversion factor will be difficult to calculate as policy makers will want to control Medicare spending and yet still ensure access to physician services.

9
The Resource-based Relative Value Scale for Pricing Physicians' Services

William C. Hsiao and Daniel L. Dunn

Numerous flaws have been found in the present system for compensating physicians, which is based on customary, prevailing, and reasonable charges (CPR). Some experts say that it is inflationary and administratively complex and that it distorts fees and institutionalizes inequities in physicians' charges.[1] The independent Physician Payment Review Commission appointed by Congress has concluded that the CPR method creates "patterns of allowed charges that embody inappropriate incentives for the use of medical services, as well as for physicians' decisions on where to locate and what to specialize in."[2] Physicians themselves think that the payment method is irrational and unfair, and that it encourages abuse.[3] Indeed, the consensus seems to be that the current payment system based on physicians' charges should be completely reformed. We describe an alternative approach to pricing physicians' services.

Conceptual and Theoretical Issues

How should the prices of physicians' services be determined? Economic theory posits that the optimal price for a service (without considering equity and social benefits) is determined in a competitive market. The problem is, the market for physicians' services does not meet the necessary and sufficient conditions for a reasonably competitive market.

On the demand side, for example, consumers have limited

This research was supported in part by the Office of Research and Demonstrations, Health Care Financing Administration (HCFA), under a cooperative agreement (17-C-98795/1-03). The opinions expressed are those of the authors and not necessarily of the HCFA.

221

knowledge on which to base their choice of physicians' services. Consumers are uninformed about the prices of physicians' services relative to other goods, and would find it costly and awkward to obtain the necessary price and quality information. Furthermore, they are incapable of assessing their own medical needs. Consumer ignorance and the asymmetry of information between the patient and the physician weaken consumer sovereignty and lead to a client-agent relationship. A physician is unlikely to be a perfect agent for the patient, however, being both an adviser and a supplier of services whose own economic interest is directly affected by the advice he or she gives.

The special nature of medical care also affects demand for some physician services. When patients are in pain or severe distress (for example, during medical emergencies or because of serious diseases of the heart, brain, and eyes), their demand for medical care is not fully voluntary and rational. Nor do they have the time and presence of mind to search for the lowest price.

As a result, physicians operate autonomously, subject to few of the checks and balances that competitive forces generate. Physicians themselves have long acknowledged their discretionary power to determine the quantity of services they provide, which is not necessarily identical to patients' demand.[4]

On the supply side, there are constraints on the provision of medical services by nonphysician medical professionals and barriers to entry into medicine. Although limits on medical school admissions and licensing requirements protect patients from unqualified providers, they also grant monopoly power to the medical profession.

In addition, health insurance distorts patient demand for medical care and lessens providers' sensitivity to the prices they charge. Third parties now pay approximately 75 percent of the total expenditures for physician services. Also important is the fact that insurance coverage varies across types of service: office visits, hospital visits, surgery, and tests. Third-party payers have traditionally covered a larger portion of physicians' inpatient hospital services than outpatient care. This uneven insurance coverage creates uneven distortions in demand.

The extent of these market failures and the resulting monopolistic power of physicians are illustrated by the widespread practice of price discrimination.[5] Although this practice has been reduced somewhat with the expansion of health insurance coverage, it still persists, as illustrated by the experience with physician assignment under Medicare and the recent proposal by the American College of Surgeons to balance-bill high-income patients.[6]

Prices for physician services are not consistent with those that would exist in a competitive market. Because consumers differ in their sensitivity to prices, some services are priced much higher than others, relative to their cost or value. Most physicians provide several types of services and their elasticity of demand varies.[7] Physicians can raise prices more sharply on those services that are less price elastic. Variations in health insurance coverage by type of service contribute further to the distortion in relative prices. Historically, surgical and inpatient physician services were insured whereas ambulatory services were not. As a result, prevailing prices are distorted unevenly by the imperfect market and offer inappropriate economic incentives to physicians. In turn, there can be adverse side effects in the consumption of complementary goods (notably hospital services), total health expenditures, efficiency, and health outcomes.

Policy makers and third-party payers throughout the world are investigating alternative methods of payment in their search for a rational and systematic payment scheme. One possibility is the negotiated-price approach used in Canada, Japan, and West Germany, which relies on political process to set prices. Another would be to base prices on the resource-input cost of providing a given service, as is done in the United States to establish prices in spheres where the market fails, such as public utilities. It is unfeasible, however, for pricing physicians' services; the existing measures of the production costs of such services in settings where physicians are salaried, such as HMOs, are still largely determined by physicians' earnings in the fee-for-service sector, which embody the distorted prices in the current system.

Our approach to physician payment has been to find a second-best alternative, the resource-based relative value scale (RBRVS). The theoretical concept behind the RBRVS is simple: In a competitive market, the long-run equilibrium price of a good should approximate the long-run average cost of its production. (We assume that the long-run marginal cost approximately equals the long-run average cost.) The RBRVS we have developed is a method of approximating the *average relative costs* required to produce a range of physicians' services.

Methodology of the Study

The purpose of our study was to investigate the resource-input costs of physicians' services and to develop methods to measure them. We began by systematically examining the factors that physicians identify as constituting their work input and other resource costs. We then developed methods to measure these components of resource costs. We accomplished these tasks. We needed the expert knowledge from economics, measurement psychology, clinical medicine, statistics, and survey research. A detailed description of our methods, data, and results has been published elsewhere.[8] Thus in this section we limit ourselves to a brief overview of our approach.

A Resource-Cost Model of Physician Services. To measure resource costs, we developed a model that postulates three basic inputs to physicians' services: (1) the total work of the service, encompassing the *time* involved and the *intensity* with which that time is spent; (2) *practice costs*; and (3) the *opportunity cost* of physician training.

These three factors determine the resource-based relative value of a given medical service:

$$RBRV_{is} = (TW_i)(1 + RPC_s)(1 + AST_s)$$

where TW = total work input by the physician. Total work includes the physician's work expended before, during, and after the service itself. Physician's work encompasses (1) the physician's time, (2) mental effort and judgment, (3) technical skill, (4) physical effort, and (5) stress due to risk. RPC = an index of relative specialty practice costs and AST = an index of amortized value for the opportunity cost of specialized training (the income forgone when physicians pursue additional years of specialty training, rather than entering practice), where i indexes services and s specialties. We measured work service by service; we measured practice costs and opportunity costs on a specialty-specific basis.

The Consultative Component. Because this study called for a variety of information, particularly from the medical field, a critical part of the work consisted of consulting with practicing physicians.[9] We organized fourteen advisory committees of physicians and also sub-contracted for support and assistance from the American Medical Association (AMA). The investigators, however, were solely responsible for the design, conduct, and intellectual basis of the study. The technical and consultative activities were undertaken as parallel and closely related tasks.

We obtained guidance on current medical practice from 100 physicians organized into fourteen technical consulting groups (TCGs). These physicians were nominated by more than thirty societies representing various specialties in a process coordinated by the AMA. We asked for three nominees for each position on the TCGs and selected from each specialty highly respected physicians in academic and community-based practices throughout the country. It was understood that their participation implied no endorsement of the study or its results.

The TCG physicians were our main source of substantive information on medical practice in the specialties, the most important services and procedures, and the typical complexity of patients seen. They also helped define physicians' work and its components, commented on methods of measurement and their validation, and evaluated the reasonableness of the results.

In addition, we took the step, unusual for a research project, of conducting a national consultative conference, in March 1988, at which individuals representing many interests—medicine, government, health services research, third-party payers, consumers, business, and unions—critically reviewed the work of the study while it was still in progress. Their comments helped us further refine our work.

The Technical Component. Because the resource costs of physician services have multiple components, many steps were involved in developing the RBRVS, most important of which was to measure the relative work that physicians invest in the services they perform. We partitioned this work into pre-, intra-, and postservice phases and obtained measures of the work involved in each phase for selected services from different specialties.

The measurement of physicians' work. In seeking to measure physicians' work, we confronted two vexing methodological problems. First, no established method existed for measuring resource inputs for physicians' services. Previous efforts had focused on two methods and encountered serious difficulties in both cases.[10] In one study, physicians were asked to rate each service with an open numeric scale. In the second study, physicians were asked to rate each service with a closed numeric scale. Both studies produced consistent ordinal rankings of the work required in performing services, but not reasonable cardinal measurements of work. In the previous studies, little attention was given to the fact that physicians perform a great variety of services, ranging from counseling patients to transplanting organs.

We first looked at the concept of physicians' work input. In the previous studies mentioned above, work was said to consist of two distinct but not mutually exclusive factors: time and intensity. We found intensity too vague a concept to define and measure and therefore asked physicians to define the components of their work. From interviews with them and pilot studies of the measurement of

225

work we postulated that the dimensions of physicians' work are (1) time, (2) mental effort and judgment, (3) technical skill and physical effort, and (4) stress due to risk.

We next explored methods of measuring physicians' work and its dimensions. Because work, mental effort, technical skill, and stress are almost impossible to measure objectively, we relied on the subjective judgments of the physicians who perform given services. After consulting with psychologists, statisticians, and economists and testing several approaches, we decided that magnitude estimation was the most reliable and valid method of obtaining subjective assessments of work and its dimensions. Unlike the open or closed numerical scales of previous studies, which yield unreasonable results, magnitude estimation rates a service in relation to a reference service, using a ratio scale rather than a cardinal or ordinal scale. Respondents can rate a service high or low as they believe necessary to reflect reality. Magnitude estimation has been used before to measure subjective perceptions and judgments, with reliable, reproducible, and valid results.[11]

In the field of general surgery, for example, we chose uncomplicated inguinal hernia repair as the reference service and assigned a value of 100 to the work it required. A surgeon who judged the work performed in a lower anterior resection for rectal carcinoma to be 4½ times that of an uncomplicated inguinal hernia repair responded with a rating of 450.

To measure work, we next developed vignettes of physicians' services and then mapped these vignettes into the *Physicians' Current Procedural Terminology*, 4th edition, familiarly known as the CPT-4,[12] which classifies physicians' services for purposes of billing. The vignettes were worded to represent the work of the typical service in a given CPT-4 code. The CPT-4 identifies more than 7,000 distinct services and procedures. Although the work of a given specialty may encompass several hundred of these codes, a far smaller number typically accounts for the bulk of its workload. We selected approximately 23 services in each of 18 specialties for in-depth study.

We then conducted a national survey of a random sample of 3,200 physicians to obtain ratings of the work in various services described in the vignettes. In accordance with the magnitude estimation method, we asked the respondents to rate the work of a service relative to a reference service. The scale was open-ended; respondents could rate each service as high or low as they believed necessary to reflect reality. For each specialty, we selected a widely performed reference service, appropriately located on the scale of work, in which work was likely to vary little from physician to physician. We also obtained measures of time and ratings of the dimensions of intensity (mental effort and judgment, technical skill and physical effort, and stress due to risk).

We then used the survey results to estimate the related work performed before and after a given service. The intraservice phase is the period during the service itself, such as an office visit, operation, or consultation. In addition, physicians spend significant time on various activities before and after a given service, such as reviewing records, communicating with other professionals and relatives of the patient, and visiting surgical patients in the hospital. Needless to say, these activities vary with the type of service and the setting in which it is rendered. We constructed a typology of pre- and postservice work and then used the survey data to estimate pre- and postservice times; appropriate rates of work per minute were systematically assigned, and the product of the two was calculated to estimate work. We summed the work before, during, and after the service to derive total service work.

Cross-specialty linkage of the RBRVS. Since each specialty rated work using a different reference standard, we next faced the task of linking the relative-value scales of different specialties. The key was to identify pairs of services from different specialties that require equal amounts of work. A cross-specialty panel of physicians first identified services that are performed more or less identically in different specialties. We termed these "same" services. They then identified pairs of nonidentical services performed by different specialties that they considered "equivalent" in work. We thus developed a grid of linked services across specialties, with at least four identical or equivalent services connecting one specialty to another. The entire network consisted of eighty-two links. Of these, forty-two were "same" services and forty were "equivalent." We then used a weighted least-squares method to standardize ratings of work across specialties.

Extrapolation. To keep the project feasible, we surveyed the work of only a few services in each specialty and extrapolated their work values to a much larger group of services. To do so, we identified small homogeneous families of services and assumed that charges represent reasonable indicators of relative work within such families. For instance, the cholecystectomy family has six closely related procedures: cholecystectomy, cholecystectomy with cholangiography, cholecystectomy with exploration of common duct, and so on. We assumed that, within such families, health insurance and other imperfections of the market have acted similarly on all the member

227

services. If so, charges for individual services within each family should represent reasonable surrogates for the total work each involves.[13]

From each family, we selected a benchmark service for which a total work value was available in the national survey. After calculating ratios of charges between the benchmark service and nonsurveyed services in the same family, we extrapolated work values by multiplying that of the benchmark service by these charge-based ratios for the nonsurveyed services.

Practice costs. Physicians' practice costs consist primarily of employee wages and fringe benefits, professional liability insurance, office rental, equipment, and supplies. The best source of information on specialty-specific practice costs is the 1983 survey of physicians' practice costs conducted by the National Opinion Research Center.[14] We updated the 1983 survey data with 1986 professional liability-insurance premiums. We then calculated these practice costs as percentages of the gross revenues of each specialty and apportioned them among the specialty's services on the basis of total work input required by each.

Opportunity costs of residency training. The length of time a physician spends in residency training varies by specialty, customarily ranging from one year for a general practitioner to seven years for a neurosurgeon or thoracic surgeon. Each additional year of specialty training imposes further economic costs on the physician. The opportunity cost of a year of training can be approximated as the difference between a resident's salary and the income the resident could earn in practice. We obtained data with which to calculate the opportunity costs of training from specialty boards[15] and from the AMA.[16] After calculating the specialty-specific opportunity cost of each year of residency and summing the total cost, we amortized the total over the average remaining working lifetime in each specialty.

A National Survey of Physicians' Work

To gather ratings of work and its dimensions from a large sample of physicians, we designed a straightforward survey instrument that could be administered over the telephone. The questionnaire was carefully pilot-tested to eliminate any misunderstandings that could bias the survey.

A stratified random sample of physicians was then selected from the AMA's 1986 Physician Masterfile, which lists every known physician in the United States, including nonmembers of the AMA. We stratified the sample geographically into ten regions by the national percentage of board-certified physicians in each specialty, and by specialty-specific proportions in each region.[17] Physicians who worked in patient care fewer than twenty hours a week were excluded, as were those in residency training or over age sixty-five, and those who lacked a current address in the AMA Physician Masterfile.

After a successful pilot test on four representative specialties— anesthesiology, general surgery, internal medicine, and radiology— the survey instrument was administered to a national sample by a professional survey firm.

We surveyed 3,164 physicians, 1,977 of whom completed interviews, for an overall response rate of 62.5 percent. Response rates ranged from a high of 69 percent for radiology to a low of 56 percent for obstetrics and gynecology. To ascertain whether the quantitative measurement of work obtained from the survey was reliable and valid, we performed statistical analyses on the data collected from the pilot study and the national survey.

Technical Findings

Our investigation of physicians' work led to three important technical findings. First, physicians' work can be defined by a systematic and rational approach, and measured by the magnitude-estimation method. Second, the relative work input for physicians' services can be defined and reliably estimated. Third, physicians' work consists of four dimensions: time, mental effort and judgment, technical skill and physical effort, and stress due to risk, and measurements of these dimensions are highly consistent with measurements of work.

In every specialty, the mean ratings of work were reproducible and highly reliable. The majority of the standard errors ranged from 4.0 to 8.0, as a percentage of the mean. To evaluate the reliability of the ratings of work more thoroughly, we used the intraclass-correlation method.[18] This method indicated the degree to which two physicians in the same specialty agree on their ratings of various services. The results appear in table 9–1, column 2. All the correlations are above 0.5; the majority are above 0.7. Although there is no universal standard specifying what value of intraclass correlation reflects reliable subjective judgments, it is commonly agreed that values above 0.6 are very good and those over 0.7 are excellent.

Although the intraclass correlation is customarily reported for reliability tests, it is less meaningful for our present purpose than the reliability measure shown in table 9–1 under "Mean of Sample of Physicians." This measurement, obtained from the intraclass corre-

TABLE 9–1

RELIABILITY OF RATINGS OF INTRASERVICE WORK BY SPECIALTY

Specialty	Number of Physicians in Sample	Reliability	
		Individual physician	Mean of sample of physicians
Rheumatology	119	0.810	0.998
Orthopedics	107	0.802	0.998
Otolaryngology	105	0.797	0.998
Oral and maxillofacial surgery	117	0.795	0.997
Thoracic and cardiovascular surgery	96	0.790	0.997
Radiology	117	0.784	0.998
Urology	115	0.778	0.998
Ophthalmology	98	0.776	0.997
Anesthesiology	117	0.720	0.997
General surgery	103	0.717	0.996
Internal medicine	101	0.713	0.996
Family practice	110	0.698	0.996
Pediatrics	103	0.674	0.995
Obstetrics and gynecology	89	0.651	0.994
Pathology	115	0.632	0.995
Allergy and immunology	112	0.626	0.995
Dermatology	106	0.522	0.991
Psychiatry	100	0.522	0.991

SOURCE: W. C. Hsiao, P. Brown, E. R. Becker, et al., *A National Study of Resource Based Relative Value Scales for Physician Services: Final Report to the Health Care Financing Administration*, publication 18-C-98795/1-03 (Boston: Harvard School of Public Health, September 1988).

lation by the Spearman-Brown predictor formula, predicts the coefficient of correlation between two sets of means of the ratings of work, had we drawn from the population of all specialists two samples of the size we actually obtained.[19] These coefficients, which range from 0.991 to 0.998, predict that the mean values for each service would be very close to each other. When different groups of experts agree this closely, it is likely that their judgments reflect reality.

It is possible, however, for two groups of experts to agree and both be wrong. We thus evaluated whether the ratings of work could be predicted from the ratings of the component dimensions of work—in order to test consistency between the whole and its parts. Separate predictions were made for each specialty, using the mean ratings of

TABLE 9–2
MULTIPLE LINEAR REGRESSIONS WITH ESTIMATED POPULATION MEAN
RATING OF WORK AS THE DEPENDENT VARIABLE

| Specialty | Residual | | | |
	Sum of squares	Degrees of freedom	Mean square	R-squared
Medical				
Allergy and immunology	.01352	13	.00104	.991
Dermatology	.03846	16	.00240	.964
Family practice	.02053	20	.00103	.993
Internal medicine	.02274	19	.00120	.988
Pediatrics	.02000	16	.00125	.988
Psychiatry	.01055	19	.00056	.989
Rheumatology	.00504	13	.00039	.999
Surgical				
General surgery	.02126	20	.00106	.996
Obstetrics and gynecology	.03727	21	.00177	.986
Ophthalmology	.01233	16	.00077	.998
Oral and maxillofacial surgery	.03691	18	.00205	.994
Orthopedic surgery	.01858	16	.00116	.997
Otolaryngology	.03813	16	.00238	.994
Thoracic and cardiovascular surgery	.01242	16	.00078	.998
Urology	.03244	16	.00203	.994
Other				
Anesthesiology	.00951	17	.00056	.993
Pathology	.00946	12	.00079	.994
Radiology	.02449	16	.00153	.993

SOURCE: See table 9–1.

work and the mean values of the respective dimensions; the regression results appear in table 9–2. The multiple correlation coefficients (R^2) for each specialty are very high for data obtained from a cross section of physicians. That is, the mean of the ratings of work can be predicted from, and are therefore consistent with, the means of the ratings of the components of work. This high a degree of consistency constitutes statistical evidence that the ratings of work are probably valid.

External objective information further validated the judgment of the physicians in our survey. We compared the data on duration of surgeries obtained from our national survey (data based on physician recall) with 1986 operating room log times from eight hospitals in two regions of the United States; the times proved very similar.[20]

There is no objective standard with which to compare our results to ascertain how well they represent reality. Thus we relied on the next-best alternative: We subjected the results to reviews for reasonableness by practicing physicians to see whether the results have face validity. For this purpose, our technical consulting groups reviewed the survey's ratings of work and its dimensions. By and large, they found the ratings to conform to the reality they had experienced in clinical practice. The TCG physicians' review, and the results of formal statistical analysis, led us to conclude that, in general, the ratings of work are reliable, consistent, and valid.

We also found that a common scale of work can be developed to measure interspecialty relative values. The weighted least-square procedure produced a "best" fitted work value for each pair of linked services, that is, the value that exhibits the least deviation between the actual and fitted values. In computing approximate confidence limits for the deviations, we found that, at the 90 percent confidence level, the fitted mean values differed from the actual mean values by less than 7 percent; this result suggests that the services we selected are good links between specialties. Further, a jackknife analysis of the regression residual sum of squares and other sensitivity analyses suggests that our choice of links did not have much effect on the process of alignment.[21] The common scale is statistically robust.

We also found it feasible to develop an RBRVS for most services and procedures, without having to study each of the 7,000 CPT-4 codes, by extrapolating the RBRVs of services studied in depth to those not studied. For most invasive, imaging, and laboratory services, our extrapolation method produces results judged by practicing physicians as reasonable and valid. For evaluation and management services, however, our method of extrapolation within families of services is probably not the best approach, because the CPT-4 descriptions of this category of services are not exact.

Substantive Findings

We found that current physician charges are not closely related to resource costs. For most evaluation and management services, ratios of current Medicare charges to RBRVs range from 0.2 to 0.5. For most hospital-based invasive services, this ratio is more than 1.0. The typical ratio for services performed by radiologists is about 1.0. In other words, relative to resource cost, evaluation and management services are compensated at a lower rate than invasive, imaging, and laboratory services. Roughly speaking, evaluation and management services are currently compensated at less than half the rate of invasive services. This finding holds true whether evaluation and management services are performed by surgeons, internists, or family practitioners.

We also found wide variation in charges-to-RBRVs ratios within categories of services, whether evaluation/management or invasive services, although it was greater among the latter. Evaluation and management services performed in hospitals, for example, are compensated at a higher rate than the same services performed in office settings. This phenomenon may be attributable to the more thorough insurance coverage of hospital-based services. But the variation within service categories also suggests that, within the same specialty, individual physicians might be differently affected by an RBRVS-based fee schedule, depending on the mix of services they perform.

We found only small differences in mean work per minute (an implicit measurement of intensity) within evaluation and management services. Furthermore, when we partition evaluation and management services by setting (hospital, office, nursing home, telephone), the differences in work per minute become minimal. Physicians' work for these services varies closely with the time spent on a patient.

Work per minute for invasive services varies greatly—from 1.9 to 19.4. For other categories of services, such variations are much narrower, ranging from 2.0 to 5.0. Moreover, average work per minute is much lower for evaluation and management than for invasive procedures; in fact, it averages less than half that of invasive services.

Pre- and postservice work appears to represent a significant fraction of physicians' total work. Although physicians are well aware that much of their time and effort are spent before and after performing a given service for a patient, there has heretofore been no systematic study of pre- and postservice work. We found pre- and postservice work to represent close to 50 percent of the total work of typical invasive services, and 33 percent of typical evaluation and management.

Impact

Current physician charges do not reflect resource costs. For office and hospital visits, the Medicare program is currently paying $25–45 for each 100 units of resource cost. For most hospital-based invasive services, this rate exceeds $100 for each 100 units. The important policy implication of this finding is that physicians are paid very generously for some services, but not for others; the economic playing field for physicians is not level. The more generous payment rates for surgery and other services, such as tests, provide incentives for greater and inappropriate utilization.

If Congress replaces the current payment system with an RBRVS-based fee schedule, there could be significant increases in fees for some office, hospital, nursing home, and consultation medical services, while some surgical fees could decrease by 10 to 35 percent. These changes in fees would affect physicians' Medicare revenues. To evaluate the potential impact on specialty earnings, we simulated an RBRVS-based Medicare fee schedule. For this analysis, we assumed that total Medicare physician payments would remain fixed ("budget-neutral") and that the RBRVS affects only the component of the fee that reflects the physicians' work (net income), but not the portion covering practice cost. The results show that the gross revenues for the typical physician in most specialties will not be affected greatly. Yet, for six specialties, revenues from Medicare could increase or decrease up to 30 percent.

Limitations of the Resource-based Relative Value Scale

The RBRVS has its limitations. For one thing, it does not take into account the quality of services. At present, it is simply not feasible to differentiate the quality of the 500,000 physicians practicing in the United States. When accurate physician-specific information does become available, however, the RBRVS could incorporate a quality index. Years of experience and certification by specialty boards have both been suggested as crude proxies for quality.

Furthermore, the RBRVS measures only resource inputs; the benefits of services are not considered. The status of current knowledge and data makes it unfeasible to incorporate benefits systematically into any relative value. Nonetheless, a rational payment system should recognize social benefits.

Nor does the RBRVS take into account patients' demand for services. In a reasonably competitive market, fees for physicians' services would approximate the resource costs required to produce them, but services for which the costs exceeded patients' willingness to pay would not be in demand by patients. Although RBRVs may reasonably represent the relative costs of different services, it is conceivable that RBRVS-based rates for some services could exceed patients' valuation of them. This problem must be solved if the RBRVS is put into practice.

Unresolved Methodological Issues

Several important methodological questions need to be resolved before the RBRVS is incorporated into payment policy. It will take considerable time and research effort to address them adequately.

First, our study relies on the CPT-4 system to classify physicians' services. Some of the limitations of that system directly affect the RBRVS. For example, we found considerable ambiguity in the CPT-4 codes for evaluation and management services; different specialties seem to use the same code to describe and bill for very different services. This shortcoming is so severe that we adopted an alternative approach to extrapolation in this category, using service time rather than charges.

Second, surgeons often charge global bills for a package of services, which includes initial examination, postoperative services in the hospital, and office visits after hospital discharge. The services encompassed by such global bills vary greatly among surgeons, however. They are not specified by the CPT-4 coding system. Until the package of services is well-defined and used by physicians, it will be impossible to generate accurate RBRVs for services that are billed globally.

Third, our current formulation of the RBRVS allocates specialty-practice and opportunity costs to each service performed by a given specialty in accordance with the work input that service requires. But because overhead costs and the costs of specialized training do not necessarily vary with the amount of work, this method of allocation may not be ideal.

The practice costs incorporated in the RBRVS incorporate only interspecialty differences; interservice and regional variations in practice costs within a specialty are not considered. For example, the practice costs of office-based and hospital-based services could differ; some services may require greater-than-average amounts of equipment or material costs. Moreover, professional liability insurance premiums, rent, and wages can differ greatly between regions. The monetary conversion factor is probably the most suitable vehicle for taking into account these differences in practice costs.

Summary

The current physician payment system is widely criticized for retaining historically distorted fees. Distorted fees, in turn, present perverse incentives to physicians and may encourage the provision of inappropriate services and more rapid inflation in health care costs. The RBRVS offers a feasible, systematic, and rational alternative that is based on resource costs, most notably physicians' work input. By removing the perverse incentives, the RBRVS could enhance cost-effective medical care and ameliorate the physician shortage in some primary care specialties.

A Physician and Market Perspective on the Hsiao Proposal

A Commentary by Joel Ira Franck

William Hsiao's proposal for a national resource-based relative value scale for physician reimbursement is a vivid example of attempting to exchange one form of failed government policy for another. In response to the debacle of massive government intervention in the medical marketplace over the past twenty-five years, Dr. Hsiao has condemned the possibility of a free market in medicine and proposed a radical scheme that may lead to total price control and governmental resource allocation of physician services in the United States.

The foundation of my critique is that if the basic principles and methodology underlying a study that purports to be "scientific" are erroneous, then the so-called statistical reliability of the study is irrelevant.

Hsiao's conceptions of the competitive ideals and realities of the medical marketplace are wrong. I know because I work in it everyday. Although this marketplace is highly regulated, physicians still face tremendous competitive pressures that should be encouraged, rather than stifled by further regulation.

Medical consumers are not ignorant. The dissemination of medical knowledge in the popular media is enormous. I am often questioned on the most technical of points by my patients. Incentives preventing a physician from performing unnecessary and costly procedures include pressure from referring physicians, second opinions, hospital complication review committees, regional peer review organizations, and finally, the specter of a malpractice suit. A damaged reputation can be a disaster for a practice.

For nonassigned Medicare claims, all copay claims, and even a few of the 100 percent covered claims, patients apply significant price pressures to doctors. This is especially true in regions of low- or middle-income status. Patients negotiate prices with me daily, and let me tell you, it is a buyer's market. Physicians, particularly specialists, are sensitive to price pressures from peers. One complaint from a patient back to a referring doctor can lead to significant economic repercussions for the specialist. Pressure to participate in insurance programs that control cost are enormous.

Advances in medical technology and knowledge yield the greatest impetus to competition. Patients frequently ask for the latest and most effective treatments, encouraging doctors to compete on those terms.

Hsiao's assertion that a "just price" matches "resource costs" in a perfectly competitive equilibrium is misstated. A basic principle of economics is that prices determine monetary costs, and not vice versa. Following Hsiao, perhaps, we should confiscate all profits from American industries, because prices do not match costs. Costs are not the effort expended in achieving a particular goal, but rather the loss of opportunities to pursue other goals with the same resources. Thus, Hsiao does not even measure economic costs in his study.

Although claiming to espouse free-market theory, Hsiao has unwittingly adopted the Marxian paradigm of the labor theory of value. According to Hsiao, "An equitable system of reimbursement should compensate services, requiring different amounts of work accordingly."[1] According to Marx, "Skilled labor is only . . . multiplied simple labor, so that a small quantity of skilled labor equals a larger quantity of simple labor. Experience shows that skilled labor can always be reduced in this way to the terms of simple labor."[2]

Adopting any intrinsic theory of value, independent of actual exchange prices, such as Hsiao's unintended application of the Marxian labor theory of value, will make rational economic calculation impossible and lead to the severe misallocation of economic resources. Even many contemporary Socialists recognize this, and long ago abandoned the labor theory of value in favor of various schemes, albeit ineffective, of instituting exchange prices via market socialism.

Subjective evaluation is the true basis for all economic exchange and is, in fact, critical in medical economics. Medical treatment and outcome are virtually never cut-and-dried. That value judgments are made in medical care every day is obvious in the choices patients make with respect to smoking, drugs, obesity, exercise, medical compliance, and the psychological costs of pain and suffering from treatment and surgery versus disease, to name but a few.

The methodological fallacies of Hsiao's study are almost innumerable. His reduction of "work" to the four factors of "time," "stress," "cognitive effort," and "technical effort" is arbitrary. The terms are never even defined. This reminds one of the reply of a

Supreme Court justice to a demand that he define "pornography": "You just know it when you see it."

The fact that Hsiao sees no relation between treatment and objective outcome or subjective results as evaluated by the patient would characterize any medical effort, including "bleeding with leeches," as "work." The factor of "stress" can variously refer to fear of iatrogenic injury or malpractice, guilt, emotional exhaustion, frustration with difficulty, time away from family, and so on, and is totally subjective. The factors of "cognitive" versus "technical" effort are meaningless. Does "cognitive" refer to the total medical knowledge applied in the given case or only the specific knowledge? To assert that the "technical" skill of a surgeon is somehow separable from his or her knowledge is just plain insulting and pure fantasy. Even "time" is not objectively verified. A short encounter can easily be skewed from 15 to 20 minutes, yielding a 33 percent increase, but it would be difficult to skew a 150-minute procedure up by 33 percent. Specialty groups have already proven that many of the time estimates of surgery are completely wrong.

"Magnitude estimation," as defined by Hsiao and used to obtain work and factor ratings, is a psychophysical technique that "yields close correspondences between physical measures of sensation and the subjective ratings of perception."[3] For example, a psychophysicist may validly use this technique to demonstrate the ranges in which humans can accurately estimate a temperature stimulus. A neurophysiologist might then use the data to discover how the nervous system accurately reflects the physical stimulus in its responses. But there is no external objective physical measure with which to compare the subjective ratings of work and the other factors studied by Hsiao. Thus, a completely inapplicable technique from another field of science is used inappropriately by Hsiao.

Even assuming that the method of magnitude estimation was applicable, he misuses it. About 100 representatives of each of eighteen out of fifty-two recognized specialties were asked in a thirty-minute phone conversation to rate five statistical categories of twenty-three services, described by one- or two-sentence vignettes, and thus were asked for 115 responses. For each specialty (say, internal medicine), a "reference service" (say, an office visit for a fifty-two-year old otherwise healthy hypertensive) was given a rating of 100 and other services rated against this. According to the textbook by Stevens that Hsiao himself relies on, as the procedures become more complex, the ratings relative to the reference service would become notoriously inaccurate.[4] Hsiao himself admits that the ratings are very sensitive and would change depending on the actual reference service chosen.

He failed to control for this by using multiple reference services across various ranges within each specialty.

No data are given to prove that the randomly surveyed physicians accurately represented the population of doctors they were supposed to with respect to details of training, intensity of practice, experience, income, and, most important, whether the respondents had significant experience in the services for which they were being surveyed. Thus, one-half of the chest surgeons surveyed admitted that they never perform any open-heart surgery and yet were asked to rate these services.

The technique of surveying "services" was totally erroneous. Instead of asking respondents to rate the average work of a given CPT-4 code, such as brief office visit or inguinal hernia repair, physicians were given a one- or two-sentence clinical vignette, alluded to previously, and asked to rate work. CPT codes were then retroactively applied to the specific clinical vignettes in order to create the relative value scale. This resulted in preaveraging the ranges of complexity of services subsumed under a given CPT code according to the preconceived notions of Hsiao's group. Is the result of blending tomatoes, cucumbers, and radishes in a Cuisinart an "average" vegetable? By way of analogy, if economists decided to survey consumers about the price of dinner, but for simplicity asked only about chicken dinners, the results would be invalid.

Hsiao's conclusions are contradicted by his own data. He claims extraordinary accuracy for a regression formula that relates work to time, stress, cognitive and technical skill, and effort. In fact, the regression factors are entirely different for each specialty. Thus, work for each specialty, and perhaps for each physician, is internally understood differently, as it is related to each of the four subfactors in an entirely different fashion. This critical flaw invalidates Hsiao's claim that he can cross-link specialties by identical or equivalent services. His own data prove that a general surgeon and gastroenterologist would relate the work of colonoscopy to time, stress, and effort differently, and yet Hsiao persists in claiming the work involved is the same. If his claim is correct, the work of economists and belly dancers could be related in the same way, and Hsiao could determine all market wages.

Hsiao's estimates of pre- and postservice work, which he asserts accounts for up to 50 percent of total work for a service, are based on arbitrary extrapolations of very limited services. The extraordinary complexity and difficulties of preoperative evaluation and postoperative care are glossed over in this analysis.

To extrapolate beyond the 372 of the 7,000 possible surveyed services, Hsiao broke down groups of services into homogeneous "families" and assumed that "charges alone explain a high proportion of the variation in work across the spectrum of services rendered by physicians." This assertion completely contradicts the whole thesis of his study and turns it into an attempt to keep reimbursement ratios for services *within* a specialty constant, but to shift overall reimbursement from one specialty to another. This, of course, was the politically attractive idea from the start.

Hsiao's attempt to factor in practice costs is erroneous as it is based on outdated information from a 1983 survey and understated malpractice estimates for surgical specialties. In his cost calculations, Hsiao assumes that practice costs are a fixed percentage of gross income and would remain so after the significant shifts in specialty incomes that he proposes. This is clearly false. A physician's costs at any given time are fixed, and, thus, lowering his gross income will significantly raise costs as a percentage of income. Thus, a 50 percent cut in gross income for a cardiac surgeon with 50 percent of current income as fixed expenses, would leave him with no net income at all.

The opportunity costs of residency are grossly miscalculated. In contradiction to the rest of his assertions about rewarding "work," Hsiao made no attempt to calculate the relative work of a more difficult versus somewhat more bearable residency. In fact, it is this last differential factor that probably distinguishes entry into different specialties most, and, from the supply side, in what specialists demand for reimbursement. Specialists who endured long and more difficult residencies naturally will demand higher reimbursement than specialists with an easier training experience.

Hsiao's assertion that a "drowning victim offered assistance by a lifeboat" is a valid model of the noncompetitive economics of medical care is completely fallacious. Probably less than 1 percent of medical care is truly immediate and life saving with no opportunity for choice or discussion. I know this because I am a neurosurgeon, whose specialty is among the most emergency-intensive.

Hsiao is, perhaps, his own severest critic. In his own words: "There is no objective standard with which we can compare our results to ascertain how well they represent reality." Hsiao alludes to Canada and Massachusetts as successful "natural experiments" in the use of RBRVS, a country and state, whose health care systems are, contrary to the popular press, in shambles.

Hsiao purports that his "scientific" method can determine a "just" price for the reimbursement of medical services by physicians. The clear implication of this is the adoption of total national price control and resource allocation of physicians' services. Hsiao is quite

241

explicit about this: "A fee schedule . . . could influence physician decisions about what services to provide . . . practice location, and specialty choice."

Adoption of the Hsiao proposal, especially as recommended by the Physician Payment Review Commission (PPRC), with a severe limitation on balance billing and focused expenditure targets, will result in a regulatory disaster. Considering that there are 440,000 physicians who utilize an average of at least 100 of 7,000 CPT codes in at least 200 geographic communities in the United States, more than ten billion, and probably closer to one hundred billion, physician reimbursement rates will have to be calculated and periodically updated utilizing the RBRVS methodology. The impending bureaucratic nightmare is mind-boggling.

Ideas have very serious consequences. If balance billing is permitted, then implementation of the Hsiao RBRVS would lead to a distorted insurance reimbursement structure for Medicare. Beneficiaries would suffer significant additional costs in order to make up for the miscalculations in the system. If Hsiao's study is indeed viewed as accurate and scientific, it will no doubt be applied to all forms of physician and health provider reimbursement, in both the government and private sectors. If balance billing is significantly limited, as proposed by the PPRC, or banned, then the economic dislocations and distortions caused by price control in the medical sector will be borne by everybody.

There is no natural constituency to offer support for the Hsiao proposal. The essence of the scheme, especially as modified by the PPRC, is to proclaim that health care is a "free good," by virtue of total price control, and then compel physicians to ration it. All patients, especially the elderly, will suffer owing to a progressive denial of access that historically has accompanied every attempt at price control. Physicians, whose integrity and independence are threatened by these proposed controls, will gradually cease to practice in that context. It is only naive self-deception that leads one group of medical specialists to think that they will benefit at the expense of another group. The 50 percent cut in medical school application rates that has occurred in recent years, and corresponding decline in quality of medical graduates, will only accelerate as the word spreads about the declining independence of the medical practitioner. The taxpayer will suffer because of the increasing economic inefficiency of price control and the additional expenses of the developing bureaucratic morass. The entire medical marketplace will sustain profoundly damaging economic distortion and misallocation of resources owing to price and resource controls. Even the Congress and executive branches of government will suffer, as the voters gradually begin to feel the effects of price controls on medical care. The only potential beneficiaries of this kind of program are the regulatory bureaucrats who might enforce the program.

It is ironic, indeed, that at a time when the world is turning everywhere to free markets—when a leading economist of the Soviet Academy of Sciences pronounces that "socialism is dead," and a leading communist Chinese economist states, "There is only one theory that works, and that is market theory"—at this historic moment, the United States, the fountainhead of free enterprise, is considering turning its back on the proper and essential role of the free market in medical care, which comprises 12 percent of its economy.

In contradistinction to the Hsiao and PPRC programs, numerous methods of introducing market incentives in order to ensure freedom of choice and efficient delivery of health care can be proposed. In exchange for deregulation, physicians must give up the cartel-like thinking and practices that, in the eyes of policy makers and economists, have reduced them to a British trade union type of mentality. Barriers to entry must be minimized by eliminating professional licensing boards and establishing reputable and competing private specialty certification boards. Closed medical staffs and the overt rejection of dealings by medical doctors with allied health professionals must come to an end. Government-granted monopoly power on the prescription of medication must end.

In exchange for accepting the forces of economic competition in the medical marketplace, the benefits of deregulation must be offered to physicians and patients. The government, in politically practical ways, should be removed from the business of health care. As an interim step, competing Medicare carriers should be encouraged within the same geographic location. With the success of introducing competition in this sector, capitation programs might be introduced. Finally, the retired should be offered a voluntary voucher system of health insurance. These measures, along with long-term planning—such as health IRAs and voluntary specified living wills, setting out what each patient wants done at the time of critical illness—would greatly diminish dependence on the government and taxpayer purse for medical care. Health care for the needy could be encouraged by tax deductions at Medicare rates to physicians and other providers, and vouchers to beneficiaries. Such an approach would by and large eliminate the need for Medicaid. With the diminishing status of government in health care would come a diminishing role for onerous regulation.

Hsiao is guilty of what has been called the fatal conceit of confusing the man-made with the natural, of attempting to interfere with the natural spontaneous order of free people exchanging values, including health care, on the open market. The replacement of prices for medical care as established on an open market by an artificial fee schedule is not what is needed, nor is it right. On the contrary, every effort must be expended on discovering and implementing mechanisms of bringing back market processes and free exchange into the economics of health care.

Correcting Market Imperfections in Physician Payments

A Commentary by Glenn T. Hammons

Janet Mitchell and William Hsiao have compared current charges by physicians for their services to the amount of work that physicians estimate is required to provide these services. Each has presented views about the market for physicians' services and made recommendations for changes in physician payment. Mitchell has concluded that the distortions in relative payments and the market imperfections causing them are relatively minor, so that relatively small adjustments in the amounts paid for some surgical and technical services are needed and a Medicare fee schedule could be based largely on current physician charges. Hsiao concluded that the imperfections of the market are pervasive, and that extensive realignment of physician fees is warranted. His work to develop a relative value scale (RVS) based on resource costs would provide a basis for that realignment through a new fee schedule based on that RVS.

I would like to comment on Mitchell's and Hsiao's comparisons of physician work to charges and on the implications for physician payment policy. I will begin by examining the results of the two comparisons of work to charges, then interpret these results in light of my views of the market for physician services, and draw implications of these findings for reforming physician payment. I would like to note that I am already "on record" with respect to certain aspects of Hsiao's work. The Physician Payment Review Commission for which I work concluded that Hsiao's study will provide reliable and valid results for a relative work scale of physicians' services. The commission recommends that, when this study is completed, improved, and revised, the relative work scale be used as the basis for a relative value scale and fee schedule to pay for physicians' services in Medicare. My views are consistent with the commission's position.

The two studies yield similar results when they compare physi-

245

cians' estimates of relative work to relative charges for these services. The methods used to develop estimates of work and compare them to charges are conceptually similar, but differ in important details. The survey from which Mitchell obtained estimates of physician work employed a closed-ended scale. Each physician was asked to equate the work of his or her specialty's most difficult procedure to 100 and then assign a number between 0 and 100 to all other procedures in the specialty. Hsiao's study used an open-ended scale. A procedure in the midrange of difficulty for each specialty was set to 100 and all other procedures were arrayed above and below that without an upper limit on any value. In an earlier study, Hsiao had found that a closed-end scale produces internally inconsistent estimates of work. Therefore, one wonders whether the Mitchell survey results suffer from the same problem.

The two studies also differ in the way that cross-linking was done. Mitchell used one service, the chest X-ray, to link all the specialties, whereas Hsiao used four to twenty services to link pairs of specialties. The use of a chest X-ray or any other single service to link specialties could introduce random error into comparisons among specialties. The use of multiple links should reduce that error. Consequently, one would expect Hsiao's multispecialty scale to be more reliable than Mitchell's scale.

In spite of these methodologic differences, Hsiao and Mitchell describe similar results when they compare charges to physician work. Mitchell finds that relative physician work and physician charges are highly correlated and that much of the variation in charges is explained by variations in work. The correlation between charges and work, however, is much higher when the surgical dummy variable is included. More precisely, charges and estimates of work are highly correlated for the pooled data of medical specialists and surgical specialists combined only if the surgical dummy is in the regression. The surgical dummy variable picks up a threefold difference between the prices for surgical procedures relative to other services. In other words, surgical services are generally paid three times as much as other services for the same amount of effort or work.

The implications of these findings depend on the interpretation of the coefficient for the surgical dummy variable representing a surgical service. The surgical dummy variable appears to be a huge "fudge factor" without which charges are *not* very well correlated with physician work for different services and procedures. To conclude that the differences captured by the dummy variable should continue to be reflected in payment rates for these services, Mitchell must find a legitimate explanation for this difference within the context of a well-functioning market. She suggests that the dummy variable may reflect large differences in practice costs or training costs between surgical and other services, or differences in the value that consumers place on the two groups of services. But she does not provide evidence or arguments for these possibilities.

Hsiao also finds a high correlation between his relative work values and current charges, and the correlation is much higher within surgical services and within evaluation and management services (visits and consults). If these groups are then further subdivided into smaller, more homogeneous groups, the correlations within each subgroup are still higher. For example, work and charges are more highly correlated within surgery and within the group of evaluation and management services than for all physician services and procedures together. Like Mitchell, Hsiao finds that the amount charged per unit of work is several times higher for surgical procedures than for evaluation and management services. This is analogous to Mitchell's positive surgical dummy variable. Unlike Mitchell, he concludes that this large unexplained difference in payment per unit of work results from market imperfections and is not justified by legitimate differences in costs or value.

In summary, both studies find that we now pay several times more for surgery than for a visit or consultation that physicians estimate to be the same amount of work. The investigators disagree, however, about the implications of these findings because of different views about the functioning of markets for physician services. The conclusions that the rest of us reach also depend on these assumptions.

Everyone agrees that there are imperfections in these markets and that they may variably affect groups of services or groups of physicians. Mitchell mentioned the effect of widespread and differential insurance coverage, and the effect of "sticky" prices—not only sticky absolute prices (charges for coronary artery bypass surgery do not fall over time) but also sticky relative prices because of the way Medicare prevailing charges have been constrained by Congress.

Everyone would agree that consumers have limited information about price and quality of medical services and limited ability to make informed choices. There is also often refusal to make choices, widespread purchase of Medigap coverage, and other impediments to the effects of market forces. And, of course, physician stocks change slowly, there are barriers to entry, and so forth.

Both agree that because of sticky prices some services such as coronary artery bypass surgery are artificially high. Mitchell would say that such "overpriced" surgical services need to be reduced, and Hsiao would agree. They would also agree that differential insurance coverage means certain classes of services may be sold in markets of different degrees of price competition, with implications for prices. And both would agree that, in this particular case, surgical services as a class should be reduced relative to other services. But how much they should be reduced depends on your explanation for the threefold surgical dummy variable. Hsiao would go much further. He argues that there are many market imperfections and all kinds of systematic and random departures from the prices you would observe in a competitive market, and current charges lack validity.

Hsiao and Mitchell differ in their views of the competitiveness of the market for physician services. If one believes that the market functions pretty well but there are a few things wrong here and there, you reduce prices for selected overpriced procedures and you may realign groups of services to some extent (and the extent might depend on how you interpret the dummy variable), but you continue to rely on the market to set prices for physician services. If you implement a fee schedule for physician services, you rely largely on current charges as the basis for relative prices in the schedule. This seems to be Mitchell's position. She argues that the huge differences in compensation per amount of physician work picked up by the surgical dummy variable may well be legitimate reflections of factors working through the market—differences in practice costs or training costs, or differences in the value that purchasers place on different kinds of physician services.

But if you believe the market does not function at all well and you wish to use a fee schedule to pay for physician services, you do not rely on current charges in setting relative fees. Rather, you search for another basis as Hsiao has done. His solution is to replace charges with estimates of long-run average costs (including physician work and overhead) required to produce these services, as if to simulate the results of a competitive market.

The market for physician services has many imperfections. It goes well beyond the problem that prices for a handful of procedures are too high. There is a major misalignment between surgical and technical procedures versus other services, and a premium or a windfall for surgery and technical procedures. I am not sure how much of it is due to differential insurance coverage or other factors. What data we have do not support the conclusion that much of the effect of the threefold surgical dummy can be explained by differences in practice costs or differences in training costs. And I do not think the differences represented by the surgical dummy reflect systematic differences in the value placed on different types of services by consumers. Without a well-functioning market—which we do not have—it is difficult to know what "value" consumers place on different physicians' services. Hsiao is correct in pointing out that the distortions of relative prices for physician services are pervasive, and that a fee schedule based on something other than physician charges is needed.

But if a resource-based fee schedule is implemented for Medicare, there are still critical decisions to be made. It will be necessary to revise and update continually a fee schedule through some combination of market and administrative mechanisms. How should this be done? Do we continue to use analytic studies like Hsiao's to set prices administratively? Could we systematically measure access to services—perhaps a reflection of market forces—and use that information to modify prices? Should we set up a negotiating mechanism between payers and providers to agree on prices?

An alternative approach is to establish a reasonably competitive market. That is philosophically very attractive but difficult to do as long as we maintain fee for service as the method of paying for (and being paid for) physician services. We can try to get more information to consumers, and take other general measures to counter sources of market deficiencies. We can try to take advantage of market forces for particular services through methods like selective contracting. But I doubt that a well-functioning market for individual physician services is within our reach.

We could instead develop a market for competing medical plans rather than for individual physician services, as Alain Enthoven has advocated. That is intellectually attractive and might be feasible if we could find competent managers to run the plan, could set up the market so it actually worked, and gave the managers tools to influence the physicians in their plans. It has potential advantages over the path we are on, for fee for service with a process for setting and changing prices has its own disadvantages and it will take a lot of effort to maintain it. But can we get there? I do not know. For now, there are many benefits from moving to a fee schedule based on resource costs, with Hsiao's work as the basis for relative prices for physician services.

Unexplained Sources of Differences in Physician Charges

A Commentary by Finis Welch

Two features of the relative value scale (RVS) are of particular interest: the procedure used to determine relative valuations and the intended use.

Physicians in various specialties were surveyed regarding the effort associated with their medical activities. The questionnaire included a list of procedures, and respondents were asked to score each procedure on the (specialty-specific) list in terms of the total effort involved in performing it. Effort was said to refer to time spent in the procedure, including preparation and postprocedural time, complexity, and stress. The score was scaled relative to a numeraire procedure (an in-office examination of a well patient) assigned a score of 100. If a respondent returned a score of 200, the procedure was assumed to require twice as much total effort as the numeraire procedure. Because all respondents in a specialty were not expected to agree on scores, the average score was used to determine the relative value of the procedure.

The RVS is intended to be used to determine relative compensation, say, for insurance payments. A procedure with an average score of 200 will receive twice as much compensation as a procedure with an average score of 100 in the same specialty.

All that remains is to determine the compensation for the numeraire procedure. In the Harvard RVS, numeraire procedures are compensated by specialty, in recognition of differences in the training costs of specialists and in the costs of supporting facilities and personnel. As an example of such an application, suppose that we modify the way professors are paid and adopt a fee-for-service system alongside an RVS calculated, perhaps, by a group of physicians at Johns Hopkins. Under this system, professors must rent their offices and hire and pay their support personnel (secretaries and research assistants) and they must pay for support facilities (for example, computers). Services involve (1) teaching courses that vary in enrollments, complexity, and time in preparation and in grading papers and exams (which may be subcontracted to teaching assistants to be paid by the professor), (2) attending conferences such as this one that vary in time requirements, in preparation of papers to be presented, discussed, or heard, in time and effort and stress at the conference, and in postconference time in revising papers and comments, (3) conducting preliminary research and writing papers for publication in peer-reviewed journals, revising and polishing them, (4) participating on university committees (to review colleagues who are considered for promotion) and national committees (to examine proposals that Medicare adopt an RVS or that the federal minimum wage be increased to $x/hr), and so on.

As noted, compensation is a fee for service in this system. It has no base salary and no expense accounts, no computing or assistance budgets. In constructing the Hopkins RVS for professors, the analysts would probably start by focusing on the professors' time requirements for various activities. On average, it might take professors of economics as much time to produce a theoretical paper as it does to produce an empirical paper, even though the theorists would view empirical papers as less consuming of intellectual effort and the empiricists would view the theoretical papers as requiring less total effort. But even if the time and effort requirements are identical on average, the costs will not be because empirical work cannot proceed without data and computational resources that are not required by work in pure theory.

Now, the fundamental question is whether compensation ought to be based on costs without reference to the quality of what is produced. In a world where individual professors negotiate their prices, compensation will respond to perceptions of quality. In a world where price is capped by an externally imposed amount, consumers can seek out those providers they assume are best, but providers cannot ration consumers by raising their prices. Some providers will be swamped and because they cannot increase their prices they can respond by selecting only the easiest cases among the many that compete for their time. Other providers whose services are not in as great demand will have to remain partly unemployed or await the overflow from the providers seen as superior by consumers. If the RVS errs in fixing relative prices, all providers will have incentives to skew their offerings toward those activities where relative prices are too high. Fixing relative prices in a specialty or discipline on the basis of providers' own time and effort does not

251

allow for differences in the relative importance of support staff and facilities.

In this case, one suspects that providers will define their services narrowly and require consumers to compensate support separately. A professor might agree to conduct an empirical study only if the purchaser agrees to pay the research assistants and computation resources separately. A physician might move an in-office procedure to a hospital, where hospital facilities and anesthetic services are billed separately. The next question is how compensation is to be fixed between disciplines or specialties.

If the Hopkins group follows the Harvard stereotype, it will select a number for each discipline as the numeraire compensation for that discipline. Activities within the discipline will be compensated as the product of the discipline's numeraire value and the activity's relative score. As an example, suppose that the numeraire for economists is 110 and that it is 100 for sociologists. In this case, activities that economists assign a relative value of, say, 200 will receive 10 percent more compensation than activities that sociologists assign an equal relative score.

Numeraire compensation, following the Harvard procedure, is determined by several factors, including time spent on training and overhead costs. The postbaccalaureate time to a Ph.D. for professors of English and history is typically twice as long as it is for professors of mathematics, so numeraire compensation would be adjusted accordingly. Chemists and biologists work in laboratories and require expensive equipment, and the numeraire rate will be adjusted for overhead costs. Unless theoretical and applied physicists are distinguished as separate specialties (and they may or may not be in fact, as individual physicists switch freely between these activities), the overhead allowance will be common to all. Once numeraire compensation is determined, the fee structure is fixed. In contrast, in an open market where prices that are too high are penalized by fewer selections and subsequently lowered, the full RVS does not have a built-in adjustment mechanism.

There is one property of an RVS that is not transparent at first blush. Statisticians call it regression toward the mean. Regardless of the details or of the rubric surrounding the Harvard procedure, it can be described as an attempt to understand existing fee structures on the basis of objective criteria that are observable in principle, such as time involved in training and in performance of procedures, together with subjective criteria that are not easily measured, like complexity and stress. The initial design in the Harvard study consisted of a detailed scheme of relative values based on time before, during, and after procedures; complexity; and stress. Later, the simpler scheme of averaging questionnaire respondent total scores was adopted.

The alternative procedure used by Janet Mitchell and her colleagues employs least-squares regression to explain observed differences in maximum allowable charge rates for procedures in terms of constructed measures of time requirements before, during, and after procedures and complexity of procedures. Since the statistical technique is often used, its properties are well known. The regression phenomenon is that extreme values are not explained as precisely as intermediate values. The least-squares technique produces a fitted value that is the prediction based on the explanatory factors. The technique is designed to preserve averages, so the average of the fitted value is also the average of the observed value. Fitted values are less disperse, however. Variance (about the mean) is a measure of dispersion and the variance of the fitted values relative to the variance of the observed values is called the regression R^2. It is the most commonly used measure of goodness-of-fit, of how well the factors considered fit the data. The R^2 number is bounded by 0 and 1 and the values reported by Mitchell and others are in the range of 0.6 to 0.7.

The regression phenomenon for least squares is defined as

$$E(Y - \hat{Y}|Y) = (1 - R^2)(Y - \overline{Y})$$

where Y is the observed value of the thing to be explained (allowable charges), $\hat{Y}$ is its prediction from the least-squares technique, and $\overline{Y}$ is the average of Y. In words, the above expression refers to a given value of Y. The greater the difference between Y and the average, $\overline{Y}$, the greater is the expected difference between the observed and predicted values. The factor $1 - R^2$ refers to variance in Y not explained by the least-squares technique. Thus, we are not surprised in the Mitchell and others study that the predictions for the most (and least) expensive procedures are wide of the mark. This systematic nature of prediction errors is to be expected.

The Harvard RVS is not an explicit statistical technique and its properties cannot be as succinctly described. It would be surprising, however, if the regression property does not hold. Consider, for example, the twelve procedures listed by Jack Hadley. The most expensive is a coronary bypass and the least expensive is an in-office visit for a healthy patient. The relative value of the coronary bypass in the Harvard RVS is 25. If the office visit is assigned a numeraire score of 100, the score of the coronary bypass is 2,500. It is not surprising that respondents to the Harvard questionnaire rated the

253

total time, stress, and complexity requirements of a bypass as greater than an in-office visit and, at first blush, a score of 2,500 seems high but not unreasonable. Compare this number to the relative prices presented by Hadley. If I fix a numeraire score of 100 for the office visit, the corresponding relative value of the coronary bypass is 22,300. It is difficult to believe that physicians would have responded with such a high score unless they were prompted to do so. Yet, if the Harvard RVS is adopted and if compensation for the office visit does not change, compensation for the bypass will fall to 11 percent of its previous level. The property of reduced dispersion appears to hold for the Harvard RVS, as for the Mitchell and others study.

My concern with the intended use of the RVS has to do with the nature of scientific inquiry. Given the history of Medicare costs, it seems reasonable to study the sources of differences in physician charges. Differences between specialties are particularly interesting, and the emphasis in the Harvard study on training and overhead costs seems like the right place to start. Even so, one might prefer something that is more tractable in terms of description and method so that future research can either replicate or contradict findings. It is disappointing that the earlier idea of examining relative charges within a discipline was abandoned in favor of the simple composite scoring technique. One hopes that underlying correlates of composite scores are being studied. But whatever techniques are used, it is important to identify those parts of observed differences in relative charges that can be explained in terms of observable inputs, like time and complexity. The difference between what is explained and what is not represents a continuing problem that may justifiably be an issue for further research. The step from the simple partition of observed prices into explained and unexplained parts to a position holding that only the explained parts are justified is long and incredibly arrogant. That, pure and simple, is what the adoption of an RVS implies.

As Rick Warren-Boulton and others have noted, if the objective is to lower payments to physicians, fees can be lowered pro rata or physicians' incomes can be taxed more severely. If an RVS is adopted on the basis of the Harvard, Mitchell, or similar studies, I can only assume that the objective is to reduce the dispersion in physicians' earnings. If that is the objective, then it and the rationale behind it should be specified for public examination and discourse.

Alternatives for Setting and Adjusting Fee Schedules

I

A Discussion

WILLIAM S. HSIAO: To sharpen the debate, I will argue that our study is very different from the Mitchell-Cromwell study, just the opposite of what Terry Hammons said. We were getting a direct measurement of the work input that physicians estimate is required for each service. Mitchell and Cromwell did not measure that. They measured two components of it, and therefore, they don't have an end result. Then they regressed their measures on the charges. And, of course, we do know that charges are highly correlated with time, and also highly correlated with complexity, even if it is measured incorrectly. In 1985, we found that.

The problem of measurement is getting the cardinal measurement of the intensity and work. So it doesn't surprise me that Mitchell and Cromwell found some explanatory power; there is a correlation between the time, complexity, and charges. But I will submit, their study did not give you an independent measurement of what work goes into performing specific physician services. And that's the core of our study. When we measure these dimensions, we are trying to test the validity and the consistency of the parts and the whole. Mitchell and Cromwell were not able to do that. So, the two studies are not comparable.

Second, because of the correlation between the charges, time, and complexity, there isn't an independent validation in the Mitchell and Cromwell study to say the current charges are not so distorted, because there is no independent variation.

Incidentally, I know we have been criticized for not including the posthospital discharge visits in our relative value. I would like to give you an explanation.

We surveyed surgeons, asking them what services are included in their current charges. We found that they did not include a

Part II of this discussion is on page 310, and part III on page 374.

255

preoperative visit or the initial diagnosis visit, but they do tend to include the posthospital discharge visit. Actually, sometimes they included it and sometimes they didn't. We compensated for the parts that physicians did not include in the global fee for the preoperative visits by excluding the postoperative visits. We think that the range of error is between 5 and 10 percent.

Let me turn to Dr. Franck, whose presentation was very eloquent.

One of his main points is the question of just price. First of all, I never used the words "just price." I don't really know what justice is, and so I always use the words "fair and rational price," and let me emphasize the point for the noneconomists in this audience. We were trying to mimic the price in a competitive market. I would like to add that I am not a Marxist.

In the competitive marketplace, the price eventually will come pretty close to the resource cost, because if the price exceeds the resource cost, competition will move in and bid down that price. And if the price is below the resource cost, of course, the firm will go bankrupt. So our conceptual approach is actually following the competitive market theory.

Concerning the patient's willingness to pay as a measurement that has certain normative value, doesn't that only have normative value when there is competition? Otherwise, you are letting the consumer surplus get extracted by the supplier. So let's recognize this basic fact: We will only use a consumer's willingness to pay in a competitive market as an optimum price.

Now, two quick points. First, before it was published, our work was reviewed carefully by roughly twenty-nine experts in five fields: clinical medicine, economics, psychology, statistics, and survey methodology. So at least that group of experts found our work to have scientific credibility.

Dr. Franck mentioned that some specialties have shown that their time data come out to be very different from ours. I have heard many rumors about how people have found something that is very different from ours and that it renders our study invalid.

I will put this challenge out. Since we let our work be completely open and exposed to the world and had it refereed by the best journals, whoever wants to say that they can prove we are wrong should also go through the same peer review process, instead of letting unproven conclusions circulate. I would just make a plea that other people's work be put on the same playing field and same plane as ours.

JOEL IRA FRANCK: Dr. Hsiao, here is the testimony of the American

College of Surgeons and the American Society of Thoracic Surgeons before the Physician Payment Review Commission (PPRC).

MR. HSIAO: I read that stack of testimonies. Now we need to get qualified people to evaluate it and give them the raw data to see how it was gathered, rather than taking the testimony itself as valid.

I certainly second what Dr. Franck has said about the need for a behavioral model for physicians to study the objective we are trying to achieve by reforming prices or controlling quantity. We are really in a world of uncertainty in making predictions about whether the resource-based relative value scale (RBRVS) is a good thing or a bad thing.

JANET B. MITCHELL: I am a little surprised to hear that there were studies that showed a strong positive relationship of time and complexity to physician charges, because I am certainly not aware of it, nor is the Department of Health and Human Services.

The reason that we got into this study to start with was not to develop a relative value scale, but to evaluate the administration's inherent reasonableness policy in which they were identifying surgical procedures that they considered overpaid and that should be subject to rollbacks. And as you know, a number of procedures have been rolled back on the basis of PPRC's recommendations.

We wanted to see whether there were some objective criteria by which one might identify overpaid procedures, since most of the evidence that we were aware of was pretty anecdotal. There was the belief that certain operations were easy today compared with twenty years ago, but there were not any good data.

We did a study of coronary bypass surgery and did find declines in operating times since the early 1970s, but, for the most part, it has been hard to get that kind of information. It is reassuring to know that higher fees for some services can be justified in terms of the amount of physician time (both during the procedure and postoperatively) and the perceived complexity (however you choose to measure complexity).

We have compared our time estimates with those from the RBRVS study, and they are so similar that it is surprising. The few instances in which the reported times differ substantially can be explained by the vignette that was used in the RBRVS study. So, like Bill Hsiao, I would be very surprised if other specialty groups could do a truly random survey of physicians and get reported times that would be materially different from those found in the RBRVS study, or our own study.

257

LEE BENHAM: Both of these studies find some services that are too high priced. Insofar as this process has gone on a while, it implies the existence of excess capacity on the provider's side for the more technical services. So the question is: What information is there on independent measures of excess capacity for providers of these procedures?

QUESTION: Some data on gastroenterology—on the number being trained and the number of procedures that were required in their training—show a very disproportionate ratio there. A lot more surgeons were being trained than seemed to be usefully employed.

How many specialists do you observe being trained *vis-à-vis* these prices? That is what it really comes down to. Do you know?

Ms. MITCHELL: I don't know.

MR. FRANCK: My impression from talking to friends in big cities is that they are crying for something to do. They are going out and giving speeches so they can find somebody else to do surgery on. That suggests to me excess capacity, but Janet Mitchell knows a lot more about that than I do. I only have anecdotes.

Ms. MITCHELL: There are some published studies showing that surgical work loads have been falling over time, because the supply of surgeons is growing faster than the number of patients.

QUESTION: If the consumer faces a price close to zero, and if we are trying to limit the amount of GNP devoted to medical expenses by arranging supply prices, doesn't this have adverse consequences in the long run? Congress apparently thinks it can save money by arranging supply prices. But it is doing nothing about the demand. The consumer still faces a price of zero, or very close to zero. How do you deal with that?

MR. HSIAO: If there is an expenditure cap and you then reduce providers' payment rates, you are probably going to have some kind of excess demand at the zero price. You may find that there's a reduction in certain supply—let's say surgery or tests—and more supply in primary care. At least the superficial impression everybody has is that we have a surplus of surgeons and a shortage of primary care physicians. So you will see a shift in the marketplace.

QUESTION: Would you also expect the more talented people to leave or not enter the industry?

MR. HSIAO: That would not necessarily be the case because the talented people will still be compensated very handsomely, either through direct payment or balance billing.

ROGER G. NOLL: I have two questions for Bill Hsiao. First, he attempts to measure forms of disutility to doctors, such as stress or work effort. If the disutility of those things is not linear, then how could he make any argument at all about who is overpaid from the results of his study?

Second, how does one decide what is a legitimate sample and what isn't? Suppose we define "doctors" as all the people in his sample, plus baseball players, and we try to measure time and stress and all that. More than likely we would identify Orel Hershiser as overpaid at $3 million a year. And the reason it is not a silly question is the point that was made in Janet Mitchell's paper: It is clear that the explanatory power of the equations keeps getting higher the more homogeneous the data.

I also worry about the other factors left out, about the specification error in the model. Any attempt to base prices on the subset of variables that are included as explanatory variables would—because of specification error—simply overlook things that are important.

MR. HSIAO: In response to Roger Noll's first question, I would say that, although we measure stress or technical skill, we are really not using that information, other than to check on the consistency and the validity of our measurement of work. So what we should focus on is this measurement of work, whether that is linear or nonlinear. With the magnitude estimation method, we found the relationship is log-normal.

On the second question, we took a random sample of physicians in a given specialty, and stratified by board certification and nonboard certification as represented in that specialty, and then we also stratified by geographical region.

10
Comparisons of the Value of Physician Time by Specialty

William D. Marder and Richard J. Willke

In a perfectly competitive market for physician services, the value of physician time would be an important determinant of the equilibrium level of fees. Even in imperfectly competitive product or service markets, the wage rates of key members of the labor force will affect prices. Thus, whatever one's view of the degree of competition in the physician services marketplace, a conceptual model of variation in physician fees depends on the conceptual model that determines the value of physician time.

A substantial body of literature addresses the question of variations in earnings (that is, time prices and labor supply) within the framework of a human capital view of labor markets (see appendix A for a brief review of the relevant literature). This perspective asserts that individuals invest in acquiring skills—that is, human capital—in order to increase their subsequent productivity and earnings.[1] The cost of these investments is the value of the opportunities that these individuals forgo. The graduate medical education, or residency training, that prepares physicians for the different specialties has long been recognized as an investment in human capital.[2] Thus, human capital acquired during residency training can be easily understood as having the potential to raise the value of a physician's time. We present further quantitative evidence of the effect of investments in specialty-specific skills on the value of physician time.

The effect of human capital investments of employees on output prices is conceptually more complicated because human capital plays a role in productivity as well as the price of time, and the net impact is uncertain. This study applies empirical techniques generally used in the analysis of human capital investments to investigate variations

The views expressed in this chapter are those of the authors and do not necessarily represent the official views of the American Medical Association.

in the value of physician time. We avoid the complicated economics of physician fees by leaving to others the "appropriate" role of the value of time in payment formulas.

Fees and the value of physician work were, however, the central focus of the effort by Hsiao and others to develop a resource-based relative value scale (RBRVS).[3] To a certain extent, the human capital perspective was built into the RBRVS conceptual model of physician fees. The RBRVS contains an "amortized cost of specialty training (AST)" adjustment, although measuring human capital stocks of physicians in different specialties was not the primary focus of the Hsiao study.[4] Consequently, relatively little attention was paid to these variations, at least in comparison with issues such as the amount of time and complexity associated with different procedures. Given the importance of the value of time, as opposed to the amount of time spent per patient contact, further investigation is warranted.

The Hsiao study not only presented estimates of the opportunity costs of specialty training but also assumed, for the purposes of payment reform, that the rate of return to training *should* be a constant across all specialties. We estimate average rates of return to investments in residency training needed to enter different specialties. In fact, we provide three estimates, depending on the treatment of leisure time of physicians. Not surprisingly, there are significant variations in average returns to investments in specialty-specific skills.

We also present a formula for amortization of specialty training costs that is based on standard labor economics concepts. We find that Hsiao's formula for AST factors does not follow from such underpinnings, and as a result, is significantly biased toward *understating* the amount of variation in the value of physician time, independent of the rate of return applied.

Data Available for the Study

Several kinds of data are needed to estimate the potential earnings of physicians in different specialties. An ideal source of information would be panel data that followed individual physicians through the course of their careers. Residency training experiences would be measured as well as earnings streams during a lifetime of practice, and retirement and mortality probabilities could be estimated as an outgrowth of panel attrition. Unfortunately, such data are not available, and all studies of the economic returns to practice in different specialties must rely on cross-sectional data (with important exceptions relating to retirement and mortality).

Following standard practice in labor economics, we used cross-

261

sectional data to construct artificial cohorts and estimated returns to specialty training on the basis of regression analysis of the effects of experience on earnings. We had access to a variety of cross-sectional data sets that measure the situation of physicians during residency (1983 and 1987 surveys of resident physicians), the early years of practice (a 1987 survey of young physicians), prime ages, and preretirement years (1987 and 1988 Socioeconomic Monitoring System, SMS, surveys of nonfederal patient care physicians). Earnings and hours worked by practicing physicians were estimated from a combined sample of respondents to three SMS surveys and the 1987 survey of young physicians (for a total of 12,878 respondents). In addition, we had access to the data collection associated with the American Medical Association's Physician Masterfile, which permitted us to estimate the demographic determinants of retirement and mortality (see appendix B for background information on the data used in this study).

Rates of Return to Specialty Training

The standard formula for determining the internal rate of return to an investment with known costs and benefits is

$$\sum_{t=0}^{T} (Y_{it} - Y_{0t}) (1+r_i)^{-t} = 0 \qquad (10.1)$$

where r_i is the rate of return that solves this equation, given that Y_{it} is the net income by year from the investment, including costs as negative elements, and Y_{0t} is the net income by year along the alternative noninvestment path, with a total time of $T + 1$ years from the beginning of the investment to the end of the return period.

This formula, in its simplest interpretation, involves income paths that occur with certainty for each year in the return period. In our application, that would mean assuming once-and-for-all retirement (or death) after year T for both the investment and noninvestment paths. Across the physician population, however, retirement or death occurs with some probability in each year of the period, but the probability differs for investment and noninvestment paths. If we assume that the expected value of income by year is the appropriate income path, adjusting for the probability of being in practice in each year, the formula becomes

$$\sum_{t=0}^{T} (P_{it}Y_{it} - P_{0t}Y_{0t})(1 + r_i)^{-t} = 0 \qquad (10.2)$$

where P_{it} and P_{0t} are the probabilities of being in practice in year t in the investment and noninvestment paths, respectively. This adjustment eliminates the need to incorporate different expected work lives or period lengths for different paths, given that T is the maximum feasible work life on either path.

The minimum amount of residency training necessary to obtain a license to practice medicine is one year in most states.[5] The minimum necessary to become board-certified in a specialty is three years. We therefore define those physicians with one or two years of residency training who are not board-certified and who are practicing in a primary care specialty as being on the noninvestment "base specialty" path Y_0. The different investment paths, or specialties, that we decided to examine represented a compromise between those in the RBRVS study and those specialties with a large enough sample to enable us to estimate age-earnings profiles. As a result, we combined all internal medicine subspecialties into one category, and divided surgical subspecialties into the following categories: ophthalmology, subspecialties requiring five or fewer years in residency for board certification, and those requiring six or more years.[6]

The empirical strategy for estimating rates of return to investment in specialty training has two principal components. First, the determinants of yearly earnings by specialty—primarily experience, sex, self-employment, and board certification—are estimated using regression analysis and the survey data described.[7] Then, predicted earnings for a typical physician in each specialty category are constructed for each year of residency and practice and weighted for retirement and mortality as in equation (10.2).[8] The number of years in residency is determined by the median years in residency for board-certified physicians in the specialty. The rate of return that equates the present value of earnings in the specialty and in the base—in other words, that solves equation (10.2)—can then be calculated.[9]

The cost-benefit trade-off of specialty training that our estimation strategy produces is illustrated in figure 10–1. The solid line represents the calculated age-earnings profile for general internal medicine from the second year of training (age twenty-eight) to age seventy-five, while the dashed line is the profile of the base specialty. The opportunity cost of training for general internists is shown as the shaded area below the base specialty-earnings profile during the early years of residency training and practice. The benefits of the investment are shown in the other shaded area above the base specialty profile during the middle and later years of practice. The rate of return to this investment is the interest rate that equates the discounted values of the two shaded areas.

This basic strategy has three variations. The simplest is to use

263

FIGURE 10–1

ESTIMATED AGE-EARNINGS PROFILE FOR BASE SPECIALTY
AND GENERAL INTERNAL MEDICINE

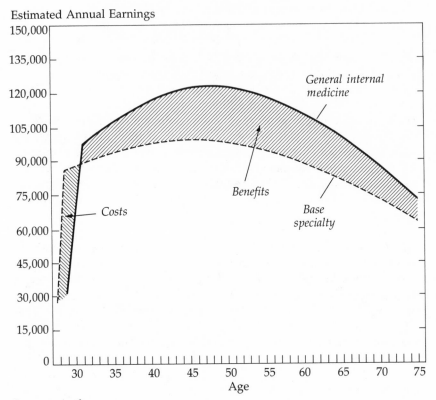

Estimated Annual Earnings

SOURCE: Author.

actual yearly earnings as the sole indicator of costs and benefits of
training. Physicians are individuals, however, whose choices are
made to maximize utility, not just income, and leisure is an important
aspect of utility.[10] There are significant variations in physician hours
of work across specialty and career stage. Residents work particularly
long hours, even in the later years of residency.[11] For those in
practice, average annual hours worked in 1987 ranged from about
2,350 for psychiatrists and pathologists to more than 3,000 for obste-
trician/gynecologists, with base specialists at about 2,870 (see table
10–1). Rates of return calculated on earnings alone are likely to
overstate the true rate of return if hours of work in the specialty are
longer than those in the base, and to understate the true rate if the
specialist works relatively short hours.

264

TABLE 10-1
AVERAGE EARNINGS AND HOURS WORKED PER YEAR
BY SPECIALTY, 1987

Specialty	1987 Earnings (dollars)		Annual Hours Worked[a]	
	Mean	Standard deviation	Mean	Standard deviation
All specialties	134,699	104,167	2,791	878
Base	90,302	49,230	2,867	886
General/family practice	91,577	59,649	2,868	907
General internal medicine	107,421	72,621	2,963	947
Medical subspecialties	158,293	131,196	2,891	981
General surgery	164,105	90,420	2,944	1,015
Ophthalmology	195,875	190,870	2,444	684
Other surgical subspecialties (0–5 years in residency)	206,970	163,982	2,844	835
Other surgical subspecialties (6+ years in residency)	204,931	135,672	2,752	817
Pediatrics	86,580	43,523	2,701	776
Obstetrics/gynecology	157,056	121,584	3,045	911
Radiology	182,438	86,111	2,592	680
Psychiatry	104,245	53,910	2,353	710
Anesthesiology	162,241	68,500	2,737	792
Pathology	136,694	59,937	2,357	553

NOTE: For physicians in SMS surveys, weighted to represent the U.S. physician population.
a. Calculated as the product of weeks worked in the previous year and hours worked in the previous week.
SOURCE: Authors' calculations.

Laspeyres-type and Paasche-type hours adjustments can be used to calculate leisure-adjusted yearly earnings and rates of return. The Laspeyres estimate uses base specialty annual hours and the specialty-specific hourly wage to create annual earnings for the base and investment specialty: $Y_{kt} = W_{kt}H_{ot}$, $k = 0, i$, where W and H are hourly earnings and yearly hours, respectively. As pointed out elsewhere, Laspeyres adjustments may under- or overstate the rates of return, but "an investment in training which appears profitable in terms of a Laspeyres estimate of real returns is nevertheless always attractive."[12] With the Paasche adjustment, earnings are calculated by using hours of work standardized to the specialty level: $Y_{kt} = W_{kt}H_{it}$, $k = 0, i$. This

265

adjustment will overstate rates of return, so that "investment in training which is revealed to be unprofitable in terms of a Paasche estimate is therefore truly unattractive."[13]

To implement these variations, we estimated two annual hours regressions, one for residents and one for practicing physicians. Each controls for specialty, experience, and sex; and the physician regression controls for employment status, board certification, and family situation. The hourly wage regressions mirrored the yearly earnings regressions. We assumed that hourly wages were constant over the relevant range of hours.[14]

Table 10-2 presents our results. Column 1 shows undiscounted opportunity costs of residency training, with no labor supply adjustments, for each specialty analyzed. They depend primarily on the length of residency, shown in parentheses. Base specialists are assumed to undergo one year of residency, so opportunity costs begin in the second year. Costs are about $40,000-50,000 per year, the difference between base specialty and resident earnings (which vary somewhat by specialty). The opportunity costs in lengthy surgical subspecialties are as high as $300,000.

Column 2 shows the estimated rates of return for board-certified physicians in each specialty; these rates are based on predicted values of actual yearly earnings with no labor supply adjustments other than for retirement and mortality probabilities. Note the great range of these estimates. Pediatricians earn only a 1.3 percent rate of return on training, with general/family practitioners (GPFPs) faring just slightly better, whereas anesthesiologists earn a 39.1 percent rate of return. The largest specialty, general internal medicine, receives a 15.2 percent rate of return, which is below pathology's 20.4 percent median rate among these thirteen specialties. It is not surprising to find a certain amount of variation in the rates of return to investments in different kinds of human capital.

The hours-adjusted rates of return are shown in table 10-2, columns 3 and 4. For most specialties, the changes between unadjusted and the Laspeyres and Paasche rates of return are not too large. Returns for GPFPs and pediatricians change very little. Returns for general internists and medical subspecialists fall somewhat because of their longer-than-average work hours, both as residents and practicing physicians. Returns for surgeons and obstetrician/gynecologists tend to fall for the same reason, even though ophthalmologists work shorter hours in practice. Returns for anesthesiologists stay very high, in that their hours of work do not differ significantly from those of the base specialty. Rates of return for radiologists, psychiatrists, and pathologists increase markedly, however. As residents and prac-

TABLE 10–2: Opportunity Costs and Rates of Return to Specialty Training

Specialty	Opportunity Costs, Undiscounted[a] (median years in residency)		Yearly Earnings (%)[b]	Laspeyres Adjustment (%)[c]	Paasche Adjustment (%)[d]
General family practice	89,708	(3)	4.1	3.9	3.7
General internal medicine	87,157	(3)	15.2	12.7	11.8
Medical subspecialties	191,682	(5)	19.4	18.5	17.4
General surgery	181,816	(5)	22.4	22.1	18.6
Ophthalmology	177,598	(5)	28.7	29.5	22.0
Other surgical subspecialties (0–5 years in residency)	177,598	(5)	34.5	29.2	23.5
Other surgical subspecialties (6+ years in residency)	295,655	(7)	18.9	18.1	14.0
Pediatrics	154,618	(4)	1.3	2.1	1.5
Obstetrics/gynecology	124,889	(4)	35.1	25.9	22.0
Radiology	144,426	(4)	30.5	46.7	50.7
Psychiatry	130,287	(4)	10.8	23.9	25.2
Anesthesiology	121,858	(4)	39.1	40.4	36.8
Pathology	140,430	(4)	20.4	50.1	58.0

NOTE: For board-certified physicians, with proportion female and self-employed set to sample means, and adjusted for probability of being in practice for each age through seventy-five.
a. Sum of earnings differences versus base specialty during years in residency.
b. Adjusted only for retirement and mortality.
c. Hours worked set to those of base specialty.
d. Hours worked for base set to those of investment specialty.
SOURCE: Authors' calculations.

titioners, physicians in these specialties work the fewest hours, with pathologists being the lowest in the (very influential) residency years. The labor supply adjustments reduce their investment costs and increase their practice earnings, resulting in the higher rates of return.

None of the rates of return shown in table 10–1 can be identified as the "best" estimate. We know that actual yearly earnings will tend to over- or understate rates of return as specialists work longer or shorter hours than the base, respectively. Laspeyres and Paasche estimates change these rates or return in the expected directions, but there is no guarantee that the correction is accurate. Paasche estimates should be an upper bound, according to Lindsay, but in some cases the Paasche estimates are the lowest of the three. This does not involve any logical inconsistency because the Laspeyres estimate could over- or understate the true return.[15]

Value of Time Assuming Equalized Returns

Algebraic Derivation. In our discussion of the rate of return formula (10.1) thus far, the incomes Y_{it} and Y_{0t} were known with certainty and the rate of return r_i was to be determined. Using the same formula, we can fix the rate of return at r_m and, given Y_{0t}, let the Y_{it} be determined.

This process is made possible by imposing the rule that the markup is a constant proportion:

$$Y_{it} = (1 + d_i) Y_{0t}, \qquad t = n, \ldots, T \qquad (10.3)$$

during the postinvestment period, given that the residency period is n years, $0, 1, \ldots, n - 1$. The markup factor, d_i, is the proportion by which specialty income is to exceed base income. Substituting in (10.1), and ignoring work life differences for simplicity,[16] we have

$$\sum_{t=0}^{n-1} (Y_{it} - Y_{0t})(1 + r_m)^{-t} + \sum_{t=n}^{T} ((1 + d_i)Y_{0t} - Y_{0t})(1 + r_m)^{-t} = 0 \quad (10.4)$$

which, with rearranging, yields

$$d_i \sum_{t=n}^{T} Y_{0t} (1 + r_m)^{-t} = \sum_{t=0}^{n-1} (Y_{0t} - Y_{it})(1 + r_m)^{-t} \qquad (10.5)$$

The right-hand side is simply the present value of the opportunity cost of training, call it $PVOC_i$, and the summation on the left-hand side is the present value of base specialty income in the postinvestment period, call it PVY_{0n}. Solving,

$$d_i = PVOC_i / PVY_{0n} \qquad (10.6)$$

Retracing our steps, d_i is that markup factor, which, when used to determine specialty income relative to the base, allows a fixed rate of return r_m to specialty training. We will show markup factors that are computed with the specialty-specific rates of return first; then we impose a common r_m and show the resulting markups and ASTs. First, however, we review how this calculation was made in the RBRVS.

Comparisons with RBRVS Methodology. The formula underlying Hsiao's methodology is similar to (10.6) but different in an important way. Hsiao calculates markup factors using the following formula:

$$d_s = PVOC_i/PVY_i \qquad (10.7)$$

where PVY_i is the present value of income in the investment specialty, not the base specialty.[17] The substitution of the present value of specialty income for the present value of base income in the denominator will lead to substantially smaller markup factors for specialties with relatively high incomes. Furthermore, the markup factor d_s calculated by (10.7) has no basis in theory. The human capital literature emphasizes the *comparison* of earnings streams in the individual's choice set. Using current specialty income as a base and adding some factor related to the costs of training involves some double counting. The specialty profile already incorporates, in the human capital sense, a return on the investment. The difference can be seen in figure 10–1, which is shaded to show the costs of the investment in the early years. The d_s factor is an allowable benefit that should be approximately where the market-determined benefit is currently shown. Equation (10.7) suggests that we start on top of the shaded benefit area.

The Hsiao approach can be compared with an amortization process. Amortizing training costs over current specialty income does not take into account the fact that specialty income already incorporates some return to that training. Their technique is really a "second-stage" amortization over a fully amortized base (if one accepts current rates of return), which will naturally lead to a smaller markup factor than the appropriate "single-stage" markup over the true base.

Since the ultimate products of their calculations are the AST factors, which are defined as

$$AST_s = \frac{1 + d_s}{1 + d_{GS}} - 1 \qquad (10.8)$$

where the markup factor in the denominator is that for general surgery, it may seem that any underestimation of the appropriate markup factors will more or less cancel out because both numerator

269

and denominator are too small. This is not the case. When we recalculated the AST_i using markup factors calculated with the correct d_i from (10.6) (using GPFPs as the base), but otherwise using opportunity costs, incomes, and retirement ages that Hsiao and others used to obtain their d_s and AST_s, we obtained a range of AST_i factors from .1120 (thoracic surgery) to $-.045$ (family practice).[18] This range of variation is about 150 percent larger than their range of .05 to $-.01$. Thus we conclude that their calculations substantially compact the true relative values of physician time when specialty training costs are amortized.

Another assumption made by Hsiao and others is that average incomes would grow by 6 percent per year. In conjunction with the 9 percent financial rate of return they allow, the effective real rate of return r_m they employ is $(1.09/1.06) - 1$, or about 2.83 percent. It is questionable whether the growth rate of income should be employed if the base specialty income grows at the same rate; however, 2.83 percent approximates the traditional 3 percent real rate of return to capital that is often a benchmark. We note these assumptions mainly for comparison with our findings about actual real rates of return to specialty training.

Also note that Hsiao and others use earnings of general internists as the alternative in the fourth and later years of training for medical subspecialists and general surgeon earnings for some surgical subspecialists. This would be appropriate only if a *marginal* rate of return to subspecialty training were being calculated or imposed, in which case the generalist earnings should be the alternative throughout the entire working life.

In order to calculate an *average* rate of return to the entire residency, however, or to calculate a *single* markup factor or AST to be applied to a consistent base, it is appropriate to use base specialty earnings as the alternative earnings during the entire residency, including subspecialty training. This procedure is consistent with a once-and-for-all specialty choice among specialty alternatives faced by medical students. The opportunity costs in table 10–1 are calculated in this way.

Our methods for comparing earnings streams in the different specialties are not too different from those of Hsiao and others. Where there are differences, however, the human capital approach to measurement problems generates a larger potential markup or amortized cost adjustment factor. The next section presents the size of these differences.

Markup Factors and Amortized Costs of Training. The construction of AST factors begins with the selection of a specialty to use as the "numeraire," the denominator in equation (10.8). Although relative values should ultimately be transparent to this choice, we used general internists as the numeraire instead of general surgeons because there appears to be free entry into this specialty and the likelihood of rents creating a scaling problem for the ASTs seemed small. At the end of this section, however, we repeat some calculations using general surgery as the numeraire to facilitate comparisons with the RBRVS results.

Table 10–3 shows the markup factors, expressed as percentages, that would have to be applied to average base specialty earnings in order to amortize the opportunity costs of specialty training over the working life of the specialist, employing specialty-specific average rates of return. Labor supply adjustments to these markup factors result in changes similar to those seen in the internal rates of return based on relative hours of work in residency and practice. In each case, the variations are quite large. The Paasche scenario provides the greatest variation in the value of time presented in this discussion—from 5.3 percent for GPFPs to 130.1 percent for ophthalmologists. This scenario implies that the time of surgical subspecialists of all types, as well as anesthesiologists, is more than twice as valuable as that of GPFPs and pediatricians.

Also shown in table 10–3 are the AST adjustments relative to general internal medicine that would result from markup factors. The figures in the Paasche scenario range from −8.9 percent for GPFPs to 99.0 percent for ophthalmologists, and are quite similar to those in the other two scenarios, although individual specialties can differ. Relative to general surgery, the total range is −42.3 percent to 25.9 percent. This spread of 68 percent is more than ten times larger than that used by the RBRVS.

The ASTs in table 10–2 do not impose equal returns to specialty training in different areas. Table 10–4, however, shows variations in the value of physician time that would be justifiable assuming 5 percent and 10 percent returns to residency training in *any* field. For yearly earnings at 5 percent, the AST increases by about 3–4 percent per year of training beyond the three years for general internists, and at 10 percent it is about 6–7 percent per extra year of training. It ranges from −0.6 percent for GPFPs to 16.4 percent for the long surgical subspecialists at the 5 percent rate of return, and −1.5 percent to 31.1 percent at the 10 percent rate of return.

At these fixed rates of return, labor supply adjustments increase the range of variation among the specialties, and the Paasche adjustments are larger than the Laspeyres adjustments. At 5 percent, the

271

TABLE 10–3

SPECIALTY TRAINING ADJUSTMENT FACTORS NECESSARY TO ACHIEVE
ACTUAL INTERNAL RATE OF RETURN

(percent)

Specialty	Yearly Earnings		Laspeyres Adjustment		Paasche Adjustment	
	Markup	AST	Markup	AST	Markup	AST
General/family practice	5.3	−9.6	5.1	−8.8	5.3	−8.9
General internal medicine	16.5	—	15.3	—	15.6	—
Medical subspecialties	57.0	34.7	58.9	37.9	59.5	37.9
General surgery	67.7	43.9	82.3	58.1	82.8	58.1
Ophthalmology	95.9	68.2	126.6	96.6	130.1	99.0
Other surgical subspecialties (0–5 years in residency)	127.9	95.7	124.6	94.8	123.1	92.9
Other surgical subspecialties (6+ years in residency)	105.0	76.0	120.0	90.8	110.7	82.2
Pediatrics	7.4	−7.8	7.5	−6.7	7.9	−6.7
Obstetrics/ gynecology	76.5	51.5	64.3	42.5	64.9	42.5
Radiology	69.4	45.4	94.6	68.8	93.8	67.6
Psychiatry	18.3	1.6	41.0	22.4	40.9	21.9
Anesthesiology	87.6	61.0	111.7	83.6	111.1	82.5
Pathology	40.8	20.8	95.9	69.9	99.1	72.1

NOTE: For board-certified physicians, with the proportions female and self-employed set to the AMA SMS sample means, and adjusted for the probability of being in practice for each year through age seventy-five. Markup corresponds to d_i in the text. Computation of AST uses general internal medicine as the reference specialty.

SOURCE: Authors' calculations.

Laspeyres range is −0.6 percent to 20.2 percent, and the Paasche range is −1.9 percent (with pathologists now the lowest) to 27.7 percent; at 10 percent, the ranges are −1.0 percent to 38.0 percent for the Laspeyres case and −1.3 percent to 52.2 percent for the Paasche case.

To facilitate comparison with the Hsiao and others study, in table

TABLE 10–4

AMORTIZED SPECIALTY TRAINING ADJUSTMENT FACTORS
NECESSARY TO ACHIEVE STANDARD RATES OF RETURN
TO SPECIALTY TRAINING

(percent)

Specialty	Yearly Earnings 5%	Yearly Earnings 10%	Laspeyres Adjustment 5%	Laspeyres Adjustment 10%	Paasche Adjustment 5%	Paasche Adjustment 10%
General/family practice	−0.6	−1.5	−0.6	−1.0	−0.7	−1.3
General internal medicine	0	0	0	0	0	0
Medical subspecialties	8.5	14.2	7.8	14.4	8.2	15.2
General surgery	6.6	12.8	9.0	16.6	12.4	22.5
Ophthalmology	6.7	12.5	9.0	16.6	17.1	30.9
Other surgical subspecialties (0–5 years in residency)	6.7	12.5	9.0	16.6	13.7	24.9
Other surgical subspecialties (6+ years in residency)	16.4	31.1	20.2	38.0	27.7	52.2
Pediatrics	4.7	8.2	4.9	8.7	6.3	11.2
Obstetrics/gynecology	2.4	4.9	4.1	7.4	5.9	10.7
Radiology	3.2	6.7	0.4	0.9	−1.2	−1.8
Psychiatry	3.0	5.5	1.2	2.4	0.0	0.2
Anesthesiology	1.2	4.1	3.2	5.8	3.8	6.0
Pathology	2.7	6.3	−0.2	−0.1	−1.9	−3.2

NOTE: For board-certified physicians, with the proportions female and self-employed set to SMS sample means, and adjusted for the probability of being in practice for each year through age seventy-five. Computation of AST uses general internal medicine as the reference specialty.
SOURCE: Authors' calculations.

10–5 we present AST factors computed with a 2.83 percent rate of return and with general surgeons as the numeraire specialty. In general, the range of adjustment factors is more than twice as large in our study, with significantly smaller adjustments for GPFPs and general internists, which we calculated at −5.2 percent and −4.3 percent, respectively, in comparison with −1 percent for both in Hsiao and others. The highest adjustment is 6.9 percent for surgical subspecialists with six or more years of training, compared with 5 percent for thoracic surgeons in their study. These groups do not

TABLE 10–5
COMPARISONS OF AST ADJUSTMENT FACTORS COMPUTED RELATIVE TO
GENERAL SURGERY
(percent)

Specialty	Hsiao et al. Result	Yearly Earnings	Laspeyres Adjustment	Paasche Adjustment
General/family practice	−1	−5.2	−6.5	−8.7
General internal medicine	−1	−4.3	−6.1	−8.1
Medical subspecialties	3	2.2	−0.8	−2.8
General surgery	0	0	0	0
Ophthalmology	−1	0.3	0	3.1
Other surgical subspecialties (0–5 years in residency)	0, −1	0.3	0	0.8
Other surgical subspecialties (6+ years in residency)	5	6.9	7.4	9.9
Pediatrics	0	−1.0	−2.7	−3.9
Obstetrics/gynecology	−1	−2.9	−3.3	−4.2
Radiology	−1	−2.6	−5.8	−8.9
Psychiatry	1	−2.3	−5.3	−8.1
Anesthesiology	−1	−4.3	−3.6	−5.6
Pathology	0	−3.0	−6.2	−9.4

NOTE: See William C. Hsiao, Peter Braun, Nancy L. Kelly, and Edmund R. Becker, "Results, Potential Effects, and Implementation Issues of the Resource-Based Relative Value Scale," *Journal of the American Medical Association*, vol. 260, no. 16 (October 28, 1988), pp. 2429–38. Hsiao et al. use 2.83 percent rate of return.
SOURCE: Authors' calculations.

differ greatly because we used a different method to calculate their opportunity costs, as decribed earlier. If we had used general surgeons' earnings as the alternative in the final two years of training, this adjustment would have been substantially larger. The opportunity cost we use is the correct one in this context.

Conclusions

This study presents new, detailed estimates for the value of physician time that are of general interest in the analysis of physician manpower issues and could be used in a resource-based relative value scale. We have benefited from access to detailed survey data on physician earnings and hours worked both during residency training and in practice. In addition, the perspective of labor economics, particularly the human capital approach to earnings variations, provided us with a vast literature from which to draw methods for studying this problem. We also had the resources to focus attention on what was a small but important part of the development of the Hsiao resource-based relative value scale.

Equilibrium in the Labor Market—Ability and Amenities Considered. Table 10–2 documents the wide range of returns to investments in graduate medical education in different specialty-specific skills. We now turn to some economic explanations of these differences. Beginning with Adam Smith, economists have expected wages to differ by amounts that would equalize the monetary and nonmonetary advantages or disadvantages among work activities and among workers themselves. Others have pointed out that prices play a large role in achieving equilibrium in labor markets as in all markets, the main difference being that the equilibrium in a labor market "achieves a matching and sorting function of allocating or assigning specific workers to specific firms."[19] Sensitivity to the special character of labor market equilibrium helps put our results into perspective.

The neoclassical view of wage differences under competition would suggest that if all physicians had identical tastes and talents and all practice opportunities had the same characterisitics, then each physician would earn the same wages. Observed variations in wage rates could be associated with different amounts of human capital investment, other worker characteristics, and differences in the characteristics of physicians' practices. In this context, should the rate of return to different human capital investments be equalized? The neoclassical response is that, *on the margin,* total returns should be equal in markets with free entry and exit in long-run equilibrium.

The key qualifiers are who is *on the margin* and how to measure *total returns.* The sorting of physicians into specialties involves inframarginal workers whose above-average returns can be viewed as rents accruing to their unique abilities. Alternatively, the market could be viewed as encompassing important nonmonetary factors that obscure real returns when only monetary factors are observed.

The results presented in this discussion and the literature cited relate to the average monetary returns to investments in human capital, not marginal total returns. The large differences in rates of return among the specialities examined are not necessarily evidence of barriers to entry into the specialties with high returns, although

275

we could not rule out this explanation. We sought an empirical test of the existence of entry barriers in the specialties but were unsuccessful in developing a feasible strategy. High monetary returns could signify low nonmonetary returns to work (as explained below). We considered measuring the ease of entry by observing the number of frustrated potential entrants—that is, by using data from the National Resident Matching Program (NRMP) to measure the size of queues for training programs in different specialties. But such an approach is not likely to succeed. The NRMP covers only a fraction, albeit a large one, of all residency positions, and its coverage varies by specialty.

In addition, we could not ignore the effect of unmeasurable dimensions of ability. These could play an important role in several specialties. In surgery, for example, some procedures are particularly difficult, and in the more "scientific" specialties like radiology and pathology only a subset of all physicians could achieve minimal competence. Coupled with the hypothesized sorting of workers in the long-run equilibrium, unmeasured ability differences could easily account for large swings in average measured returns.

Other things being equal, unpleasant working conditions will be associated with higher earnings. Are the specialties with high measured rates of return also those with the most dissatisfied physicians? Preliminary work on reported satisfaction levels of young physicians suggests that anesthesiologists are among the most dissatisfied physicians and that in general there is a negative correlation between physician income and some measures of satisifaction. Are the low average returns to training in pediatrics a result of the satisfaction derived from providing well-baby care? We do not know, nor do we now have a feasible empirical strategy to resolve the issue.

In summary, there are substantial variations in the rate of return to investments in human capital in the several specialties examined in this study. Differences in the average rates of return to specialty training are not, however, inconsistent with long-run equilibrium in the market for physician services or physician labor. Differences in the ability of inframarginal workers and variations in the amenities of practice are consistent with the sorting and matching that are to be expected in labor market analyses. We cannot, however, rule out disequilibrium explanations for our results. Some of the specialties that are associated with high return on investment are on no list of candidates for barriers to entry (for example, pathology), but others appear to have significant queues for first-year residency slots. There is no straightforward empirical test to disentangle this issue.[20]

Policy Considerations beyond the Economics. Whether we believe that measured differences in the returns to training in physician specialties represent equalizing differences and the long-run equilibrium or reflect anticompetitive barriers to entry is irrelevant to the policy debate under way. The implication of the RBRVS study is that payment differentials should be associated with the amounts of human capital invested but *that there should not be differential rates of return* to training investments in different specialties.

Which rate of return represents a politically acceptable level? Our suggestion for the benchmark specialty would be the return to investments in general internal medicine. This specialty and pediatrics display the characteristics that even a skeptic would expect to observe under free entry. Between 1980–1981 and 1987–1988 the number of first-year residency places in internal medicine training programs increased by 5.1 percent and positions in pediatrics went up 3.3 percent, whereas the total number of first-year places declined 3.8 percent. Neither specialty is known for its high earnings potential. The large percentage of women in pediatrics and the difficulty in differentiating returns to human capital investments from potential sexual discrimination suggest that general internal medicine (11.8–15.2 percent) provides the better benchmark rate of return for policy calculations.

Our approach to measuring the opportunity costs of training in different specialities generated estimates that are similar to those of the RBRVS study. Our construction of equalization factors, amortized values of specialty training, did not. We developed an alternative view of the markup factor and the amortized value of training that was based on the human capital approach. The results from this approach indicate that much larger adjustments are warranted as a return to the investments of forgone earnings and leisure time of resident physicians.

These adjustments (ASTs) were developed on the assumption that policy makers are committed to equalizing average monetary returns to specialty-specific investments. That is a policy decision, not an economic one. Similarly, the use of these ASTs is driven more by policy concerns than economic ones. The economics of their derivation, however, suggests that the AST is relevant as an adjuster for the value of physician time, not the nontime inputs in the production of physician services.

Appendix A: Literature Review

Our study is based on a review of the literature developed since World War II on analyzing physician incomes. One of the original studies of variations in physician earnings found physician incomes in 1929–1934 to be 16.5 percent higher than those of dentists after adjusting for differences in investment costs.[21] Subsequent studies using 1955–1965 data and 1966 data reported substantial profits to investment in medical training, even at a 10 percent discount rate.[22]

These studies ignored the labor-leisure choices associated with choice of a profession. Lindsay contended that income comparisons must be adjusted for differences in hours of work across professions, and he reexamined the three studies mentioned above in that light.[23] His adjustments significantly reduced the apparent profitability of medical training in each study, but generally did not eliminate it. In a study of 1969 earnings data Mennemeyer found that physicians continued to have a higher rate of return to training than any other profession, not adjusting for hours differences, but that dentists had equivalent or higher hours-adjusted rates of return.[24]

A more recent calculation of internal rates of return for physicians, dentists, and lawyers, relative to college graduates, for the 1967–1980 period (both adjusted and unadjusted for hours of work differences) found unadjusted rates of return for general practitioners were in the 16–19 percent range for this period, while adjusted rates were 12–15 percent, both without strong indications of a trend. Rates of return for all physicians were approximately 2–3 percent lower. Lawyers had much lower rates of return, generally 6–7 percent, and dentists were comparable to physicians, with 14–16 percent rates of return, both adjusted and unadjusted.[25]

All of the above studies, aside from Mennemeyer's, construct the net present value of income solely from average income (mean or median) in a single year, assuming that income is constant over one's entire working life. Hsiao and others followed this procedure with the addition of a constant growth factor. When calculating a rate of return to training, this method is deficient in two major ways. First, income is decidedly not constant over one's working life—expected physician income almost doubles between the initial years of practice and the peak earning years. The shapes of the earnings profiles, and differences in these shapes across professions, can have important effects on net present value and rate of return calculations. (The Mennemeyer study addresses this problem, although in a limited way. Mennemeyer also took pains to estimate retirement and mortality differentials.) Second, the use of cross-sectional rather than longitudinal data to construct expected earnings profiles results in an earnings structure that may represent the current state of the profession, but does not truly reflect the rate of return to training for any given individual or cohort. Economy-wide or industry-specific pro-

278

ductivity growth can cause a cross-sectional age-earnings profile to appear flatter than an individual's expected profile would be. Because our work is based on cross-sectional data, we are able to address the first criticism effectively but not the second. Unfortunately, longitudinal data on physician incomes have not been collected.

In previous work, we investigated the changing returns to medical education during 1974–1985 and estimated returns to specialty training in each of twelve broadly defined and exhaustive specialty categories.[26] In that study, we applied Lindsay's hours adjustment model to the choice of medicine versus baccalaureate education, but we undertook no hours adjustment in our analysis of specialty training investments. Our results were qualitatively similar to those of other studies that used hours adjustments. Medicine remained a profitable investment in human capital but the returns were not extraordinary (approximately 16 percent in 1985). This study extends our previous work by reestimating returns to specialty training with more recent data and paying careful attention to the hours adjustment across specialties.

Appendix B: Data Sources

This appendix provides background information on the cross-sectional and longitudinal data that were used in this study.

Surveys of Resident Physicians. In 1983 and again in 1987 the AMA undertook mail surveys of random samples of resident physicians.[27] The questionnaire collected individual physicians' responses to items such as salary, hours, types of work, working conditions, and educational indebtedness. These samples were pooled and used in the regression analysis of yearly and hourly earnings and yearly hours worked during the residency stage of the physician's career.

Socioeconomic Monitoring System (SMS). The AMA Socioeconomic Monitoring System (SMS) is an ongoing telephone survey of physicians that collects data on the characteristics of medical practice and health policy issues related to patient care. This system produces a stratified random sample of nonfederal patient care physicians, excluding resident physicians. The core survey collects data from approximately 4,000 physicians, and the autumn survey collects data from approximately 2,800 physicians. The SMS collects individual physicians' responses to a variety of questions, including hours spent in different practice activities and annual net income from medical practice. These data can be used to analyze the pattern of earnings in different specialties. For this study, we pooled the respondents from three SMS surveys: fall 1987, spring 1988, and fall 1988. Average hours and earnings by specialty for this pooled sample are shown in table 10–1.

AMA/ERF Survey of Young Physicians. The earnings of physicians in the first years in practice are a key element in determining the returns to specialty training. This is particularly true for those physicians who undertake the minimum amount of residency training. In order to improve the precision of our estimates of earnings for these early years, we added to the SMS data results of a survey of young physicians conducted as part of the AMA/ERF Study of the Practice Patterns of Young Physicians funded by the Robert Wood Johnson Foundation. This survey collected data similar to the SMS data from a group of 6,000 young physicians (who had been in practice for two to six years and were younger than forty). The additional information on the early years in practice represents a significant improvement over previous estimates of the returns to specialty training.

Physician Masterfile (Retirement and Mortality). Established in 1906, the AMA Physician Masterfile contains current data for all physicians in the United States, including both members and nonmembers of the association. The Masterfile contains a variety of data on each physician, including his or her age, sex, medical school, year of medical school graduation, licensure, specialty, specialty board certification, place of practice, type of practice, and current mailing address. Much of the information in the Masterfile comes from the census of Physicians' Professional Activities, a mail survey of all physicians in the United States that has been conducted every four years since 1969. Between census years, a weekly update system keeps the Masterfile current. We used historical files for each individual to identify which physicians retired or died during 1970–1986. These data were used to estimate multivariate retirement and mortality equations.[28] The earnings and hours streams estimated with the cross-sectional data are adjusted to reflect expected work life in the different specialties.

Appendix C: Markup Factor Formulas

This appendix details the calculation of markup factors d_i shown in table 10–4 in the case using annual earnings adjusted for the probability of being in practice. If r_m is the mandated rate of return to

280

specialty training investments, then the goal is to determine an income path Y_{it} that provides this rate of return. Thus, we must solve

$$\sum_{t=0}^{T} P_{it}Y_{it}\,(1 + r_m)^{-t} = \sum_{t=0}^{T} P_{0t}Y_{0t}\,(1 + r_m)^{-t}$$

for Y_{it} under the assumption that in-practice probabilities P_{0t} and P_{it} are specific to the path chosen. Furthermore, separate these into the investment period, years $0, \ldots, n - 1$, and postinvestment years n, $\ldots, T$, and rearrange.

$$\sum_{t=0}^{T} (P_{0t}Y_{0t} - P_{it}Y_{it})(1 + r_m)^{-t} = \sum_{t=n}^{T} (P_{it}Y_{it} - P_{0t}Y_{0t})(1 + r_m)^{-t}$$

The left-hand side expression is the present value of the opportunity cost of the investment, henceforth $PVOC_i$.

If Y_{it} is defined as a fixed percentage above Y_{0t} during the postinvestment period

$$Y_{it} = (1 + d_i)Y_{0t}, \qquad t = n, \ldots, T$$

we can substitute for Y_{it}:

$$PVOC_i = \sum_{t=n}^{T}(P_{it}(1 + d_i)Y_{0t} - P_{0t}Y_{0t})(1 + r_m)^{-t}$$

$$= d_i \sum_{t=n}^{T} P_{it}Y_{0t}(1 + r_m)^{-t} + \sum_{t=n}^{T}(P_{it} - P_{0t})Y_{0t}(1 + r_m)^{-t}$$

and solve for d_i:

$$d_i = [PVOC_i - \sum_{t=n}^{T} (P_{it} - P_{0t})Y_{0t}(1 + r_m)^{-t}] / \sum_{t=n}^{T} P_{it}Y_{0t}(1 + r_m)^{-t}$$

Observations on the Value of Physician Work Time

A Commentary by Jody L. Sindelar

Marder and Willke add much to our knowledge of the market for physicians. The wealth of data they provide and the care they have taken in structuring the empirical analysis give us considerable insight into the earnings of physicians and the rate of return (ROR) to different specialties. The raw data indicate that there is great variation not only in the mean level of income by specialty, but also in the standard deviation across specialties (this could, however, be due to their aggregation of several specialties into a few broad categories). Further, there is quite a range of average hours worked by specialty, from a low of slightly more than 2,400 hours per year for ophthalmologists to a high of 3,045 hours per year for obstetricians/gynecologists. There is more variation, however, in income within specialty.

Marder and Willke find substantial variations in the raw rates of return (ROR) by specialty and also in the ROR after controlling for the several factors (for example, board certification, percentage female, and self-employment). ROR calculations here refer primarily to monetary aspects of ROR, which are calculated on the basis of amortizing income over the base of the opportunity cost of residency.

A thorny problem in calculating rates of return is that hours worked may be endogenous (we return to this issue later). Whether hours worked are endogenous or exogenous should imply different methods for calculating rate of return. To handle this problem, Marder and Willke calculate ROR using a variety of assumptions. Their results range from a low of 1 percent for pediatrics to highs of 39 percent for anesthesiology and 58 percent for pathology.

The variation by specialty may be due to barriers to entry in a specialty; limitations on substitution among specialists and across physician versus nonphysician personnel; supply constraints, including age at which skills atrophy; riskiness of the occupation; and compensating variation due to a variety of working conditions, including irregularity of hours, the type of patients one treats (for example, geriatric versus pediatric), and so on. Self-selection may also play a role. Dranove and Satterthwaite point out only one of the many types of self-selection: self-selection by ability into specialties.

If the variations in returns across specialty are surprising, the levels of returns are startling. In previous studies of returns to education in general, RORs have been estimated to decline with increased years of education. Typically, there is a relatively high rate of return to finishing high school, a smaller return to college, and an even lower rate of return to a Ph.D. Yet, in the case of additional training for physicians across specialties, this relationship does not appear to hold. It does hold, interestingly, within specialty. That is, in those specialties where one could have either four or five years of residency beyond the basic training, for example, the rate of return within specialty declines with additional years. But it does not decline from the base specialty to progressively longer residency, as one might expect.

Results from the Marder and Willke chapter raise several interesting questions: why is the return to specialty training so high, and why do we not see the normal decline in ROR that occurs with additional education? Although the chapter does not attempt to answer these questions, the empirical results can perhaps give insights into these issues. The results indicate, for example, that women are paid less and those self-employed are paid more, other things being equal. The magnitude and the significance of these effects, however, differ by specialty. These findings are consistent with differences in self-selection, barriers to entry, or compensating wage differentials by specialty. Further examination of earnings regressions and inquiry into how and why there are variations in income by characteristics of the physician could prove to be informative.

Technical Issues

The concepts behind calculations of both the ROR to training and the "markup" for a relative value scale are fairly straightforward and simple. The implementation, however, is not. In particular, choices have to be made on how to conduct the calculations given the constraints imposed by the data, and the choices must reflect the underlying theory.

Cross-Sectional Data. The most appropriate data for calculating

RORs of specialties would be longitudinal data that follow specific individuals over their lifetimes. Only cross-sectional data are available, however. Thus, one must use cross-sectional data to mimic longitudinal data. By using a cross section of individuals of various ages, one basically assumes that young physicians will learn and earn like older physicians in the same specialty. One relies on a "synthetic cohort" to yield reasonable estimates. Yet it may be incorrect to assume that today's young physicians will earn and work like today's older physicians because of changing social factors (for example, labor force participation of spouses), market, and policy factors (for example, managed care, diagnosis-related groups, and health maintenance organizations). Further, specialties may vary systematically in the extent to which older cohorts are representative of younger cohorts (for example, in some specialties advances in technology may obviate the need for some skills more rapidly than in other specialties).

The problems of cross-sectional data are obvious, and unfortunately they are unavoidable as no large sample longitudinal data exist suitable for these purposes. While use of synthetic cohorts is unavoidable, outside information could perhaps be used to give guidance as to the direction of the potential biases introduced both for ROR calculations in general and for potential biases by specialties.

Length of Training and of Amortization Period. Marder and Willke argue that the point at which the base and specialty earnings paths cross is, in theory, the appropriate place to think of as the end of the opportunity costs and the beginning of the net positive earnings period for specialties. Although they calculated RORs using this crossover point, they estimated the markup and AST factors in a slightly different way—by using the end of training as the point at which opportunity costs are assumed to stop. However, opportunity costs may extend beyond formal training. For example, the specialist may earn less immediately after training than a physician with less specialty training but more years of work experience. Thus, the crossover point and the end of the residency do not necessarily coincide. So to calculate the markups appropriately, one would want to use the crossover point but consider everything up to that point as opportunity costs, and everything after that point as returns.

The choice of the point at which costs are assumed to end changes the estimate of the opportunity costs and the amount of remaining work life over which to amortize these costs. These effects could, in principle, be important. Although there may be little difference on average between the two calculation methods, there could be some biases across specialties.

Endogenicity. Marder and Willke also address the important issue of the endogenicity of labor supply choices. As their data indicate, specialties have different average hours worked per year and different years of post-training work. The variations by specialties in hours worked per year and age of retirement may be endogenous. A shorter work life, for example, may be due to an income effect. If it is an income effect, and a choice by physicians, would the government want to amortize the physicians' training costs over the shorter work life that occurred because physicians were highly paid and had the luxury of retiring earlier? Such an increase in pay by the government would yield an even higher hourly remuneration to those already highly paid. On the other hand, if the earlier retirement is due to an exogenous factor, such as obsolescence of abilities—say, deterioration, with age, of the necessary manual dexterity—then the government's perspective may be different. So the government needs to consider the endogeneity of labor supply in determining how to structure its payment for physicians and calculate ROR. If the reasons for labor supply differentials are largely exogenous to physicians' labor supply decisions, then policy makers might want to include the differentials in their calculations. If they are endogenous, presumably they would not want pay differentials to reflect such choices.

Marder and Willke deal with this problem of endogenicity in their empirical analysis by calculating RORs with alternative assumptions about hours, giving something akin to a minimum and maximum rate of return. The empirical results suggest that the assumptions about hours matter empirically. Unfortunately, we do not yet have enough information to determine whether labor supply decisions are affected more by endogenous or exogenous factors and whether the degree of endogenicity varies systematically by specialty. Thus the alternative calculations are very useful.

Geographic Variation. One drawback of the Marder-Willke study is that no adjustment has been made for geographic regions or urban/ rural designations. Thus some bias may be built into the calculations. For example, one specialty may be more likely to locate in an urban setting than another but may have similar opportunity costs. Whether the government wants to pay a higher return to those specialties that systematically locate in an urban setting is an open question. Again, the answer may depend on whether it is a life style choice of the physician or a necessary aspect of the specialty itself.

285

Nonpecuniary Consideration. No data are available on the nonpecuniary aspects of specialties, with the exception of the number of hours worked. Thus all the calculations by Marder and Willke, like those of Hsiao, are monetary. Although calculations of nonpecuniary aspects cannot be made, discussions of these could be helpful and could point out potential biases and problems. In the literature, the discussion of nonmonetary aspects of life typically revolves around the post-training period, for example, compensating wage differentials owing to variations in prestige, riskiness, or hours of the job. Training has potentially systematically differing nonpecuniary aspects as well. One of the most obvious is the differing number of hours per week worked across specialties during residency. With diminishing marginal utility of income, the greater hours of work in some residencies would result in systematic underestimates of their nonpecuniary costs, even after controlling for hours worked. This would occur because of the nonlinearities in utility. Such factors may be important to consider in determining policy.

Applications to RBRVS Calculations

In calculating the markup factor or AST, Hsiao and others are amortizing opportunity costs over a measure of post-training work life. They use earnings by a specialty as the base. This introduces several problems, one of which is the endogeneity of hours and years of work life. That is, their base incorporates decisions on labor supply that are endogenously determined in part by the pay level. Another is that earnings include the "effort" part of "work" as well as the hours part. Hsiao and others try to differentiate between these two in their "work" calculations. By including them both in the base over which to amortize, they would underestimate the return to "high-effort" specialties. In this case, "high effort" means both more hours as well as more "effort" per hour. That is, the larger earnings base over which to amortize opportunity cost is higher because of greater stress or whatever other factors yield higher pay. By including pay for these factors in the base, Hsiao and others are violating their principle of stipulating greater returns for greater effort. According to the Hsiao formula, these physicians would be undercompensated in the new payment regime.

Thus the ASTs of Hsiao and others are not calculated appropriately and according to their own criteria. Even if the AST is calculated in a way that corresponds to an appropriate underlying theory, however, there is no obvious compelling theory that yields the multiplicative form.

Broader Relevant Policy Issues

In calculating ASTs, Hsiao and others imply that RORs across specialties should be equalized in order to mimic the market. Although this could be a mimic of the market outcome if all other factors were properly controlled for, all other factors are not controlled. Specifically, most nonpecuniary aspects of the specialties are ignored. Thus the goal of equalized monetary returns is not appropriately based in a market theory.

A related policy consideration is that in changing the relative payments across specialties one goal might be to increase the supply of physicians to some specialties and decrease it to others. Given the long training periods, however, even small changes in supply could take many years. It is unlikely, however, that policy makers would wait that long in their evaluation of the policy outcomes. Although the fees set to each specialty would be largely in the hands of the government, the training costs could vary over time, both by changes in specialty patterns and by related government policies (for example, the move in New York to restrict the hours worked by residents). Thus the AST would have to be recalibrated as secular changes take place in the residencies. To coordinate the changes in residency with the changes in pay—both to reward the appropriate cohort and to bring forth the appropriate supply—would be very difficult.

11
Fee Schedules and Utilization

Mark V. Pauly

No one is happy with the current method of determining what Medicare will pay toward the cost of physician services. The current customary, prevailing, and reasonable (CPR) system pays different amounts for the same service to different physicians. More to the point, it does not yield price levels that bring forth a set of services we know to be appropriate at costs we know are minimized. Although there are many who believe that the current system is not right, and although it is easy to criticize it, no one is quite sure what would represent a better alternative. One possibility is to have *relative* payments for different services based largely on the amount of time a procedure typically takes, with some ad hoc adjustments for subjectively evaluated complexity and possibly for training time. This approach is embodied in the resource-based relative value system (RBRVS).[1]

In this chapter, I wish to explore some of the possible consequences of implementing an RBRVS-based system and alternative systems for setting Medicare payment levels. A special concern is the possible impact of RBRVS, and other systems, on the volume of physicians' services of different types. Perhaps not surprisingly, there will be considerable ambiguity about what those impacts will be, and even more ambiguity about whether any given impact can be judged to be an improvement over the current state of affairs. I therefore also explore a kind of "reverse spin" by asking what assumptions about objectives, physician behavior, and patient behavior *would* lead to the greatest likelihood that RBRVS will improve matters.

Doctors may accept Medicare payments as payment in full for 80 percent of their total charge, or they may choose to bill the patient for more than the 20 percent coinsurance. That is, they may accept

I am grateful to Ted Frech and John Eisenberg for helpful comments. Background research for this chapter was supported by Health Care Financing Administration grant number 99-C-99169/5-01. All opinions expressed are those of the author.

assignment or may decline assignment. A complex relationship exists between what Medicare pays, the price the doctor receives, and the price the patient pays out of pocket. In the first part of the chapter, I will consider the case of doctors who accept assignment and who sell to patients who do not pay the copayment out of pocket. The effect of RBRVS and other payment policies for doctors who "balance bill" will be treated later, as will the effect of beneficiary payment of the copayment.

Objectives for the Physician Payment System

The original design of the Medicare payment system was based on the notion that Medicare should reimburse in a way that would just allow the beneficiary to pay the going price in the market for doctor services. That concept has eroded over time, in part because in many markets Medicare is the 800-pound gorilla, unable (even if it wanted to) to leave the market as it found it. In larger part, the gorilla has become more and more dissatisfied with the amount and type and cost of the bananas it is being supplied and has taken steps to unlink itself from a market it feels is not doing what it wishes.

But what is the objective behind physician payment strategies Medicare has tried to pursue? There has been a vacillation between two concepts of what the objectives of payment ought to be. In some respects, Medicare appears to adopt a government contract pespective, imagining that there is some set of medical services it wants to buy (and distribute to Medicare beneficiaries). It wants to buy the right quantity and quality of those services (where quality includes, among other things, "access"), at the lowest possible price.

The paradigm for accomplishing this task is bidding; in an idealized setting, bidding permits a buyer who does not initially know what the lowest cost for some service is or which sellers can produce at that cost to identify both pieces of information.[2] Although real world bidding arrangements may not be perfect, they may be good enough for government work.

The most serious challenge for implementing bidding-type arrangements for Medicare assignment would be the necessity, finally and at long last, that someone specify exactly what it is that Medicare wants to buy. The Health Care Financing Administration (HCFA) would have to take the responsibility of saying how much care is appropriate, for how many beneficiaries, and with what degree of quality and ease of access. Specifying how much implies, of course, that you also say how much is too much, and why.

Once having specified, say, how many lens replacements for

cataracts it wants to buy from how many doctors at what locations, Medicare could simply accept the lowest set of bids consistent with this specification. Or, more realistically, the result could be approximated by gradually reducing the current fee levels until the level of services offered, the level of quality, and the conditions of access meet the specified objectives.

In the past, policy makers have frequently suggested that the volume and intensity of care doctors provide for Medicare patients is inappropriately high. It is relatively easy to blame doctors for providing services that are possibly inappropriate, especially when the standard of appropriateness is flexible. It is a much more daunting task for the HCFA to take the responsibility itself for specifying defensible limitations to the aggregate use and quality of care.

Information on the effectiveness of services, which is currently the subject of a great deal of research, is a necessary but not a sufficient condition for implementing a bidding-type system. In cases where bidding would seem eminently feasible and desirable, as in the case of laboratory tests, Medicare has not yet been able to get a system under way. Nevertheless, a bidding system serves as a benchmark of a system that could bring about whatever level of volume and intensity that Medicare desires, and at minimum cost. I will comment later on the possibilities for approximating a bidding system in practice. For the present, it serves as a standard, both for the HCFA and for providers, to which RBRVS or any other system may be compared.

An alternative concept is that the objective of physician payment should be to achieve *incentive neutrality*. Rather than specify particular volume objectives, the notion here is to establish a payment system that yields a physician the same real net income regardless of what types of services are rendered. "Real net income" incorporates both net money income and the amount of time spent performing the service. The idea, then, is that the physician who cares at all about patients will choose the set of services that make the patient as well off as possible, given the knowledge the physician has and given the patient's expressed desires. Put slightly differently, with no distortive financial incentives, the physician will be presumed to act as the *perfect agent* of the patient with regard to volume and intensity, given the knowledge the doctor has of the patient's preferences. Incentive neutrality is less desirable than an ideal bidding system, but it seems to represent the less comprehensive objective of current physician payment policy.

In this sort of system, if it could be achieved, there might be no need for the HCFA to specify what *its* objectives are, since the system would automatically choose what is best for beneficiaries, as based on doctors' undistorted views. The HCFA could then declare victory in the war on Part B costs and pull out of the battle, since henceforth whatever outcome occurred would, by definition, be the right outcome. The problem is that even the incentive-neutral system is not feasible, as the following analysis demonstrates.

Relative Prices in a No-Demand-Creation World

Let us begin with a simple model of real-income-maximizing physicians who cannot or will not engage in demand creation. Instead, there is a finite quantity that patients demand of each of S Medicare services. Also for simplicity, assume that demands for the different services are independent. The physician is assumed to maximize a "real income" utility function in money income Y and leisure L:

$$U = U(Y, L)$$

The production function is given by $Q = Q_M + Q_N = g(W)$, where W is physician hours worked (equal to $24 - L$ per day), Q is total quantity, Q_M is Medicare quantity, and Q_N is non-Medicare quantity. Let P_M be the Medicare price, and let $Q_N = Q(P_N)$ be the non-Medicare demand curve as a function of the non-Medicare price. Medigap insurance is assumed to eliminate the effect of copayment. We initially assume that all physicians are participating, so that the price Medicare pays determines the price the physician gets. We also initially assume that Medicare demand for any service, though finite, is larger than the amount doctors will supply. Then equilibrium requires that the following holds for every service i:

$$P_M^i = \left(\frac{u_L}{u_Y}\right)\left(\frac{1}{g_i}\right) = MR_N^i$$

where MR_N^i, the marginal non-Medicare revenue from service i, equals

$$P_N^i + \left(\frac{\partial P_N^i}{\partial Q_N^i}\right) Q_N^i$$

This expression indicates two alternative measures of cost in equilibrium: the (money) value of the leisure that must be sacrificed to produce one unit of service and the opportunity cost of using that time to produce services for non-Medicare patients. The term $(1/g'_i)$ is the marginal time cost per unit of output that Hsiao and others estimate as part of the RBRVS project.[3]

We also need an equilibrium condition across services. We can assume that the money value of a unit of lost leisure (u_L/u_Y) is the same for all services. For every pair of services i and j, we then require that

$$\frac{P_M^i}{P_M^j} = \frac{g_j'}{g_i'} = \frac{MR^i}{MR^j}$$

This can be rewritten as

$$P_M^i g_i' = P_M^j g_j' = MR^i g_i' = MR^j g_j'$$

This equality says that Medicare price received per unit of leisure time sacrificed to produce a service must be equal across services, as must marginal private revenue per unit of time. In other words, work time must yield the same net money return per minute in all uses. This is, it should be noted, an *equilibrium* condition; in the long run it *must* hold, and in the short run the system *must* be moving toward it, if the assumptions made in the model are valid. In this equilibrium, price automatically equals cost for any Medicare service supplied in positive amounts; of course, if price equals cost it is also proportional to cost.

Note, however, that this system is implausibly unforgiving. If Medicare should set the price for some Medicare service slightly below the norm, its supply will completely disappear. If it should set some price a little too high, only that service will be supplied. It seems implausible that any real-world government payment system could be that accurate, and yet we do not see Medicare services disappearing from the market. What part of the model must we modify to add realism?

There are two possibilities. One possibility is to adjust some dimension of quality to bring about equilibrium. When Medicare underpays, the content of the service rendered to beneficiaries is adjusted until cost is made to equal price (rather than the other way around). The other possibility is to assume that Medicare beneficiaries are not willing to demand all the services that doctors are willing to supply at the posted prices. Although there is probably some quality adjustment, I suspect that there is currently an excess supply (insufficient demand) for most Medicare services for most physicians. All that excess supply means here is that, if a Medicare beneficiary sought some additional Medicare service, most doctors would be quite willing to render it at current reimbursement levels. I believe that there is such willingness (indeed, eagerness) to supply in today's market. Conversely, if Medicare prices currently do not all bear the same relationship to time costs (the empirical premise on which the whole RBRVS process is built), there *has* to be excess supply for some services, and possibly for all services. With this modification, the new equilibrium statement is that the equilibrium equality condition must hold only for those services for which there is unsatisfied Medicare demand. For the other services, there is excess willingness to supply, and quantity is constrained by demand. We assume that for every physician, there are at least some such "excess supply" services.

Let P_M^S be the Medicare price of a service in excess supply, and P_M^E be the Medicare price of an "equilibrium" service (taking the same amount of time) for which there is excess demand or for which Medicare demand just equals supply. We now analyze the effects on volume of changing P_M^S and P_M^E. Suppose P_M^S is reduced for some service i that is in excess supply. As long as the price is not reduced below P_M^{Ei}, the conclusion is simple: There will be absolutely no effect on Medicare volume. The only consequence of a price reduction will be to reduce the income (and profit) of the physician. Whether the service is inexpensive or costly, relative to time, there is *no* volume impact. The reason is that, since the price exceeds the amount needed to bring forth enough supply to meet demand, a drop in price, although it may reduce the quantity physicians want to supply, will not cause volume to fall, since demand rather than supply determines volume.

Things are different for changes in P_M^{Ej}, the price of a service j that initially is in equilibrium or in excess demand. If the price for such a service is decreased, the volume of the service will unequivocally be decreased, since a doctor who is maximizing net real income will not supply a unit when the price falls below the marginal cost. Supply is constraining. If the price is increased, volume will increase as physicians move along their supply curves—unless demand becomes constraining. Moreover, if the Medicare price cuts reduce Medicare volume, the price in the private market will also be cut, in order to encourage larger amounts of the now more profitable private business. That is, there will be "negative cost shifting." In this case, there need be no concern that physicians will raise prices to others to make up for lower Medicare prices.

These points can be illustrated diagrammatically. We begin with the conventional model of a physician who provides services to Medicare and non-Medicare patients. In figure 11–1, the physician is assumed to face private demand curves $D(P_1^N)$ and $D(P_2^N)$ for services 1 and 2, respectively. For simplicity, we assume that each service takes the same amount of doctor time and the same level of practice

FIGURE 11-1
Effect of Price Changes on Physician Volume with Unlimited
Medicare Demand

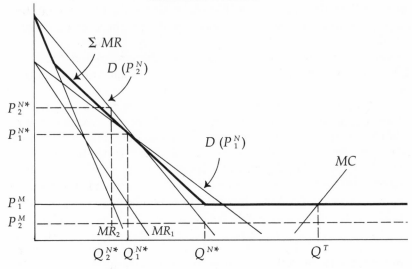

inputs. The conventional model here is one in which the public demand at the price the government sets is large enough to permit the doctor to sell as much as he wants of any service to Medicare beneficiaries.

If there were just one Medicare service with price P_1^M, and if "MC" represents the marginal cost (including the subjective value of lost leisure), the equilibrium is one in which the marginal revenue for each private service MR_1 and MR_2 is set equal to P_1^M. The private prices are those corresponding to those levels of marginal revenue, or P_1^{N*} and P_2^{N*}. The total quantity of private services is given by the intersection of a (horizontally) summed private marginal revenue curve (or the heavy line ΣMR) and P_1^M, and the total Medicare quantity is the difference between Q^{N*} and Q^T.

Now suppose there is another Medicare service with a lower price (per unit time) of P_2^M. The conclusion in the conventional model is straightforward but implausible; the doctor should supply none of this less profitable service to Medicare beneficiaries. He should concentrate instead on the more profitable service 1.

To avoid this absurd conclusion, we need to assume that there is a limit to the demand for Medicare services. If the user price is in effect zero, this limit comes from patient unwillingness to accept

294

FIGURE 11–2
The Effect of Price Changes on Physician Volume When Medicare Demand Is Limited

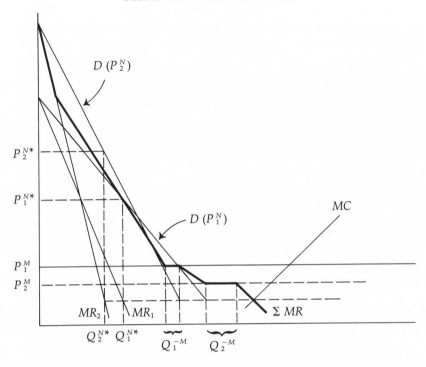

services that are uncomfortable or time-consuming. Suppose that the limits are $\overline{Q}_1^M$ and $\overline{Q}_2^M$ in figure 11–2. In setting prices and quantities, the doctor moves down the upper segment of ΣMR until MR equals P_1^M, then produces $\overline{Q}_1^M$ units, resumes movement down the next segment of ΣMR until MR falls to P_2^M, and then supplies service 2 to Medicare patients. When the Medicare demand constraint on service 2 is binding, the seller moves to the third segment of the ΣMR curve and reduces private market price until $MR_1 = MR_2 = MC$.

Now suppose that P_1^M is cut and P_2^M is increased. The overall shape of the MR curve is changed because the segments $\overline{Q}_1^M$ and $\overline{Q}_2^M$ will be moved, but the intersection of ΣMR with MC need not be changed. So there need be no change in final private market price or in quantities of Medicare or non-Medicare services. As long as Medicare's prices for both services are sufficiently high, changing those prices has no effect on private prices or on Medicare or non-Medicare quantities; only physician income is affected. The condition needed

295

for this to happen is that no Medicare price falls below equilibrium marginal private revenue.

The message, then, is that if doctors maximize real income and do not create demand, changes in prices serve only to redistribute rents for those services for which $P_M > P_M^E$. They do not affect actual resource costs, either for physician services or other services that may be complements or substitutes for those services. But for those services for which $P_M \leq P_M^E$, price cuts do reduce volume, and price increases increase volume.

A change in relative prices will have an effect in this model only if it forces price for some service down so low that it falls below the equilibrium price. But the most fundamental point this model makes is a simple one: the main problem with current Medicare prices is not that relative prices are distorted. Rather, it is that virtually all prices are just too high. The simplest strategy is to reduce all prices, regardless of their relationship to cost, and to continue doing so until shortages begin to develop. The least complicated approach would be to begin with current relative prices. Since the quantity Medicare could reasonably desire as appropriate cannot exceed demand, such a strategy moves things in the right direction. Conversely, without getting the overall price level right, there is no obvious particular merit in adjusting relative prices to any specific level.

If beneficiaries do pay coinsurance out of pocket (in contrast with what has been assumed so far), then quantities would rise for services having their prices reduced (for example, surgery) and would drop for the evaluation services having their prices increased. For people who think there should be less surgery, the message from these models will be disappointing: either there will be no change in surgery, or its rate will rise.

Adding Demand Creation—Justification and Possibilities

It is probably fair to say that the preceding model wholly misses the main rationale behind RBRVS: that is, to offer doctors different incentives in their role as agent/adviser for the patient. And these incentives will matter only if the doctor can and will affect the quantity of services patients receive, that is, if the doctor can and will create demand. In other words, physician incentives will matter only if patient demand does not wholly determine outcomes. The case for RBRVS rests foursquare on the postulate of demand creation. Without demand creation, RBRVS has no economic rationale; its only rationale is a notion of "equity" among doctors. Perhaps more important, its potential effects on volume depend on how changing relative prices will change the amount of demand that doctors are willing and able to create.

The empirical evidence for demand creation is imprecise and contradictory.[4] Demand creation is a flimsy foundation on which to rest a policy of immediate movement to an RBRVS. However "logical" it may seem, the evidence that the doctors will create demand in response to economic incentives has, in my opinion, about a fifty-fifty chance of showing any such effect, much less an effect of practical as well as statistical significance. The foundation of the case for RBRVS rests on a possibly true but unconfirmed hypothesis.

Not only is the empirical evidence weak, but even the theory behind demand effects is ambiguous. The judgments about what volumes of different services *ought* to be provided is, at base, a subjective one. In particular, the judgment that beneficiaries receive too many invasive services and too few evaluation services is still only that, a judgment. But even if one has a view of how one would want volumes to change, there is no theory to tell us unequivocally how to change relative prices to get us from here to there.

What determines whether volume will increase for services for which prices are increased and fall for those for which prices are reduced? The answer, in theory, is ambiguous. The behavioral theory used to understand demand creation is the "sophisticated target income" theory.[5] This theory imagines that a doctor suffers a subjective utility cost from manipulating information supplied to patients, but is willing to do so, up to a point, for a sufficient financial reward in terms of real net income from selling additional volume. The trade-off between the value of this subjective cost and the value of the financial reward is critical.

The ambiguity in this model comes about primarily because a price change has different theoretical effects on physician incentives to create demand. A budget-neutral cut in price has two conflicting incentives—on the one hand, the physician will want to use fewer of the services that are less profitable than before and more of the more profitable ones. This is a *substitution effect*. That is, as the profit from one service rises relative to another, net money income can be increased by inducing more of the more profitable service and less of the less profitable service. (Note that "more profitable" here is relative to the previous level of profitability; the more profitable service could still be less profitable in absolute terms than the other service.) On the other hand, if Medicare cuts the price on a service that is an important part of the doctor's total business, the price cut will cause income to fall, unless the doctor can increase demand for other services. If income falls, the physician may create demand for the new lower-priced service to get income back closer to the initial (target) level. This is an income effect. It is not possible to determine a priori which effect will predominate, and so we cannot determine whether aggregate volume will rise or fall.

Whether a given price change will increase or reduce volume depends on the degree of concentration, in the physician's practice, of the services with increased or reduced prices. The fundamental influence pushing the volume of a service up when its price is cut is an income effect. If avoiding demand inducement is a normal good, there will be less inducement for services of all types if the doctor's total income rises and, conversely, for declines in income.

To take one clear case, if relative prices are changed in such a way that the doctor's income, were he to produce the same volume, is unchanged, then we would unequivocally expect him to desire to increase the more profitable services and reduce the less profitable ones. In contrast, if a doctor's practice consists in large part of services with falling prices, the income effect toward more inducement could be strong enough to offset the dampening (substitution) effect of lower profitability. A neurosurgeon, for example, will surely recommend more office visits and other cognitive services for which the relative price rises under the Hsiao versions of RBRVS. But if these services are a small part of the doctor's total income, so that, even after they are expanded, his or her income has still fallen, then the income effect may well cause new demand creation for the invasive (surgical) services.

This is not the end of the story, of course, since consumers may not be willing to accept increases. If fees are raised for office visits, it is not obvious that consumers will be eager to accept doctor advice to make more revisits. And if they do not, then income will fall and it will be less likely that the volume of services for which prices were cut will fall.

Nevertheless, in a budget-neutral world, it remains true that volumes are most likely to move in the expected direction if each doctor's total income does not change much. Rather than redistribute income across specialties, it might be better to make specialty-specific adjustments in relative prices. (This ignores long-run manpower effects.) For instance, a reduction in surgical fees would be accompanied by a larger increase in surgeon office fees than would be true, say, for internist office visits.

But if volumes increase for some services (if in unpredictable ways) in some specialties, will they not fall for others, so at least total Medicare costs will be about the same? Maybe, but maybe not. If the services that have been reduced in price are those that tend to be concentrated in particular specialties, whereas those with increased prices tend to be diffused over all specialties, it is quite possible for aggregate volume to rise. Moreover, total Medicare costs depend not only on what happens to Part B services and expenditures, but also on what happens to complementary Part A services. If invasive procedures are more likely to be associated with inpatient care, and if some such services can rise, there is a real possibility of higher total Medicare costs after a shift to RBRVS in a budget-neutral way.

This is only a possibility, to be sure, and one that I personally would not make my pick if I had to bet on an outcome. But that is precisely the point; given current knowledge and current theory, basing prices on RBRVS is a gamble, with very high stakes.

Incentive-Neutral Fees

If we cannot tell for sure which direction volumes will follow after a change in relative prices, can we at least describe the set of fee levels we would eventually want to achieve in order to remove incentives for both demand creation and nonprice demand rationing in situations of excess demand? Advocates of RBRVS apparently imagine that getting prices proportional to relative cost is at least arguably a movement in the right direction.[6] Is this necessarily so?

To answer this question, we need to look at what would be a set of incentive-neutral prices. The first point to note is that, for net income to be independent of the volume of any particular services, it is not enough for price to be merely proportional to marginal cost: Price must be equal to marginal cost for each service. Only then will the doctor be virtually indifferent to small changes in volume.

Of course, if prices are equal to marginal cost in this competitive-like equilibrium, they are also proportional to marginal cost. But proportionality alone is not enough. If prices exceed marginal cost in an equiproportional way, that means that the financial incentive to create demand is *uniform* across procedures. But it also means that doctors have a financial incentive to deviate from perfect agency behavior by encouraging more quantity than is in the patient's true best interest.

Demand Creation—A Best-Case Scenario

There is, in general, no necessary gain from equalizing the incentive to create demand. But is there a special case in which equalizing incentives *does* help?[7]

First, we need to think about the reduction in patients' well-being caused by demand creation and about the physician's perception of that reduction. If the change in relative prices related to RBRVS works as planned, it will even out the incentives for demand creation. More demand, it is anticipated, will be created for evaluation services, and less demand will be created for invasive services. Any demand creation (in the economic sense of demand creation) reduces patient/consumer welfare. The critical normative question, then, is whether the reduction in demand creation for invasive services does enough good to offset the harm caused by more demand creation for evaluation services. Under what circumstances would there be strong reasons to believe that the gains offset the losses?

To answer this question, we obviously have to transform demand creation, in the sense of quantity deviating from the quantity that in truth maximizes the patient's welfare, into a measure of patient welfare. How this transformation occurs depends on how demand creation is limited. Demand creation by doctors can be limited either externally or internally. External limitation has been investigated by Dranove, who imagines that some consumer/patients do detect demand creation and react to it by switching doctors.[8] This behavior in turn limits the amount of profitable demand creation a doctor will undertake.

The alternative model, as noted earlier, is the sophisticated target income model in which a doctor is assumed to suffer a subjective cost when the "accuracy" of advice deviates from what the doctor regards as the most accurate advice. There are (at least) two interpretations of what generates that disutility. One is that the doctor suffers disutility in proportion to the deviation of actual advice from accurate advice, measured in a technical way.[9] That is, it is the physician's desire to provide technically correct care that imposes the subjective cost. That he is not doing what he was taught is what bothers the doctor. Another interpretation imagines that the physician cares about the level of utility the patient receives.[10] In this case, the doctor must know not only the health consequences of different therapies, but also the determinants of the patient's demand for care, such as income, insurance coverage, and time cost.

Now consider two services that require the same amount of time. Equilibrium in the sophisticated target-income story requires that the ratio of the doctor's marginal profit to marginal disutility of demand creation be equal for the two services. This implies in turn that, if one service has a higher price relative to cost than the other, it will have a higher marginal disutility than the other service.

If only substitution effects matter, and if the maginal disutility to the doctor is simply a transformation of the patient's marginal utility, then there will be a gain to the patient from an RBRVS-based equalization of profit per unit of time. The reason is that a reduction in the price of the high-priced service causes a fall in demand creation, which reduces harm to the patient's utility by a larger amount (at the margin) than the damage caused by the increase in demand creation for the services with increased prices. In short, if the doctor's disutility is the patient's utility, equalizing incentives for demand creation makes sense.

How plausible is this case? I have already suggested that it imposes a substantial information burden on the doctor. If he makes decisions only in terms of health effects on patients, then a budget-neutral change in relative prices need not improve patient utility. For instance, doctors may view "hard sell" suggestions for many repeat office visits or benign tests as not harmful to the patient's health. But such services, because of their time cost, may well be of high subjective cost to the patient, higher than the utility cost of invasive services.

Of course, if doctors must guess about nonhealth "costs," but do nevertheless take them into account, this only leads to noise in the prediction about the patient utility consequences of price-induced demand creation. It will still be true that, *on the average*, the marginal effect on patient utility will be greater for services with a high profit.

This approach has a serious implication for procedures rendered to people with Medigap coverage that cannot do harm and that have no time cost. Clinical laboratory tests of specimens already drawn, for example, would fall into this category. Demand for such services will be pushed out as far as is possible. Doctors will, the model predicts, say anything and do anything to get patients to accept such tests. In contrast, the "professional standards" model would not predict that demand would be created to the maximum.

If demand for such "harmless" services is pushed out to the maximum, the implication then is that changing the price doctors receive for those services will, paradoxically, have no effect whatever on their volume, even though there is massive demand creation, as long as demand for those services is independent of the volume of other services.

The most realistic (but most complicated) model would be one that blends these elements. Doctors would take into account the disutility from additional risk to the patient, nonhealth "costs" imposed on the patient, and their discomfort at deviation from what they regard as best practice, and would trade all of this off against the additional net revenue from creating demand. Then the critical factor in determining whether high-priced services that carry high physician disutility from demand creation are also services of high patient disutility is the relative importance of those concerns. The most likely outcome, of course, is that this mixture varies across services. Not all higher-profit services will be doing more marginal damage than all lower-profit services, even though on average marginal damage is positively related to profit.

What is needed is obviously better empirical information on patient utility and the reasons behind doctor motivation for demand creation (which, remember, may not exist at all). We know little about the former and nothing about the latter. In the interim, changing relative prices to equalize profitability has a chance to do some good, and is unlikely to do harm on average. But an empirically based, carefully monitored program that investigates the consequences of a variety of changes in relative prices is much superior to a program that does something for the sake of doing something because there is pressure for "effective" action, regardless of what the effect will actually be.

Modifications to the Basic Model

The basic model can be modified in two ways: (1) by asking whether a reduction in price can ever cause an increase in volume in a no-demand creation model with services that mix demand and supply constraints; and (2) by considering the effect of changes in relative prices when some doctors do not accept assignment or do not participate.

Suppose that when the price of a specific service is reduced it drops below the level at which demand can be satisfied. For some doctors, the service is now "unprofitable," given the opportunity cost in terms of lost private sector revenues or lost leisure. Suppose too that other services that are rendered to patients who seek this service are also demand-constrained. Relative to the preferred service, these services may be too time-consuming, too costly, too uncomfortable, or even too dangerous for patients to accept, but they do carry positive marginal profits (as do all demand-constrained services).

Changing what Medicare pays by cutting price for some specific service may then alter the implicit arrangement between provider and patient as follows. In return for agreeing to accept more of the services that impose too high a time, discomfort, or risk cost, the patient will be provided with the now-unprofitable-preferred service. In effect, patient and doctor agree to a set of services that extract more revenue and more profit from Medicare.

In reality, the bargaining will obviously not be so overt. Instead, the arrangement will probably become part of the package of services a physician offers to all patients, as his or her preferred style of care. The change can also be seen as a substitution of a higher time cost form of the service. The critical point is that this sort of "demand inducement" is not in any way inconsistent with a neoclassical model of physician supply. No manipulation of information, and no patient ignorance is involved; patients *gain* from this change, in comparison with the only other feasible alternative of no care from this physician. In effect, the provider response to Medicare's reduction in what it pays is to shift cost to the patient, not in the form of higher money cost (since that is ruled out by the assumption that assignment is accepted), but in the form of higher nonmonetary cost.

What will happen in a no-demand-creation model if the doctor does *not* accept assignment and relative Medicare fees are changed? To answer this question fully, one would need a model of the decision to accept assignment and the decision to set the gross price. For a doctor who is already declining assignment but who has the ability to raise his or her gross price, the immediate consequence is obvious: a cut in what Medicare pays will increase the amount the patient is balance-billed (even if the gross price falls a little). Since Medigap does not usually cover all charges in excess of the Medicare reasonable charge, the net effect of an increase in user price is likely to be a decrease in quantity demanded, to accompany this shifting of money cost to the beneficiary. Because the gross price falls, the doctor will also wish to reduce the quantity of services delivered to Medicare patients, since those services will now be less profitable than services rendered to private patients. It is just that the gross price will not fall dollar for dollar in response to a cut in Medicare payments; this is where no assignment differs from the assignment case.

The normative evaluation of this case under the neoclassical no-demand-creation assumption is therefore relatively straightforward. As Medicare pays less for some service, it causes costs to be shifted to the consumers of the service; conversely, increases in payments for other services make consumers of those services better off. A balanced-budget change in relative reimbursements therefore helps some beneficiaries (those who will consume the price-increased services) and hurts others (those who will consume the price-reduced services). Without more information, it is impossible on economic grounds to tell which state is preferable. We can say, however, that there is no particular rationale for the shift to new relative prices, just as there is no rationale against it.

In contrast to the assignment case, the "demand effect" on what patients want is larger, and the supply effect on what doctors want is smaller. In a regime of excess supply, there could be a larger effect on volume for balance-billed services than for services for which assignment is accepted. But, here again, the main conclusion has to be that we do not know enough to make even reasonable guesses.

Conclusion

There is a good chance that movement to a resource-based system of relative prices will, after a great deal of sound and fury, signify nothing except a redistribution of monopoly rents or quasi rents among doctors. There may eventually be a change in the specialty choices of physicians, but the most likely short-run response, in the models examined in this chapter, is little or no change in aggregate expenditures or in service volumes.

This prediction is surrounded by enormous variance, however. Depending on a host of unknowns (How important is the effect of relative prices on doctor desire and ability to create or destroy demand? How concentrated will relative price changes be across practices? and, What will happen to the nonmonetary price patients pay?), things could change drastically, but in wholly unpredictable ways. There is a possibility that net patient utility will increase, but no guarantee here, either.

It is not clear that there is anything terribly broken about how Medicare sets doctors' payments that we know how to fix by jiggling relative prices. The de facto payment limitation in the current arrangement which RBRVS will replace (as most physicians are bound by the prevailing charge limit) means that the charge that this older system is inflationary is no longer true. The current system is, for the great majority of doctors, a fee schedule. It does have the virtue of familiarity, but the defect of complexity. Just as "an old tax is a good tax," so an old level of relative payments, because providers have adjusted to it, may well beat the consternation that radical change will cause; on the other hand, an old tax or an old payment method that no one understands may not be so desirable after all.

The current pattern may be arbitrary, it may be untidy, and it may be unfair in the view of those who get less than they would under some other alternatives. But we cannot reject the hypothesis that the recent growth in Part B spending was driven by demand, or by declines in relative user prices (both more assignment and Medigap growth) and changes in technology, both of which make beneficiaries better off. It is not that we *know* that the growth was justified, either; the proper strategy is not to base policy on an assumption that either outcome is known with certainty. Rather, proper policy faces uncertainty squarely in the face and devises arrangements that offer no guarantee of perfection after the fact, but are the best compromise with uncertainty.

In designing such policy, the most important uncertainty to recognize is the uncertainty that relative prices are a critical part of the problem. The intuitively persuasive argument from armchair economics for equalizing relative net revenues turn out to be most relevant in a perfect (but unrealistic) market economy in which no public intervention is needed. The world in which relative profitability does differ in equilibrium is a world that we know very little about—except that "reasonable" policies can produce bizarre results. Policy almost never is based on certainty, but the ambiguity here is great enough that a process of experimentation and demonstration might be wise.

The least uncertainty attaches to a proposition not about relative prices but about absolute prices. It is at least arguable that almost all Medicare prices are too high, in the limited sense that they are higher than the lowest prices needed to get doctors to supply to Medicare beneficiaries what Medicare thinks they should get. An announced policy of modest and prespecified limits on overall fee-level growth or total Part B spending may, in an analogy with Milton Friedman's advice to the Federal Reserve, be the best strategy in an uncertain world. If policy makers are bold enough to want to fine-tune in a static-filled world, they ought to specify what they want to buy and what they do not want to buy. Then prices can be designed to produce a good outcome.

Too Much Too Late for Too Little

A Commentary by James B. Ramsey

Why are we in this mess, and why are we paying attention only to incentive schemes and payment schemes and the like? Is there something that we have forgotten, that we should rethink perhaps, that is far more serious than those aspects to which we have currently been paying—I would claim—excessive attention?

So what is our problem? What is the medical malaise? Simply put: We spend too much for too little, and it is always too late. The real complaint is that we feel that we are not getting what we are buying. For example, we have very high infant mortality rates. Health is poor for many people. Although we have enormous technological opportunities, they exceed our ability to pay. Since our reach exceeds our grasp, we get a little irritated.

What are some of the possible diagnoses? I think we can forget physician monopoly rents. The numbers of physicians have been increasing. The real incomes of physicians have been roughly constant for years. Although you could make a small case here and there for monopolistic elements among physicians, I don't think it is a serious issue.

Can the problem be increased relative costs due to low capital-labor substitution opportunities? Think of actors, economists, and doctors, for example. They are all in the same category: Their relative costs rise over time.

Legislative costs are another possible culprit. Intervention by various governmental and state agencies produces mechanisms or procedures that raise total medical costs to patients. In addition, there is the problem of liability insurance rates, which are much higher in some areas than others; both directly and indirectly through higher levels of tests the insurance problem does contribute to the cost escalation. The costs associated with the "supply-induced demand effect" are minor; besides, this concept neither explains the

306

data nor is it easily distinguished from the standard demand-supply interaction.

But what about the evidence from the RICE-Colorado experiment, which involved changes in Medicare payments? Payments went down in some areas and went up in others. There was apparently a big effect on volumes. On reading the research on this "experiment" I sometimes wonder whether my colleagues live in the real world.

Suppose that the government paid outside economists $200 per day. Now, suppose that Congress, in its infinite wisdom, decided that economists are earning too much money, the price is too high, and so we're only going to pay economists $100 a day. Can you imagine what would happen to hours billed? They would double. Would the actual amount of work change? Probably not. Would the individuals who actually do the contracting obtain the results they normally obtain? Most likely yes. It would all be the same.

Don't you think that doctors will figure out clever ways to get around the devices that Medicare authorities try to put in their way? Doctors will discover how to charge the price they think is right, or that they can negotiate with their client. So, although this may not be the entire explanation, a lot of this sort of thing goes on, especially in the short term.

Another diagnosis is the subsidized demand effect. Well, this one is a tough one. If you subsidize something, people are going to consume more of it. The cheaper something is, the more anyone is happy to use it profligately. So if we add subsidies of whatever form, whether we use the approach taken in Britain or Canada, or the more privatized approach that we take in this country, there are income and substitution effects. If you lower the real price to consumers, especially later in life, they will inevitably buy more medical care.

This difficulty puts us on the horns of a dilemma. If we subsidize something, then we've just got to expect that more will be spent; total quantity demanded will rise.

Obviously, the ideas discussed so far do not really explain the problem. We are getting there, but we haven't done it yet. Two important items do show up, however. First, we tend to neglect increases in the quality of care. This is a partial winner in the "cost sweepstakes." If you measure costs without measuring quality, then you are going to overstate cost increases. If one observes medical practice today versus only twenty years ago, there have been huge improvements. There has been an increase in quality, and that would help to explain price increases but only partially.

There has also been, of course, a great expansion of the extensive high-technology frontier. A small amount of high-cost procedures do have to be offset by a large number of low-cost procedures to bring the average price down. At the rate at which technology is moving forward, it is increasing our ability to provide very costly procedures far beyond what we are really able to afford to pay to each person who might benefit from them. Many years ago, we used to give up under certain circumstances and simply let people die quietly. Now we can ensure that they survive for a long period of time, but the process uses a lot of medical resources. We just don't have the total resources to deliver such procedures to everybody who could benefit from them.

None of these ideas really hit the deep-seated malaise or the underlying problem that people are worrying about when it comes to Medicare payments. The missing factor is the patient's own reaction to incentives with respect to his or her responsibility for his or her own health. Very few people ever discuss this concept, but it is a vital issue. Personal responsibility for health care has been changing over the past fifteen to twenty years, and this needs to be documented. There has been a sharp decline in responsible behavior.

George Bernard Shaw said that when we are sick, doctors ought to pay us. His idea was that doctors are meant to keep you healthy, so that when you are sick they have failed, and therefore they ought to give you a rebate. Well, he got it wrong. He overlooked the fact that our health depends in large part on us—on how we maintain our health or destroy it. For example, the burden on the New York health facilities has increased substantially in the past few years, not because of Medicare payments, but because of what people are doing to abuse themselves.

Take a drug addict who, having spent $200 on heroin, refuses to spend another dollar or two on a needle. The potential effects of such neglect are, as we all know, horrendous and impose extraordinary costs on the health care system. Although that is a dramatic example, it does point out the extent to which people have begun to neglect their own health.

There is a complementarity between the ambient state of health and the efficacy of medical treatment, the frequency of medical treatment and the benefits to be received. That has two implications: one is that if there were a higher level of ambient health, if there were less abuse of one's own health, then the total health care costs being paid for by Medicare and other agencies would drop off because there would be less demand for that care. In addition, the efficacy of treatment would be far higher, and therefore, once again, the costs would be less. Treatment would be less difficult or less intensive.

We need to look at this problem from the patient's perspective and ask what incentives might lower the patient's demand for health care and raise the potential return from investment in medical care expenses when they exist. For example, someone who is healthy will have a far better recovery rate, use less resources, both in the hospital and outside, for a procedure as simple as an appendectomy.

This suggestion is not merely prevention in the traditional sense. It boils down to the complementarity between ambient patient health and the efficacy of medical treatment. Living in New York City, one cannot escape this phenomenon. Large numbers of people are consuming incredible medical resources from the city of New York. Why? Because of Medicare benefits? Because the prices of medical services are wrong? Because there is demand creation by physicians? No. The enormous burden on the New York medical system and the health authorities stems from the fact that they are being flooded by people who are suffering from the side effects of drug addiction and indifference to basic health care.

Alternatives for Setting and Adjusting Fee Schedules

II

A Discussion

COMMENT: Mark Pauly rightly points out that nothing earth-shaking happened with the resource-based RVS, but there are two positive aspects to it. One is a sort of "rub the tummy, feel good" aspect in the short run, that this is a way for Congress, in essence, to cut fees and feel good about doing it as they are improving the efficiency of the system.

And there is no doubt about it. They will cut fees. I don't think we will have budget neutrality. They will think that surgical and procedural fees are too high and perhaps interns and general practitioners are making enough. So in general there will be some change in relativity and we will feel better about doing something that we ought to do.

Another positive effect is the long-term effect of redistribution in terms of specialty. If you believe that there is some physician-induced demand, then it is probably more procedure oriented, more high-tech, maybe more surgical oriented than primary-care oriented. What you will get is a reduction in these types of services in the long run.

So, in the short and moderate run, the RBRVS will not have much impact other than you'll be able to do something politically that you might not be able to do otherwise and, in the long run, perhaps you'll see some improvement in the efficiency and cost-effectiveness of the system.

COMMENT: What is striking in one of the tables presented by William Marder and Richard Willke is the great variance in hours worked, not just the mean but also the variance. That may have important implications for where the marginal (as opposed to average) return is, by specialty. In other words, the higher the variance, the lower the

Part I of this discussion is on page 255, and part III on page 374.

marginal return. And so examining the variance from the income earned would be useful.

Another point to note concerns supply response. To a first order of approximation, the mean hours worked are a reasonable proxy for excess demand. One could therefore look at the specialty choices to see if there is a tendency for people to go into the specialties with the greater hours worked or the lesser variance around a high salary.

As for barriers to entry, the core thing in getting into a specialty is getting into a residency. And what's happening to the distribution of residencies by these various specialties? The number of residencies is controlled by hospitals, and the rate of return to hospitals by kinds of specialties may well be different from the rate of return to doctors by kinds of specialties. So if one observes that because of relatively few residencies there is a high return to certain kinds of specialties, the reason may be that the hospital reimbursement formula is not giving the hospital an incentive to have enough residents in that field. The return to the specialists in that field will then go down. That particular form of barrier to entry is really worth exploring.

WILLIAM D. MARDER: You are absolutely right about the residencies. The young doctors, over the past ten years, have tended to go more into the primary-care specialties. That is partly because there is a greater proportion of female physicians in the younger cohorts.

We have done a little work using data from the American Medical Association over the past ten or twelve years, looking at cohort effects, using synthetic cohorts built that way, and found some effects similar to that reported in the more general labor literature, but on a smaller scale. Young doctors starting out tend to earn a little bit less than their forebears would have, if you extrapolate their forebears' profile back a little bit. But they seem to begin catching up after six or seven years in practice. So, on the basis of some limited evidence, we don't think that cohort effects on earnings are that big.

COMMENT: But you were just comparing the general practitioners and general internists with surgical. That comparison is not going to get very far. The comparison that might get you somewhere is among the surgical specialties. This substitutability between the surgical and nonsurgical specialties may have less responsiveness, but within surgical categories they would be more responsive to income.

QUESTION: Here is a theoretical and practical question for Dr. Pauly. We don't know what the price should be for a medical procedure, as you pointed out. How can you specify—without knowing the price a priori—what the cost is?

MARK V. PAULY: Well, there are two ways to do it. (I don't think the resource-based relative value scale tries to measure marginal cost. It does some other things.) One way is to try to determine, empirically, what the cost function looks like for different services, and for services in total, and then estimate the supply function and pick the point on the supply function where you've decided that you want to be. Deciding where you want to be ultimately is what we have politicians and administrators at the HCFA for, for public insurance anyway.

The other strategy is the bidding strategy, or the bidding analog that I was trying to hint at. Without knowing what the cost function is, but, in a sense, knowing what you want to buy, you announce prices, you see whether the offers exceed or fall short of the quantity you want to buy, and when the volume of offers equals the volume you want to buy, that is the price that equals marginal cost at that volume.

COMMENT: The bottom line, then, is that Medicare must make an arbitrary political decision—we want 3,000 bypass operations this year. If there's another patient who needs it, that's too bad. We want 3,000.

MR. PAULY: My message is, if the Physician Payment Review Commission is not willing to do that, they should stop whining and complaining.

MR. MARDER: Because a number of speakers have talked about how changing physician fee structures might ultimately affect the supply of physicians within different specialties, I would just like to point out some of the arithmetic of that. Medicare pays about one-third of the fees for physician services, so if you change the fee in that Medicare sector you are having a small impact on physician net income.

We looked at the impact of future income prospects on specialty choice in some previous work and found it is statistically significant. It makes economists feel good to find those coefficients, but they are small, and it takes a long time for those things to play out.

THOMAS G. MCGUIRE: Demand prices and supply prices are flying around here, and at times Mark Pauly talks as if equilibrium is demand constrained, but doesn't some of his analysis depend on it being supply constrained?

If you cut the price, you don't need demand inducement to get more quantity. It could just be a demand response to the lower copayment on the part of patients. The question is, don't we always want to be on the supply-constrained equilibrium rather than the demand-constrained equilibrium, because we know we are too far out on demand curves? There may be some inducement, which makes matters worse. So, if we can, we want to be supply constrained.

And then the question is, how do we find it? What is the evidence of Medicare that would suggest, for different services, where we are more demand or supply constrained, and shouldn't we look at participation rates as perhaps an indicator of where demand constraints are more likely to be binding and cut prices where participation rates are very high?

MR. PAULY: First, I was thinking of the world of participating physicians with Medigap coverage, so that the demand was not sensitive to what Medicare was permitting the physician to charge. In a world where there's balance billing, you can have demand side effects. But the assumption that demand is largely independent of the price the doctor gets is not so unreasonable for much of Medicare.

Second, I agree that the supply-constrained world is the world you want to be in. After all, it is a way of controlling moral hazard without having to use deductibles and copayments. We should move from what is, in my view, largely a demand-constrained world at the moment, to a supply-constrained world.

Now, it is never crystal clear because there is always somebody on the margin; there is always some doctor who won't render service because Medicare isn't paying enough, and so it is a matter of how many doctors refuse to accept Medicare payment as payment in full, and what our social judgment is about that.

The relevant question to ask is how many physicians would be willing, at the current level of prices they get from their Medicare business, to render nontrivial increases in volume for a particular service without requiring higher prices? Would a typical neurosurgeon be willing to do more surgery on Medicare patients at current Medicare fees, if there were 10 percent more people who needed it? Could there be 10 percent more coronary artery bypass grafting at what Medicare currently pays? Ten percent more cataracts? Is there excess supply? For that matter, would there be, on the part, say, of internists and general practitioners, a willingness to render many more office visits at current prices? Or are internists on the margin, where they would say (or think), "I'd like to recommend that you come back for another office visit, but Medicare doesn't pay me enough, so I won't be able to do that for you."

The empirical documentation of how much excess supply there is at current prices would be a good step in the direction of figuring out which way absolute and relative fees ought to go.

H. E. FRECH III: I disagree with Mark Pauly and Tom McGuire. We don't want a supply-constrained system—or at least we don't want one under more or less standard fee-for-service medicine. A supply constraint takes the decision-making power away from the consumer. There is little or no incentive for the physician to care about consumer tastes and preferences, values of risk, life style, or anything like that, and it gives the medical profession and the physicians lots of power.

So I would not like that kind of a system. Luckily, we don't have that now. For most doctors in most locations, except where balance billing has been outlawed, the system is not supply constrained. There's not much nonprice rationing. If we drastically reduce prices and restrict balance billing, there will be nonprice rationing and I would count that as bad from the point of view of the consumers. Under such a system, the consumers' values would have little influence on the system, which, after all, is doing things to them.

But there is a sensible way to have a supply-constrained system, and that's with competing preferred provider plans and health maintenance organizations, where they can develop reputations for how they constrain supply, and they compete with each other so they don't have an incentive to restrain supply in ways consumers disapprove of.

JOSEPH P. NEWHOUSE: The issue may be an empirical one. Tom McGuire's comment presumes that if you are supply constrained, reductions will come in the services that consumers value least, and Ted Frech's concern is that that may not be the case, that the reductions may be random, or may occur in services the doctors don't like giving.

COMMENT: The issue is who will not get services if we are supply constrained, and how will those people who don't get them value what they are forgoing.

MR. PAULY: The ideal is some sort of arrangement in which consumers can choose which set of supply constraints under which they want to operate. Then the real issue is, when we talk about Medicare, what are we talking about? Can we envision that sort of world in which Medicare's got to produce budgetary savings fast? And how can we do that in the least damaging way?

Now I do have to admit I was thinking of the second arrangement, but I would certainly be willing to contemplate a kind of voucher, a competing health plans arrangement, even for elderly people. And as I get closer to that age, it seems more relevant to me.

12
The Effects of a Medicare Fee Schedule on Beneficiary Out-of-Pocket Costs and Physician Payments

David C. Colby and David A. Juba

Reform of the Medicare physician payment system appears likely in the near future. Medicare's current payment system—which is based on the customary, prevailing, and reasonable charge (CPR) methodology—facilitates gaming[1] and contributes to inflation.[2] Many argue that geographic and specialty variations in payments for the same services are not justified,[3] as they produce undesirable effects on the physician's choice of specialty and practice location. Others complain that the determination of payments under CPR is complex and confusing for both the beneficiary and physician.

In the past, Congress legislated incremental changes in physician payments. It froze payment levels, developed a participating physician program, reduced payments for overvalued procedures and increased them for primary care, established fee schedules for specific services, and limited balance billing. Now, comprehensive changes are being proposed.[4]

In its 1988 report to Congress, the Physician Payment Review Commission (PPRC) endorsed the concept of replacing the CPR system with a fee schedule that would be based primarily on resource costs.[5] In December 1988, the House of Delegates of the American Medical Association supported Medicare's use of a fee schedule based on a refined and fully developed resource-based relative value scale

We thank Paul Ginsburg, Roger Reynolds, and Ted Frech for comments on earlier versions of this chapter; Roz Lasker, Ann Mongoven, and Maureen Molloy for their work on global surgical services; and Herschel Goldfield for his work on practice costs. The views and opinions expressed here are those of the authors, and no endorsement by the Physician Payment Review Commission should be inferred.

COLBY AND JUBA

(RBRVS).[6] William Hsiao and his colleagues have developed the initial resource-based relative values that might be used or modified as the basis for a fee schedule.[7]

In April 1989, the PPRC recommended the adoption of a Medicare fee schedule (MFS), which incorporated the following specifications:[8]

- estimates of relative work from the Hsiao study, when available, including estimates for evaluation and management services[9]
- a uniform global service definition for surgery
- an additive formula for incorporating practice costs into the MFS[10]
- no adjustment for the opportunity cost of specialty training
- geographic multipliers reflecting variation in the prices of non-physician inputs[11]
- charge locality boundaries conforming to metropolitan statistical areas (MSAs) and nonmetropolitan areas of each state
- continuation of the participating physician program and its payment differential
- Medicare payment at the fee schedule amount regardless of physicians' submitted charge
- a limit on physician's submitted charges

We present findings from simulations that compare payments and beneficiary liabilities under CPR during 1988 and under the MFS. Payments per service under the MFS are a product of several factors: the PPRC's relative value scale, geographic and other adjustment factors, and a monetary conversion factor. The simulations incorporate conversion factors that are budget-neutral and thus make total payments to physicians under the MFS the same as under CPR.

The simulations limit submitted charges to 120 percent of the fee schedule amount. Although the commission has not recommended a specific limit on submitted charges, the 120 percent limit was chosen for illustrative purposes because it falls between the limits that Congress previously set for overvalued procedures and radiology procedures. This limit does not affect estimates of the impact of the MFS on Medicare allowed charges, program payments, or beneficiary coinsurance. It does affect estimates of the MFS impact on beneficiaries' balance bill liabilities and physicians' total practice revenues.

The simulations assume no change in the behavior of physicians and Medicare beneficiaries in response to the fee schedule. Thus no adjustment is made for possible shifts in physicians' assignment rates or participation decisions, or for possible changes in the volume or mix of services sought or received by beneficiaries.[12] (See the appen-

317

dix to this chapter for a description of our simulation methods and data base development.)

The Medicare Fee Schedule

Implementing a budget-neutral MFS would substantially increase payments for some procedures and substantially reduce payments for others. This change would occur because relative charges for some procedures (the basis of the CPR system) are different from relative resource costs (the basis of the MFS).[13]

An exhaustive analysis of MFS effects on payments for each procedure in the simulation is not feasible. Since a small number of procedures account for a disproportionate share of total Medicare program payments for physician services, MFS effects on selected procedures should illustrate the effects on all procedures in those categories.[14]

Table 12–1 shows Medicare-allowed charges for seventeen selected procedures under the two payment systems.[15] The allowed charges for office and hospital visits would increase by 24–34 percent under the MFS.[16] The allowed charges for specific surgical and diagnostic procedures (for example, hernia repair, CAT scan, and electrocardiogram) would decrease by approximately 30 percent.[17] The MFS effects on selected procedures probably would be typical of the effects on other evaluation and management (EM) services, surgical procedures, and diagnostic procedures.

Medicare program payments for all evaluation and management services in the simulation would be 28 percent greater under the MFS, payments for all surgical services would be 17 percent less under the MFS, and payments for all imaging services would be 21 percent less under the MFS than under the current CPR system.

Effects on Beneficiaries

Implementing the Medicare fee schedule with a 120 percent charge limit would affect beneficiaries' spending for coinsurance plus balance bills. The simulations examine only the impact of the MFS on beneficiaries' coinsurance plus balance bills for Medicare-covered physician services. Beneficiaries would face greater total out-of-pocket costs than are shown here.[18]

General Effects on Beneficiaries. The Medicare fee schedule would have a significant impact on balance bills but no impact on coinsurance for all beneficiaries as a group. Because the MFS is budget-neutral, it does not change the average coinsurance. For beneficiaries

318

TABLE 12–1

National Mean Payments for Selected Procedures under
Medicare Fee Schedule and CPR Payments

Procedure		CPR (dollars)	MFS (dollars)	Change (percentage)
	Evaluation and Management			
90050	limited office visit	23	28	24
90060	intermediate office visit	28	35	26
90250	limited hospital visit	26	33	28
90260	intermediate hospital visit	30	40	34
90620	comprehensive consultation	93	104	12
92014	eye exam and treatment	42	39	−6
	Surgery			
27130	total hip replacement	2404	1985	−17
27244	repair femur fracture	1299	1198	−8
33512	coronary artery bypass	3894	2828	−27
35301	rechannel of artery	1573	1172	−26
44140	partial removal of colon	1256	1072	−15
49505	repair inguinal hernia	588	414	−30
52601	prostatectomy (*TUR*)	1128	921	−18
66984	remove cataract, insert lens	1467	1164	−21
	Diagnostic			
52000	cystoscopy	105	110	5
70470	contrast CAT scans of head	113	82	−27
71010	X-ray exam of chest (1 view)	12	10	−16
93000	electrocardiogram, complete	35	25	−28

NOTE: Fees are for procedures performed by the most common specialty in the most common place of service.
SOURCE: PPRC simulations.

in the aggregate, balance bills, as well as the total of balance bills plus coinsurance, would decline significantly. Although coinsurance would remain the same, balance bills would decline by 66 percent and the total of balance bills and coinsurance would decline by 25 percent (table 12–2). We should note that the exact magnitude of the decline in balance bills depends on physicians' responses to the fee schedule. Those responses are difficult to predict.

Effects by Beneficiary Category. The impact of implementing the MFS with a 120 percent limit on submitted charges varies across categories of beneficiaries, as shown in table 12–2. Changes in coinsurance for beneficiaries in the different categories would be moderate, with the exception of changes by area of residence. In very large metropolitan areas, beneficiary coinsurance would decline by 12 percent; conversely, in small rural areas, it would increase by 6 percent. Nonetheless, the average spending on coinsurance by beneficiaries living in small rural areas would still be lower than the average spending by beneficiaries in very large metropolitan areas.

Under the MFS with a 120 percent limit on submitted charges, beneficiaries' balance bill amounts would decrease significantly.[19] The percentage decrease in balance bills for beneficiaries in different economic and demographic categories would be approximately equal. Given that no changes in assignment decisions by physicians are incorporated in the simulations, the balance bill reductions may differ from those reported in table 12–2.[20]

Beneficiary spending for coinsurance plus balance bills would decline because of the limit on submitted charges. The decline would not be uniform, but would vary only slightly across categories of beneficiaries. For example, the liabilities of beneficiaries who are sixty-five to seventy-four years old would decline more than the liabilities of those aged eighty-five or older.

The ownership of Medigap policies would make only one slight difference in the impact. The percentage change in Medigap-adjusted coinsurance from CPR to MFS is the same as shown in table 12–2. Medigap premiums, typically between $500 and $700 per year, would remain the same for most beneficiary categories. They might change by geographic areas, however, as payments and coinsurance change to reflect the fee schedule's geographic multipliers.

Effects on Individual Beneficiaries. The impact on individual beneficiaries varies from the average impact for all beneficiaries shown in the previous tables. Tables 12–3 and 12–4 describe the distribution of coinsurance plus balance bill liabilities among beneficiaries.

TABLE 12–2

CHANGES IN BENEFICIARIES' LIABILITIES FOR COINSURANCE PLUS
BALANCE BILLS UNDER THE MEDICARE FEE SCHEDULE
(120 percent balance bill limit)

| | Percentage Change from CPR | | |
Beneficiary	Total	Balance bill	Coinsurance
All	−25	−66	0
< 65 yrs	−22	−70	1
65–74	−27	−66	−1
75–84	−24	−65	0
85+ yrs	−20	−66	4
Males	−25	−66	−2
White	−26	−66	−2
Nonwhite	−19	−68	−2
Females	−26	−66	1
White	−25	−66	1
Nonwhite	−18	−68	1
Area[a]			
Very large metro	−32	−69	−12
Large metro	−23	−66	−1
Small metro	−25	−66	2
Large rural	−24	−66	4
Small rural	−25	−66	6
Income (% poverty level)			
Below	−22	−67	4
100–149	−24	−66	2
150–199	−23	−65	2
200–299	−25	−66	0
300 and over	−27	−66	−3
Hospitalized			
Yes	−26	−67	−1
No	−23	−64	1

NOTE: Excludes enrollees who did not have claims and Medicaid beneficiaries.

a. Areas are assigned by beneficiary's residence. Very large metro areas include counties in MSAs with a population of five million or more; large metro areas include counties in MSAs with a population of one million; small metro areas are all other metropolitan counties. Large rural (nonmetropolitan) counties have a population of 25,000 or more; small rural includes all other nonmetropolitan counties.

SOURCE: PPRC simulations.

TABLE 12–3

PERCENTAGE OF BENEFICIARIES BY LIABILITIES FOR
COINSURANCE PLUS BALANCE BILLS

(120 percent balance bill limit)

Expenses ($)	$ 0	1–100	101–250	251–500	501–1,000	> 1,000
Coinsurance						
CPR	0	63	18	11	6	2
MFS	0	61	20	12	6	2
Balance bills						
CPR	28	52	11	5	3	2
MFS	39	53	5	2	1	0
Total[a]						
CPR	0	51	22	13	9	5
MFS	0	56	22	12	7	3

NOTE: Excludes enrollees who did not have claims and Medicaid beneficiaries.
a. Total is the sum of coinsurance plus balance bills.
SOURCE: PPRC simulations.

Table 12–3 shows that the MFS with a 120 percent submitted charge limit would reduce the fraction of beneficiaries paying large balance bills. For example, fewer beneficiaries would have balance bills greater than $500 under the MFS (1 percent) than under CPR (5 percent). A comparison of coinsurance plus balance bills shows that the proportion of beneficiaries paying more than $500 would also decline under the MFS, whereas the proportion paying less than $100 would increase. The changes in the distribution of total liabilities are due primarily to the limit on submitted charges.

Table 12–4 provides additional data on changes in beneficiary liabilities for coinsurance and balance bills. Although some beneficiaries would have slightly higher liabilities than they do under CPR, about 71 percent of the beneficiaries would have lower liabilities under the MFS than under CPR. For 80 percent of the beneficiaries whose liabilities would increase, the increase would be $25 or less.

Effects on Physicians by Specialty

The effects of the MFS would not be uniform across specialties or among physicians within a particular specialty.[21] Differences in the impact of the MFS across specialties would be due largely to changes in relative values and differences in service mixture. MFS effects within specialties reflect differences in service mix among physicians as well as the effects of the geographic multiplier.

TABLE 12-4
PERCENTAGE OF BENEFICIARIES BY CHANGES IN
COINSURANCE PLUS BALANCE BILLS
(Medicare fee schedule with 120 percent limit)

Change from CPR ($)	With Decreases	With Increases
1–10	23	18
11–25	12	6
26–50	11	3
51–100	9	2
101–251	9	1
251–1,000	6	0
> 1,000	1	0
Total	71	30

NOTE: Excludes enrollees who did not have claims and Medicaid beneficiaries.
SOURCE: PPRC simulations.

Total payments to physicians whose practices consist largely of EM services would increase under the MFS. Conversely, total payments to physicians whose practices consist largely of surgical or diagnostic procedures would likely decline. Estimated MFS payments to physicians in medical specialties would be 20 percent greater than comparable payments under the CPR system; payments to surgical specialists would be 11 percent lower; and payments to pathologists and radiologists would be 25 percent and 21 percent lower, respectively, under the MFS.[22]

Although the effects of the Medicare fee schedule are similar for the two hospital-based specialties, radiology and pathology, they vary among surgical and medical specialties. For example, changes in total payments to surgical specialties in the simulations range from a 6 percent increase in payments to otolaryngologists to the 16 and 20 percent reductions in payments to ophthalmologists and thoracic surgeons, respectively. The increase in total payments to family practitioners (38 percent) would be more than twice the increase in payments to internists (17 percent).

Differences in service mix explain some of the variation in MFS effects among specialties. Surgical specialties for whom EM services represent a greater fraction of total payments would likely realize smaller losses in payments under the MFS. For example, reductions in payments to otolaryngologists would probably be smaller than reductions in payments to thoracic surgeons. Nearly 50 percent of

TABLE 12–5
CHANGE IN MEDICARE PAYMENTS BY SPECIALTY UNDER THE MEDICARE
FEE SCHEDULE

Specialty	Percentage Change
Medical	20
Internal medicine	17
Family practice	38
Dermatology	1
Surgical	−11
Ophthalmology	−16
General surgery	−10
Orthopedic surgery	−7
Urology	−5
Thoracic surgery	−20
Otolaryngology	6
Obstetrics/gynecology	2
Hospital-based	N.A.
Radiology	−21
Pathology	−25
Anesthesia	N.A.
Other physicians[a]	4

N.A. = not applicable.
NOTE: Does not include balance bills.
a. Other physicians includes physician specialties with data problems and those not evaluated in the Hsiao study: cardiovascular disease, clinic, general practice, gastroenterology, nephrology, neurology, neurosurgery, plastic surgery, psychiatry, and pulmonary disease.
SOURCE: PPRC simulations.

payments to otolaryngologists are for medical services, whereas only 43 percent of payments are for surgical procedures. The corresponding figures for thoracic surgeons are 5 percent and 93 percent, respectively.

Differences in the proportion of total payments from medical and surgical services could explain some of the difference between MFS effects among medical specialties. For example, medical services account for a somewhat greater share of total payments to family practitioners (88 percent) than to internists (79 percent). Of all the medical specialties, family practitioners would experience the greatest increase in payments under the MFS.

The elimination of specialty distinctions in payment for total work by procedure could also contribute to the disparity between

MFS effects on total payments to internists and family practitioners. Implementing the MFS would increase the level of payments for EM services for physicians in all specialties. At the same time, it would close the gap between Medicare payments for EM services by internists and family practitioners that exist in the CPR payment system.

Geographic payment policy explains only a small fraction of the MFS impact on total payments to a specialty. Effects attributable only to changing relative values (pure RVS effect) would be approximately the same as the combined effects of the RVS and the geographic payment policy reported in table 12–5.[23] One exception might be family practice, whose membership is relatively concentrated in rural areas. For that specialty, the geographic policy could increase average payments by as much as 5 percent.

Within-Specialty Effects. Under the MFS, total payments to some physicians in a specialty would increase, while payments to others would decrease. This would be true in varying degrees for all specialties in the simulations. For example, while total payments to most physicians in the medical specialties would increase, payments to approximately 14 percent would decrease. Likewise, while total payments to most surgeons would decline, total payments to approximately 26 percent would increase (see table 12–6). Even among the hospital-based physicians, who would be subject to the greatest reductions in total payments, MFS effects would vary widely. In the simulations, total payments to 10 percent of radiologists and 14 percent of pathologists would increase.

Two factors explain the variation in MFS effects within a specialty: service mix and geographic payment policy. The impact of service mix (the pure RVS effect) was isolated by comparing payments to physicians under two fee schedules: a national average charge fee schedule and the MFS, both adjusted for geographic differences in nonphysician practice costs. The greater the variation in service mix among physicians in a specialty, the greater would be the variation in effects of the fee schedule among them.

Table 12–7 reports the proportion of physicians in each specialty who would realize a change of a given size in their payments owing to the pure RVS effect. If service mix was homogeneous among all physicians in a specialty, the distribution of physicians would be relatively concentrated, with most physicians realizing approximately the same change in payments between the two fee schedules. Conversely, if service mix varied among physicians in a specialty, the pure RVS effect on payments would likewise vary.

The distributions of the impacts of the RVS would be concen-

TABLE 12-6
DISTRIBUTION OF PHYSICIAN PRACTICES BY PERCENTAGE CHANGE IN PAYMENTS FOR TOTAL MFS EFFECT

Specialty	Loss				Gain			
	> 50	26–50	11–25	0–10	0–10	11–25	26–50	> 50
Medical	0	2	5	7	16	25	30	16
Internal medicine	0	1	5	8	19	28	29	10
Family practice	0	0	1	3	6	17	37	36
Dermatology	0	9	20	16	12	19	15	8
Surgical	0	13	39	23	13	8	3	2
Ophthalmology	0	13	60	18	6	2	1	0
General surgery	1	15	28	24	16	9	5	2
Orthopedic surgery	0	4	31	32	21	8	3	0
Urology	0	8	22	32	17	18	2	2
Thoracic surgery	0	41	36	11	3	3	0	6
Otolaryngology	0	2	13	22	17	24	16	6
Obstetrics/gynecology	0	4	21	20	25	14	8	9
Hospital-based	1	31	48	9	4	5	1	1
Radiology	1	29	51	8	5	4	0	1
Pathology	5	45	21	15	2	6	5	1
All physicians	0	9	23	15	13	15	14	9

NOTE: Practices are weighted by payments under the MFS. Percentage loss or gain under MFS are with respect to 1988 allowed charges under the CPR system, exclusive of balance bills.
SOURCE: PPRC simulations.

326

TABLE 12-7

Distribution of Physician Practices by Percentage Change in Payments for Pure RVS Effect

Specialty	Loss > 50	26–50	11–25	0–10	Gain 0–10	11–25	26–50	> 50
Medical	0	0	2	6	11	45	36	1
Internal medicine	0	0	2	4	12	60	22	0
Family practice	0	0	0	0	0	3	93	4
Dermatology	0	0	3	47	36	12	2	0
Surgical	0	3	53	30	8	4	2	0
Ophthalmology	0	0	86	11	1	1	0	0
General surgery	0	0	59	22	9	6	3	0
Orthopedic surgery	0	0	25	64	8	2	1	0
Urology	0	0	9	76	12	1	2	0
Thoracic surgery	0	35	46	10	2	6	0	0
Otolaryngology	0	0	1	30	40	22	4	3
Obstetrics/gynecology	0	0	15	40	20	17	10	0
Hospital-based	0	22	73	5	0	0	0	0
Radiology	0	20	75	5	0	0	0	0
Pathology	0	42	56	2	0	0	0	0
All physicians	0	4	29	18	10	20	18	1

Note: Practices are weighted by payments under the MFS. Percentage loss or gain under the MFS are with respect to national average charge fee schedule with geographic adjustment.
Source: PPRC simulations.

trated for some specialties: family practice, ophthalmology, radiology, and pathology. Service mix would not be an important cause of variation in MFS effects within those specialties. Within other specialties (for example, internal medicine, thoracic surgery, and otolaryngology), the distributions would be more dispersed.

MFS Effects on Total Practice Revenues. Payments by the Medicare program are an important source of practice revenue, but they are not the only source. Revenues also come from balance billing for Medicare services and other payers. Consequently, the effect of the MFS on total practice revenues from all sources would be less than the effect on the Medicare portion alone (table 12–8). The magnitude of the effect would depend on the proportion of revenues derived from Medicare. Estimates of that proportion vary from 4 percent for obstetrics/gynecology to about 20 percent for family practice, to 40

TABLE 12–8

PERCENTAGE CHANGE IN PRACTICE REVENUES FROM MEDICARE AND
ALL SOURCES BY SPECIALTY

(Medicare fee schedule with 120 percent balance bill limit)

Specialty	Medicare[a]	All Sources[b]
Medical		
Internal Medicine	17	4
Family practice	38	6
Dermatology	1	N.A.
Surgical		
Ophthalmology	−16	−8
General surgery	−10	−5
Orthopedic surgery	−7	−3
Urology	−5	N.A.
Thoracic surgery	−20	−9
Otolaryngology	6	N.A.
Obstetrics/gynecology	2	0
Hospital-based		
Radiology	−21	−7
Pathology	−25	N.A.

N.A. = not applicable.
a. Medicare program payments are exclusive of balance bills.
b. Includes revenues from all payers. Medicare assignment rates are assumed to be unaffected by MFS and 100 percent of balance bills are assumed to be collected. Estimates of non-Medicare revenues are unavailable for some specialties.
SOURCE: PPRC simulations.

percent or more for ophthalmology and thoracic surgery.[24] Fee schedule effects on physicians' revenues from all payers reflect this variation.[25] The MFS effects range from increases of 4 percent and 6 percent in total practice revenues of family practitioners and internists to a 9 percent reduction in total practice revenues of thoracic surgeons. These changes would be larger if private insurers also adopt a similar fee schedule.

Effects on Physicians by Geographic Area

The MFS is adjusted by geographic multipliers so that fees in different localities vary with differences in an overhead-only index of nonphysician input costs. Implementing the MFS would redistribute Medicare payments from metropolitan to rural areas (table 12–9). The reduction in payments to physicians in all metropolitan areas combined would be small (3 percent) in contrast to the increase in payments to physicians in all rural areas combined (14 percent).

In each of the defined geographic area categories, payments to surgical specialists would decline under the MFS, whereas payments to medical specialists would increase. The one exception would be in very large metropolitan areas, where payments to medical specialists would decline slightly.

In each geographic area, total Medicare payments to some physicians would increase under the MFS, whereas payments to others would decrease (table 12–10). Across all areas combined, payments to approximately half of all physicians would increase, whereas payments to the other half would decline. The proportions would be different, however, in the five defined metropolitan and rural area categories.

In the large and small rural areas, total payments to a majority of physicians would increase. The proportionate increases would be in the moderate-to-large range in most cases. The patterns of increases and decreases are somewhat more symmetric in the large and small metropolitan areas. The proportion of physicians whose payments would increase would approximately equal the proportion whose payments would decrease in these areas. In very large metropolitan areas, where decreases in total payments in the aggregate would be greatest, most reductions would be small to moderate. Furthermore, total payments to many physicians in very large metropolitan areas would increase under the MFS.

Summary

The CPR system for physician payment has been widely criticized, and now it appears that the system will be reformed. William Hsiao

TABLE 12–9
CHANGE IN PAYMENTS UNDER THE MEDICARE FEE
SCHEDULE BY GEOGRAPHIC AREA

Area[a] and Specialty Group	Percentage Change
Very large metro	
Medical	−1
Surgical	−25
All physicians	−14
Large metro	
Medical	17
Surgical	−12
All physicians	−3
Small metro	
Medical	26
Surgical	−7
All physicians	3
Large rural	
Medical	30
Surgical	−6
All physicians	12
Small rural	
Medical	37
Surgical	−7
All physicians	14

a. Very large metro areas include counties in MSAs with a population of 5 million or more; large metro includes counties in MSAs with a population of one to five million; small metro areas are all other metropolitan counties. These areas accounted for 14, 37, and 33 percent, respectively, of Medicare-allowed amounts in 1988. Large rural (nonmetropolitan) counties have populations of 25,000 or more; small rural includes all other nonmetropolitan counties. These areas accounted for 9 and 7 percent, respectively, of Medicare-allowed amounts in 1988.
SOURCE: PPRC simulations.

and his colleagues have proposed that the resource-based relative value scale be adopted for this purpose. If implemented, a fee schedule based on the original methodology suggested by Hsiao would lead to a large redistribution of Medicare revenues among physicians.[26] Family practitioners would receive 60–70 percent greater revenues, whereas thoracic surgeons would receive 50 percent lower revenues. The direction and magnitude of this impact has been confirmed by others.[27]

The Medicare fee schedule as proposed by the Physician Payment Review Commission is an alternative method for determining pay-

TABLE 12-10
DISTRIBUTION OF PHYSICIANS' PRACTICES BY PERCENTAGE CHANGE IN PAYMENTS UNDER THE MEDICARE FEE SCHEDULE, BY GEOGRAPHIC AREA

Area[a]	Loss				Gain			
	> 50	26–50	11–25	0–10	0–10	11–25	26–50	> 50
Very large metro	1	24	29	12	12	12	7	3
Large metro	0	8	25	17	17	16	12	5
Small metro	0	6	21	16	16	16	15	10
Large rural	0	4	16	12	13	14	23	18
Small rural	0	2	19	8	13	15	20	23
All areas	0	9	23	15	13	15	14	9

NOTE: Physician practices weighted by payments under the MFS.
a. Very large metro areas include counties in MSAs with a population of 5 million or more; large metro areas include counties in MSAs of one million population; small metro areas are all other metropolitan counties. Large rural (nonmetropolitan) counties have populations of 25,000 or more; small rural includes all other nonmetropolitan counties.
SOURCE: PPRC simulations.

331

ments for physician services. The adoption of the proposed Medicare fee schedule would redistribute Medicare revenues. In general, medical specialties would gain, whereas surgical specialties would lose Medicare revenues. Medicare revenues would rise in rural areas and would fall in urban areas. Nevertheless, the impact of the MFS on procedures, specialties, and geographic areas would be considerably smaller than the impact produced by the original RBRVS.

Appendix

This appendix describes the simulation methodology, including data development and the calculation of the Medicare fee schedule payments. In the simulations, Medicare CPR payments and beneficiary liabilities for a large sample of Medicare claims from 1988 are compared with estimated payments and liabilities for the same services under the MFS. The simulations examine differences between CPR-allowed amounts and the fee schedule payments aggregated over beneficiaries in various age, location, and income categories as well as over physicians in different specialties and geographic areas.

Data. We based our simulations on two large files of Medicare claims information from the 1986 Medicare annual data (BMAD) system: BMAD III, which includes all claims for a 5 percent sample of Medicare providers, and BMAD IV, which includes all claims for a 5 percent sample of beneficiaries. We also used the 1986 BMAD I procedure file, a summary of local charges and other data for all claims filed during that year.

To forecast the impact of a fee schedule, one must examine a significant portion of the claims information on the two primary data files. The physician simulation file contains BMAD III data for all services provided by more than 19,000 physicians drawn from the top twenty-five Medicare specialties in terms of allowed charges received (see table 12–11).[28]

Together, these specialties account for approximately 94 percent of Medicare expenditures on physician services. Of the most important specialties, only anesthesiology is excluded from our analysis because of difficulties with data. For each specialty in the simulations, the included procedures cover at least 80 percent of their total Medicare-allowed charges.

The beneficiary analyses are based on BMAD IV records for a stratified random sample of more than 82,000 beneficiaries selected from the BMAD IV 5 percent sample of beneficiaries. The simulation excludes those beneficiaries who are dual Medicare/Medicaid benefi-

TABLE 12–11
Simulation Specialties, 1986 Approved Charges
for Physician Services

Procedure Codes in Data Set	Specialty[a]	Millions of Dollars	Percent	Cumulative Percent
Internal medicine	3,360	16.4	16.4	66
Ophthalmology	2,486	12.1	28.5	22
Radiology	1,779	8.7	37.1	98
General surgery	1,620	7.9	45.0	203
Cardiovascular disease	1,245	6.1	51.1	51
Clinic	1,215	5.9	57.0	427
Orthopedic surgery	1,082	5.3	62.3	96
(Anesthesiology)	(931)	(4.5)	(66.8)	—[b]
General practice	923	4.5	71.3	100
Family practice	843	4.1	75.4	68
Urology	754	3.7	79.1	55
Thoracic surgery	679	3.3	82.4	66
Gastroenterology	420	2.0	84.5	23
Podiatry	360	1.8	86.2	183
Dermatology	341	1.7	87.9	43
Pulmonary disease	263	1.3	89.2	34
Neurology	259	1.3	90.4	33
Psychiatry	245	1.2	91.6	11
Pathology	226	1.1	92.7	12
Otolaryngology	224	1.1	93.8	133
Miscellaneous	214	1.0	94.9	164
Nephrology	201	1.0	95.8	37
Neurosurgery	192	0.9	96.8	65
Obstetrics/gynecology	152	0.7	97.5	61
Chiropractic	102	0.5	98.0	1
Plastic surgery	101	0.5	98.5	161

a. The specialties are ordered by total allowed charges.
b. Anesthesiology is not included in the simulations because of difficulties in computing average allowed charges for a single episode of surgery from Medicare claims data.
Source: Health Care Financing Administration, BMAD I, 1986.

ciaries and those who did not file claims. The analysis file contains all BMAD IV records of claims submitted by the sampled beneficiaries for physician services.

The Health Care Financing Administration (HCFA) and the Social Security Administration provided basic information about demographic and economic characteristics of the sampled beneficiaries (sex, race, Medicaid eligibility, Social Security benefits and location), while preserving their confidentiality. The relationship between these characteristics and total income was estimated using the 1986 Current Population Survey.[29] Poverty status was then imputed for beneficiaries in the simulation from the CPS-derived formula. The poverty status for 10.5 percent of the sampled beneficiaries could not be determined. Those beneficiaries are included in the impact analysis by every category except income.

The 1983 Physician Practice Cost and Income Survey was used to estimate the ratio of practice costs to gross revenue. After cleaning the data, we calculated practice costs for office space, wages and fringes of employees, equipment and supplies, professional liability insurance, and residual items. Physician fringe benefits were included in net revenues rather than in practice costs. These estimates were updated to 1986 with adjustments for the growth of practice costs, especially in professional liability insurance premiums.

Aging the 1986 Data to 1988. Between 1986 and 1988, Congress mandated reductions and other limits on Medicare charges for overvalued procedures and established Maximum Allowable Actual Charge (MAAC) limits on the submitted charges of nonparticipating physicians, as well as different Medicare Economic Index (MEI) adjustments for primary and nonprimary care. In order not to confuse the effects of a fee schedule with effects of these legislative changes, we inflated baseline 1986 prevailing charges on the simulation files to 1988 levels, subject to limits for overvalued procedures and the different Medicare Economic Index updates for primary and nonprimary care. Submitted and customary charges for 1988 were estimated by applying the physician services component of the all-urban Consumer Price Index to 1986 BMAD III and BMAD IV submitted charges subject to MAAC limits. Physician participation and assignment rates were not aged.

Computing Work Values. The Hsiao phase I report of September 1988 provided work values for about 1,400 procedures. By December 1988, the Hsiao team revised the work values for EM and other codes, and eliminated some values for other codes. Their December supplemental report was used to extrapolate values and simulate impacts.

We found it necessary to estimate work values for more codes than the Hsiao study provided in order to have a comprehensive analysis of the impact of the fee schedule. We developed thirty-six families of services and procedures from the categories of CPT codes. The families used for these extrapolations are broader than those used by the Hsiao team. In order to estimate work values, we calculated extrapolations based on average Medicare submitted charges and the implicit work/charge relationships within each family.

We adjusted the total work values for surgical global services before estimating the fee schedule. The definition of surgical global services in the Hsiao study is narrower than that used by most Medicare carriers. Using the results of PPRC's Medicare Carrier Survey, we adjusted the total work values for surgical services so that they corresponded to the global service policy used by each carrier. This adjustment reduced the extent to which payments for surgical procedures would be reduced under the fee schedule, when compared with estimates published by Hsiao and earlier ones from the PPRC.

The simulations are based on the relative total work values for evaluation and management services reported by Hsiao and his colleagues in their supplemental report to the HCFA (December 1988). The PPRC recommends revising the coding system for EM services by incorporating time in the definitions for levels of service. Since the commission needs additional data to calibrate the system and a consensus process to develop definitive coding definitions, however, this reform was not incorporated in the current simulations.

Computing Medicare Fee Schedule Payments. Under the MFS, payment for a service includes compensation for total work (TW) and practice costs. Payments for each procedure are computed as follows:

$$PAYMENT = [(TW \times CFW) + (PC \times GM \times CFC)]$$

where PAYMENT = fee schedule determined payment, TW = total work per procedure, CFW = work-conversion factor, PC = estimated practice costs, GM = geographic multiplier, and CFC = cost-conversion factor.

The estimated practice cost for each service is the product of two specialty-specific factors: the ratio of practice costs to gross revenue and the national average CPR-allowed charge for the procedure.[30] The estimated practice cost is adjusted by geographic multipliers derived from those developed by Zuckerman, Welch, and Pope.[31] Geographic-adjusted practice costs are multiplied by a conversion factor (*CFC*) to achieve budget neutrality with respect to total practice costs before the geographic adjustment.

The total work portion of the payment is determined by multiplying *TW* values per procedure by a conversion factor (*CFW*) set to ensure budget neutrality with respect to CPR-allowed charges net of estimated practice costs. The fee schedule payment for a service is the sum of the payment for *TW* and the geographic-adjusted practice costs.

A Comparison of Three
Simulation Efforts

A Commentary by Roger A. Reynolds

The simulation results presented by David Colby and David Juba represent a third generation of estimates of the impact of a Medicare payment schedule based on a resource-based relative value scale (RBRVS). The first set of simulation estimates, developed by William Hsiao and his colleagues, were published at the time the original Harvard RBRVS report was released.[1] The second-generation simulations were those I produced at the American Medical Association (AMA) primarily to help our physician constituents evaluate the RBRVS and develop a policy stance toward potential Medicare payment changes.[2] These simulations have certain characteristics in common and have further improved our understanding of the implications of basing Medicare payments on an RBRVS.

All three simulation efforts employed the same data base and rested on the same fundamental assumptions: that the volume of different services will not change in response to changes in Medicare payment levels and that implementation of a new payment schedule will be budget-neutral. The data in all three cases derive from the 1986 Part B Medicare annual data (BMAD) files. In addition, the technical approach to producing estimates has been nearly identical in all three studies.

The Hsiao simulation concentrated on the changes in Medicare payments by procedure and in the average total payments by specialty implied by the original Harvard RBRVS. This work drew wide attention to the RBRVS because of the large losses projected for several specialties, such as thoracic surgery and ophthalmology, and the large gains projected for general and family practice.

After replicating the Hsiao results, the AMA study extended the

The views expressed are those of the author and do not necessarily reflect policy of the American Medical Association.

analysis of the effects of an RBRVS-based Medicare payment schedule to the distribution of changes within specialties and geographic differences in the impact on physicians. The results showed a wide dispersion of effects in all specialties, although nearly three quarters of physicians would experience only small gains or losses. The results also showed substantial differences across and within regions and in urban versus rural areas, but extremes were not as great as those for specialties. Rural areas were projected to experience a small gain at the expense of urban areas when the RBRVS was adjusted using the geographic Medicare economic index (GMEI).[3]

The simulation results raised several questions about the original RBRVS because the losses in some cases were large enough to suggest that Medicare payments might not be adequate to cover physician overhead. As a result, the Physician Payment Review Commission (PPRC) modified the approach used to determine overhead payments in the original Harvard study.

This accounts for the difference in the results presented by Colby and Juba and those reported previously—namely, that the magnitude of changes in Medicare payments to physicians are generally smaller in the former. Average losses among radiologists and pathologists, however, appear to remain relatively large and virtually unchanged from earlier results. Also note the greater redistribution of Medicare payments from urban to rural areas than I found in my study. This result apparently derives from the greater geographic details on the BMAD tapes available to PPRC than on the public versions that made it possible to identify urban and rural physicians more precisely.

The effects on beneficiary out-of-pocket costs had not been explored in previous simulations and this represents an important contribution of the Colby and Juba analysis. The pattern of changes projected for beneficiary coinsurance payments is not surprising since it is mainly driven by changes in Medicare-allowed charges. The changes in balance bills require closer inspection, however. These results derive from a new assumption that must be made about how submitted charges change in response to Medicare payments. The assumption made by Colby and Juba was that submitted charges would not change following the imposition of a new payment schedule.

This represents one extreme of the possible assumptions that might be made. It would be valid if the market for physician services was highly competitive and the Medicare share of the market was small, or if supply to the Medicare market was perfectly elastic. The other extreme of assumptions that might be made is that the submitted charges change by an identical amount to changes in Medicare-allowed charges, so balance bills remain constant. This assumption is more apt for an imperfectly competitive market for patients with Medigap insurance or for a situation of inelastic supply. Necessarily, changes in balance bills would be larger if this assumption was applicable. In practice, the actual results will probably fall between the two extremes, so changes in balance bills will be larger than those reported by Colby and Juba.

A second feature of the beneficiary impact analysis is that it couples the effect of a 120 percent balance bill ceiling with the effect of a new payment schedule. Since the balance bill ceiling is a distinct and separable policy from the new payment schedule, it would have been interesting to distinguish the effects of these policies in the distributional analysis. It is also of interest to examine the influence of balance bill limits on physicians since the current simulations were confined to the impact of payment schedule changes without a similar balance bill limit.

Although the simulations to date have provided insight into an RBRVS and its implications, they have a common weakness: They deny that beneficiary and physician behavior will respond to payment changes. In particular, the assumption of a no-utilization change veils the simulations in significant uncertainty.

According to empirical evidence that I have obtained on the supply of physician services to Medicare beneficiaries for each of six main types of services, utilization does vary significantly with Medicare payment levels. Medicare carrier localities were the units of observation. Laspeyres-type indexes of the volume of services and the average allowed charge level were created from BMAD for each type of service and linked with other potential predictors of the volume of services.

After considering a range of more complex specifications of the determination of Medicare volume, a simple supply function was chosen. The supply of services to Medicare beneficiaries is specified to be a function of the average allowed charge, input prices, and the number of patient care physicians in the locality. Input prices are measured by GMEI. In treating this as a supply function, I assumed that the average allowed charge can be regarded as a constant marginal market price. This follows from the observation of extensive assignment of Medicare services. Regression estimates were obtained by ordinary least squares. The possibility that the allowed charge should be treated as endogenous was ruled out with a formal specification test. A logarithmic functional form was used for each variable in the regressions, so the coefficient estimates may be interpreted as elasticities.

The regression estimates are provided in table 12–C1. The regression estimates are similar in several qualitative senses for all types of services and conform to basic economic predictions for supply functions. First, the volume of services to Medicare beneficiaries increases with Medicare-allowed charges; however, the hypothesis that supply is inelastic for visits and consultations and for radiology services cannot be rejected. The highest supply elasticities are for surgery and pathology services. Second, supply decreases with input prices. The input price elasticities vary from 1.7 to 3.2, with the highest elasticity occurring for surgical services. Third, physician supply maintains a constant ratio with the volume of each type of service. Finally, the fit of these regressions appears reasonably good, with the exception of the anesthesiology results. The good fits, however, are not unexpected given the extent of aggregation over services. The greater unexplained variations for anesthesia services than for other services are primarily due to the use of anesthesia units as the main volume measure. Anesthesia units are probably more akin to an input than an output measure, even though they are the basis for most billing for anesthesia services.

These results suggest that volume would decline if the original budget-neutral payment schedule calculated on an assumption of fixed volume is maintained. In other words, a budget savings might

TABLE 12–C1

REGRESSION RESULTS FOR MEDICARE VOLUME OF
PHYSICIAN SERVICES BY TYPE OF SERVICE

Type of Service	Allowed Charge	Input Prices	Number of Physicians	R^2
Visits and consultations	0.30	−2.11	1.01	0.80
	(1.00)	(4.60)	(27.61)	
Specialized medicine	1.75	−2.17	1.11	0.81
	(4.62)	(4.64)	(25.18)	
Surgery	2.45	−3.16	0.97	0.89
	(14.84)	(9.52)	(27.48)	
Radiology	0.20	−2.11	1.22	0.69
	(0.49)	(3.42)	(19.17)	
Anesthesiology	0.84	−2.59	0.86	0.33
	(4.64)	(2.36)	(7.57)	
Pathology	2.41	−1.71	1.03	0.68
	(7.63)	(2.69)	(15.30)	

NOTE: *t*-statistics are given in parentheses.
SOURCE: AMA Center for Health Policy Research, 1989.

actually be realized, since the volume of visits and consultations would increase only slightly whereas the volume of other types of services would decline by a relatively greater amount. A truly budget-neutral implementation of a Medicare payment schedule based on an RBRVS would require some increase in the overall level of Medicare-allowed charges, as measured by a Laspeyres index.

It follows that average gains for general/family practitioners and medical specialists would be larger than those reported in existing simulations. Losses for radiologists would be smaller, but those for pathologists would be greater. Among the surgical specialties, the direction of payment change would vary depending on their combination of visits and surgery.

Of course, these results are not definitive. They fail to explain increases in the Medicare residual over time. Nonetheless, the usefulness of behavioral information in filling in some policy gaps is obvious. A good deal of caution will still be in order even when we feel we have truly refined analyses of behavioral responses to allowed charge changes. Economists can provide reasonable predictions within the range of existing observed experiences. The RBRVS may take us beyond our experience to date, however, so our predictions may still not be very good.

13
The Content and Rationale
of PPRC Recommendations
to Congress

Paul B. Ginsburg

The Physician Payment Review Commission has developed a comprehensive set of proposals to rationalize the pattern of payments to physicians by Medicare and to slow the rate of increase in program costs. To rationalize payments, the commission proposes a Medicare fee schedule based primarily on resource costs. To limit beneficiary financial liability, it recommends limits on balance billing. And to control the growth in Medicare expenditures for physicians' services, it proposes the use of expenditure targets, increased research on the effectiveness of medical services, the development of practice guidelines, and improvements in utilization and quality review.

Since its inception in 1986, the commission has been studying the pattern of Medicare payments to physicians. The more it learns, the stronger its conviction becomes that the pattern of relative payments based on screens for "customary, prevailing, and reasonable" (CPR) charges has serious problems. It conforms neither to patterns that would promote efficiency in medical practice nor to those that one might infer to be fair among physicians or among beneficiaries.

Studies by the commission and others have shown that the current pattern of payments departs substantially from estimates of the resource costs of providing physician services. For example, the

This chapter is based on the executive summary of the Physician Payment Review Commission's 1989 Annual Report to Congress. Certain sections have been expanded to provide additional explanation of the rationale for the recommendations. Other sections have been deleted because they are covered elsewhere in this volume (chapter 12) or because they are not an integral part of the commission's payment reform recommendations. The reader seeking more details should refer to the full report.

Hsiao relative value study indicates that physicians systematically receive less payment for evaluation and management services in relation to physician time and effort than they receive for invasive and imaging procedures. The variation in payment patterns from locality to locality appears to be erratic in that it does not correspond to variations in practice costs.[1] A fee schedule would permit changes in payments for both relative values and geographic variation that would more closely approximate differences in resource costs. A fee schedule would also be simpler and less expensive to administer, and it would make the program easier to understand for both beneficiaries and physicians.

Much of the rapid increase in Medicare outlays for physicians' services reflects the rising utilization of services per enrollee. From 1980 to 1988, physician services per enrollee increased by 7 percent per year.[2] But the evidence suggests that many services delivered to patients have little or no value; expert consensus regards medical benefits as either negligible or smaller than the medical risks involved. The most promising way to control program costs is to reduce the provision of such services.

To do this, the medical profession must know which services can be expected to benefit the patient and must have a means of identifying and selectively reducing those of little or no benefit. To implement this approach, it will be necessary to increase their knowledge of the effectiveness and appropriateness of medical practices and for physicians, patients, managers of care, reviewers, and regulators to increase their use of that knowledge.

Over time, a Medicare fee schedule might help to reduce the growth of spending through a more rational set of incentives to physicians and through improvements in coding. Although a reduction in the excessive profitability of some services and procedures might reduce their use, this could be offset by responses to increases in payments for other services. The effects of a fee schedule on volume are uncertain, however, especially in the short run, and it would be unwise to count on it to solve the problem of inappropriate services.

The commission recommends three policies to slow the growth of expenditures and to reduce the provision of inappropriate services: (1) give physicians collective incentives to slow growth in expenditures through expenditure targets; (2) increase research on the effectiveness of care and develop and disseminate practice guidelines; and (3) improve utilization and quality review by carriers and peer review organizations (PROs). These proposals are outlined below.

The Medicare Fee Schedule

RECOMMENDATION: *The current CPR payment system should be replaced with a Medicare fee schedule (MFS) based primarily on resource costs incurred in efficient medical practice.*

A fee schedule consists of a relative value scale (RVS), which indicates what each service or procedure is to be paid relative to others; a conversion factor, which translates the relative values into dollar amounts of payment; a geographic multiplier, which indicates how the payment for a service is to vary from one locality to another; and, in some cases, specialty multipliers. A Medicare fee schedule also requires a policy regarding assignment and balance bills, a transition, a process for updating all aspects of it, and a system for monitoring effects.

Relative Value Scale. An RVS that is based on resource costs must reflect both the physician work (time and intensity of effort) and practice (nonphysician input) costs of each service. It cannot be specified without a system of uniform and well-specified service codes. The commission has developed specifications for each of these components of the Medicare fee schedule.

Physician work. The commission has carefully studied the research into relative value scales by William Hsiao and his colleagues at Harvard University. Its staff has examined the methodology and reanalyzed much of the raw data collected in the study. It has consulted with outside experts and has heard testimony from many organizations representing physicians, beneficiaries, and others, most of which have had their own experts and leaders examine the study. The results of this exercise have led the commission to conclude that many parts of the study will have to be revised and expanded, but the basic methodology of the study is sound.

RECOMMENDATION: *The Hsiao study's estimates of physician time and effort should be used as the initial basis for the physician work component of the RVS in the Medicare fee schedule.*

Hsiao has defined physician work as time, mental effort and judgment, technical skill, physical effort, and stress from iatrogenic risk. His team has estimated work by surveying a sample of practicing physicians in each specialty on the time and work involved in performing various services and procedures. The estimates of work for

344

each specialty are combined into a single scale by linking across specialties services that are considered the same or equivalent. Data on charges are used to extrapolate from the surveyed services and procedures to those not directly studied. By assuming that time is not the only cost element that is relevant to an RVS and by basing estimates of the subjective elements on the judgments of practicing physicians, Hsiao has measured costs in a manner likely to be acceptable to a broad spectrum of physicians. But the Hsiao estimates of work must be refined and expanded before they can be used as a basis for the RVS in the Medicare fee schedule. The principal tasks are

- to devise a more precise measurement of work before and after direct contact with the patient (pre- and postservice work)
- to identify additional services to incorporate into the cross-specialty linkages
- to refine the methods of estimating physician work for services not included in physician surveys (extrapolation)
- to collect additional data on several specialties surveyed in phase I of the study and on estimates of physician work in additional specialties
- to resolve the remaining problems relating to particular services

Much of this work is already under way.[3] Professor Hsiao has begun to test better ways of measuring pre- and postservice work and to extrapolate from surveyed services to others. When these methods are refined, he will survey specialties not included in phase I, extend the surveys of certain specialties to cover additional services and procedures, and resurvey selected specialties.

These steps are expected to refine the estimates of work considerably, but relative values for individual services may still contain inaccuracies. To correct these inaccuracies, the commission plans to use consensus panels to revise intraspecialty relative values, particularly for those developed through extrapolation and for those covered by closely related codes (for example, upper gastrointestinal endoscopy with or without biopsy). It also plans to establish a process by which medical specialty societies and other organizations can raise concerns about relative values for specific services. As an example, organizations representing thoracic surgeons suggest that the description in the Hsiao study of coronary artery bypass surgery does not reflect recent changes in the procedure that have increased the time required. After consultation with Professor Hsiao, other medical associations, and independent experts, the commission would judge whether revisions should be made.

Practice and training costs. The commission has not found the estimates of practice and training costs developed by Professor Hsiao to be a suitable component for the Medicare fee schedule. Instead, it has developed its own estimates of practice costs and has recalculated the RVS to incorporate them. It plans to refine its estimates of practice costs further.

RECOMMENDATION: *Practice costs (expenses for nonphysician inputs) should be incorporated into the RVS through an additive formula.*

The original formula used by Professor Hsiao distorted relative values because it constrained the ratio of the valuation of physician work to practice costs for each service so that it would be the same under the resource-based relative value scale as under CPR payment. But this implies that whenever the valuation of physician work changes, practice costs change by the same percentage. Although practice costs might respond somewhat to changes in the valuation of physician work over time, the one-to-one correspondence is extreme. This constraint led Hsiao to overestimate the impact of a fee schedule on different specialties.

An additive formula corrects this problem by holding practice costs for a service constant while the valuation of physician work changes. It also makes it easier to integrate geographic multipliers and to update the conversion factors over time. The commission has recalculated the RVS based on the Hsiao estimates of physician work using an additive formula to integrate practice costs and its own estimates of the ratio of practice costs to total revenues by specialty.

Under this method, the ratio of practice costs to total revenue for a specialty was used to divide the current average submitted charge for each service into a physician work component and a practice cost component. The practice cost component was held constant while the physician work component was changed to conform to the Hsiao estimates of relative work, the assumption being that under current patterns of charges the ratio of the valuation of the physician input to practice costs is the same for all services within a given specialty. Thus, when physician work is revalued on the basis of the Hsiao estimates, the ratio for each service changes while the ratio for the entire specialty stays the same.

An alternative approach considered by the staff of the Health Care Financing Administration would be to hold the aggregate practice costs of each specialty constant and to estimate the practice costs for each service by allocating this amount in proportion to physician work. This would not change the pattern of redistribution across

346

specialties under a fee schedule, but would change the relative prices within a specialty. Without data on the allocation of a physician's practice costs among the services produced, we have little basis for choosing among these alternatives.

RECOMMENDATION: *To the degree that it is technically feasible, practice cost factors used in the RVS should apply to categories of services rather than to specialties.*

As is clear from the above discussion, specialty-specific cost factors do not take into account differences in the types of nonphysician inputs used for different services. Since physicians in some specialties provide an array of services with substantially different ratios of physician work to practice costs, different practice cost factors should be used for different kinds of services in order to more accurately relate practice cost allocations to the inputs actually required. Furthermore, if the specialty-specific cost factors being used are based on historical data, they might incorporate differences in amenity levels induced by the distortions in relative payments under CPR.[4]

The commission is using data from its own survey of physicians and from other sources to estimate practice costs for categories of services, such as office visits, office technical procedures, inpatient surgery, and so on. Practice cost factors would apply across all or most specialties. Procedures that employ expensive specialized equipment will require a unique practice cost factor.[5] The commission has been working with several organizations to collect the data it needs to develop that factor.

RECOMMENDATION: *The cost of professional liability insurance should be separated from other practice costs. It can either be integrated into the RVS through a separate practice cost factor or be reimbursed directly to physicians.*

Insurance coverage for malpractice represents a large component of practice costs, although it varies substantially by specialty and by geographic area. To ensure that the Medicare fee schedule takes into account differences among risk classes and localities, either a separate practice cost factor should be used or Medicare should reimburse physicians for a portion of their premium, depending on what proportion of their services is delivered to Medicare beneficiaries. Under either approach, the federal government would have a stake in investigating the merits of premium-setting practices and in developing policies to reduce the costs of malpractice (both premium costs and the costs of defensive medicine).

347

RECOMMENDATION: *The RVS should not include an additional factor for the opportunity costs of specialty training.*

Human capital models suggest that additional years of specialty training may make physicians more productive. The relevant question to ask in designing a fee schedule, however, is how does this additional productivity manifest itself? If it permits a physician to perform a procedure more rapidly, then the additional productivity could be rewarded by a payment based on the average amount of time to perform a procedure. If it permits physicians to perform more difficult procedures, and the difficult procedures are valued more per unit of time than easy procedures, the additional productivity could also be rewarded. There are two instances in which the productivity would not be rewarded: first, if the training resulted in a service that was more effective but not recognized as a different service by the coding system, and second, if coding is based roughly on time, as in visits, and the additional training permits a saving in time.

The commission decided not to recommend a factor for specialty training, as proposed by Professor Hsiao, because it felt that the first two examples were likely to be more prevalent. There would be too many cases in which specialty differentials would violate the principle that physicians should be paid the same when the service is the same. Another concern was the potential for double counting, because physicians participating in the Hsiao study tended to rate services requiring additional specialty training as requiring more work per unit of time. Most of the vignettes rated by physician respondents encompassed a range in which some of the services require much of the additional specialty training whereas others do not. The respondents rate the former as requiring more skill than the latter.

Coding. Two reforms in coding are required for a relative value scale based on resource costs. They apply to evaluation and management services and surgical global services.

RECOMMENDATION: *The coding system for evaluation and management (EM) services should be revised so that visits are classified on the basis of time as well as site of service, type of patient, and referral status.*

Physicians cannot accurately use the current codes for EM services because the levels of service (brief, intermediate, or comprehensive, for example) that differentiate each type of visit (that is, established patient office visit, initial consultation) are not precisely defined.

Interpretation varies not only among individual physicians, but also by specialty and by region. This makes it difficult to assign accurate values to current visit codes in a relative value scale based on resource costs.

The analyses of the commission and of Professor Hsiao suggest that the physician's time is a good predictor of the work involved in each type of visit. The relationship between time and work is similar for physicians in different specialties and in different parts of the country. Thus, if time was incorporated into the definitions of levels of service, more accurate relative values could be assigned to these services. This would help physicians use EM codes properly and give carriers a better way of determining whether physicians are billing correctly for these services.

If time was incorporated into the definitions of levels of service, physicians would not receive a uniform payment per hour. Since the commission's analysis suggests that the relationship between work and time varies depending on the site of service, type of patient, and referral status, physicians would receive a different payment for providing different types of visits that last the same amount of time. The analysis also suggests that for a particular type of visit, the relationship between total work and patient contact time is not proportional, so those physicians providing more visits per hour of patient contact time would receive more payment.

Many details need to be resolved before time can be incorporated into an EM coding system. In a joint endeavor with the American Medical Association (AMA), the commission plans to convene a consensus panel made up of physicians from all leading specialties that provide EM services and include carrier representatives and beneficiaries. The panel would help design a revised coding system, drawing on data from the commission's log-diary visit survey and from the Hsiao study and would report to both the commission and the AMA's CPT Editorial Panel.

RECOMMENDATION: *The legislative mandate to HCFA to group evaluation and management codes for payment purposes should be delayed until the reform of coding for these services is completed.*

The legislative mandate to "group codes for payment purposes" by January 1, 1990,[6] is no longer an appropriate way to proceed. The goal of this mandate is to control the misuse and abuse of the coding system under the current payment method. But the commission's analysis indicates that this goal would be better accomplished by integrating precise definitions for codes with relative values that more closely approximate relative resource costs. The commission therefore recommends that this legislative mandate be delayed until coding reform is completed.

RECOMMENDATION: *Global payment for surgery should be based on the policy developed by the commission for defining which services associated with an operation are to be included in the payment for the operation. This policy should be adopted by all Medicare carriers when the Medicare fee schedule is implemented.*

Surgical services have long been billed on the basis of a global fee, which means that the operation, many perioperative procedures, and EM services are all included in the fee. Medicare pays for surgery on a global basis, but each carrier uses a different definition of which services are to be included in the global payment and which are to be paid separately. A national RVS requires a uniform definition that is clear, fair, and easy to administer.

After reviewing the recommendations of a consensus panel of surgeons and carrier representatives that was convened by the commission, the commission has developed such a global fee policy. Under this policy, the global fee will include preoperative hospital visits on the day of surgery and the day before, postoperative visits for ninety days after the operation, and intraoperative procedures by the principal surgeon that are considered usual and necessary. Services to be paid separately include the surgical consultation (examination and discussion at which decision to have surgery is made), nonoperative procedures not specified as included, and reoperations for complications.

Estimates from the Hsiao study for relative work for surgical procedures must be revised to reflect this uniform definition of the global fee. The definition used in the Hsiao study is narrower than most carriers' definitions today. A survey of carriers suggested a difference averaging 10 percent. The commission's simulations included in this report have adjusted for this.

Specialty Differentials. Under current policies of many Medicare carriers, payment varies according to the specialty of the physician.

RECOMMENDATION: *Specialty differentials should not be incorporated into the Medicare fee schedule.*

The payment for the same procedure code should be the same across specialties unless the work provided by different specialties is sub-

350

stantially different. The commission's proposed coding reform of EM services should make this situation less common.

In some cases, physicians in different specialties provide different services under the same code, but would receive the same payment under the Medicare fee schedule, because distinct codes that would capture these differences accurately do not exist. These legitimate reasons for differences in payment, when substantiated, should be recognized by establishing new codes and setting relative values to reflect differences in resource costs. Such coding changes would be included in updates of the relative value scale.

Specialty-specific Relative Value Scales. Medicare currently pays for the services of anesthesiologists and radiologists on the basis of relative value scales specific to those specialties.

RECOMMENDATION: *The Medicare fee schedule based on resource costs should determine payments to all physicians, including those currently paid under specialty-specific relative value scales.*

Most carriers have long used various versions of the relative value guide (RVG) developed by the American Society of Anesthesiologists to pay for anesthesia services. The RVG bases payment on time, the difficulty of the operation, and patient condition. The Omnibus Budget Reconciliation Act of 1987 (P.L. 100-203 [OBRA87]) directed the secretary of health and human services to develop a standard version of the RVG for use by all carriers. This policy has recently been implemented.[7] The RVG is resource based and has been in use for some time. The commission will consider it as an alternative to the intraspecialty relative values developed by the Hsiao study. The cross-specialty linkages from the Hsiao study would be used to integrate the RVG for anesthesia with the rest of the RVS.

Currently, services provided by radiologists are paid on the basis of a fee schedule developed by the Health Care Financing Administration in consultation with the American College of Radiology. The commission will evaluate whether the relative value scale underlying this fee schedule improves upon the Hsiao study's intraspecialty relative value scale in its ability to reflect resource costs. If this should be the case, the commission would integrate these relative values for radiology into the overall RVS using the linkages developed in the Hsiao study.

Geographic Multiplier. The relative value scale described above should be applied uniformly throughout the nation, but the actual payment rates in different localities need not be uniform.

RECOMMENDATION: *Payments under the MFS should vary from one geographic locality to another to reflect the variation in physicians' costs of practice. The cost-of-practice index underlying the geographic multiplier should reflect variation only in the prices of nonphysician inputs.*

In response to a mandate from Congress, the HCFA has sponsored the development of an index to estimate differences in practice costs faced by physicians in different localities. This index is based not on the actual practice costs incurred by physicians in different areas, but on the prices that they face for the various nonphysician inputs that they use.[8]

The physician's time and effort should be valued uniformly throughout the nation. Thus, if physicians in two regions of the country provided the same services to Medicare beneficiaries, they would earn the same net income from those services. This principle may not be consistent with an attempt to simulate a hypothetical labor market for physicians' services. The commission was influenced by the recommendations of many organizations of physicians and senior citizens expressing their sense of what is fair and workable and by the observation that most Canadian and European fee schedules do not vary fees geographically, in part to ensure access to care in those areas less desirable to professionals.[9]

The cost-of-practice index developed for the HCFA by the Urban Institute and the Center for Health Economics Research measures variation in prices for rent and salaries of nonphysician employees.[10] It is based on the assumption that medical equipment, medical supplies, and "other" items are purchased in national markets and therefore the index does not reflect variations in their prices. The index also includes a component to reflect the opportunity cost of physician time and effort. It is measured by the earnings of employed professionals. Under the commission's recommendation, this component would be assigned a constant value.

Price indexes such as this one may not accurately reflect the costs of practice in rural areas, however. Rural physicians may face higher prices for equipment maintenance, for example, an item assumed to have uniform costs. In addition, rural practices may have some diseconomies from fewer opportunities to purchase rather than provide support services. The commission has collected data on the costs of rural practice and will analyze them to determine if an additional adjustment for rural practice is called for.

PAUL B. GINSBURG

RECOMMENDATION: *The Medicare fee schedule should encompass a uniform policy on the delineation of charge localities.*

To apply the geographic multiplier, a new set of boundaries would have to be drawn for charge localities. At present, each carrier has the discretion to draw locality boundaries within its area of responsibility, and carriers use very different principles to identify charge localities. In concert with the HCFA and its carriers, the commission plans to develop a uniform policy that will be flexible enough to allow carriers to suggest to HCFA what adjustments would better reflect unique local circumstances.

Assignment and Balance/Extra Billing. A Medicare fee schedule would have to incorporate a policy decision concerning assignment and balance billing. The current maximum allowable actual charge (MAAC) limits would no longer fulfill their purpose under a fee schedule. Given all of the changes in payments resulting from the Medicare fee schedule, a limitation based on what physicians charged for a service in the second quarter of 1984 would no longer be appropriate.

RECOMMENDATION: *Charges for unassigned claims should be limited to a fixed percentage of the fee schedule amount. This policy would replace the existing MAAC limits. The commission does not have a recommendation for the specific percentage to be used.*

The commission advocates that limits be imposed on charges for the same reason that it advocates a fee schedule based primarily on resource costs: That is, the market for physicians' services does not function well enough to provide financial protection for Medicare beneficiaries. The PPRC Survey of Beneficiaries found that the balance bills are shouldered by low-income beneficiaries as well as those better able to pay them. Indeed, when area of residence was held constant, income of the beneficiary did not have a significant effect on the probability of a claim being assigned.[11] The commission does not recommend mandatory assignment at this time, however. Mandatory assignment would be unacceptable to many physicians and inconsistent with the commission's goal of orderly change.[12]

There are two precedents in OBRA87 for limits on charges. Charges for the services of radiologists were limited to 125 percent of the amount specified for the service by the radiology fee schedule in 1989, 120 percent in 1990, and 115 percent after 1990. The other precedent involves physician charges for overpriced procedures for which the prevailing charge was reduced. These charges were limited to 125 percent of the new prevailing charge plus one-half of the difference between the allowed charge and the MAAC in 1988, and to 125 percent of the reduced prevailing charge thereafter.

RECOMMENDATION: *Balance billing should not be permitted for any Medicare beneficiary whose cost sharing is paid by Medicaid.*

This recommendation would make it necessary to clarify the provision in the Medicare Catastrophic Coverage Act of 1988 (P.L. 100–360). Under this provision, state Medicaid programs must pay Medicare cost sharing for beneficiaries seeking this assistance who are not otherwise eligible for Medicaid, but who have incomes below the federal poverty level. The current legislation covers Medicaid payment of deductibles, premiums, and coinsurance, but does not require physicians to accept the Medicare-allowed charge as payment in full, as they do for other Medicare beneficiaries covered by Medicaid. Since the commission views these persons as Medicaid beneficiaries, the policy on balance billing that applies to all dual eligibles should apply to them.

In principle, the commission believes that assignment should be required in situations where the beneficiary has no meaningful choice of provider, but it is not yet able to clearly delineate those services for which patients rarely have a meaningful choice of provider. Therefore, the commission is not prepared to issue a specific recommendation on this issue at the present time. In the future, it will assess the feasibility of identifying services for which patients rarely have a meaningful choice of physician. The commission will also be examining the burden of coinsurance and balance billing for medically or financially vulnerable beneficiaries.

RECOMMENDATION: *The Participating Physician and Supplier Program (PAR) and its payment differential providing higher fees to participating physicians should be continued under the Medicare fee schedule.*

The PAR program appears to have increased the assignment rate through its 5 percent payment differential, by facilitating beneficiary efforts to identify physicians who will accept assignment, and by freeing physicians from restrictions associated with unassigned claims. The commission supports efforts to encourage physicians to accept assignment, but the PAR program would be more effective if it were more widely publicized among beneficiaries.

Conversion Factor. The conversion factor transforms the RVS into a schedule of dollar payments.

RECOMMENDATION: *The Medicare fee schedule is a fundamental payment reform. Decisions on payment updates should be made independently of this basic reform.*

The commission has assumed that the initial conversion factor would be set at a level such that Medicare outlays projected under the fee schedule would equal those projected under the current payment system. This "budget-neutral" conversion factor for the initial year would separate the fundamental reform embodied in the MFS from issues such as the resources available for medical care for the elderly and the appropriate level of payment to physicians. These aggregate concerns would be addressed separately, through an update to prevailing charges for all services. With this aggregate update in place, fees for each service under the MFS would be established using a budget-neutral conversion factor. Updates in the conversion factor would be based on expenditure targets (see below).

Transition. A transition period is needed to give physicians and beneficiaries time to adjust. It would permit some of the advantages of the Medicare fee schedule to be gained before the definitive version of it is available, would allow for midcourse corrections, and would increase the chances that private payers will change their policies as Medicare changes are being implemented. The transition should begin soon, but with relatively modest initial changes in payment; it should use improved data as they become available, and should avoid disruptions or increases in Medicare's administrative burdens.

RECOMMENDATION: *A transitional stage should begin in 1990, with the implementation of the full Medicare fee schedule planned for 1992.*

In one plan that would meet these objectives, this transitional stage would initially retain customary and prevailing charge screens. For each charge locality, a projected fee schedule amount would be calculated for each of the 300–500 services and procedures that account for the largest dollar volume of Medicare claims. For each service/locality combination, the percentage difference between the fee schedule amount and the average allowed charge under current policy would be calculated. In the case of EM services, however, where accurate relative values for particular codes would not be available until coding was reformed, percentage differences would be calculated for categories of service, such as office visits and hospital visits.

For the first year of the transitional stage, the prevailing charge of each service would be changed by one-fifth of this percentage difference. Thus, if office visits are to increase by 28 percent under the Medicare fee schedule, for example, the prevailing charge for each visit code would increase by 5 percent during this first year. For the second year of the transitional stage, the Medicare fee schedule would be revised to reflect all the additional relevant data that would become available. Prevailing charges would be adjusted by an additional one-fourth.

Under an alternative plan for the second stage, payments could be a blend of each physician's average allowed amount for the service in 1990 and the projected Medicare fee schedule amount. This alternative would make it possible to eliminate prevailing and customary charge screens during the second year and incorporate new boundaries for localities.

Implementation of the transitional stage would begin about six to nine months after enactment of the legislation. After two years of experience, the full Medicare fee schedule would be implemented, along with coding reforms. The commission staff is planning to hold discussions with the policy and operations staffs of the HCFA to revise the details of this proposed transition plan.

Monitoring Access. Although the Medicare fee schedule is expected to improve the quality of care and to increase access by beneficiaries on the whole, payments for particular procedures and particular localities may be set too high or too low. Also, no one can accurately predict how physicians and beneficiaries will respond to changes in relative payments.

RECOMMENDATION: *The Medicare program should devote greater effort to monitoring access to care and the degree of financial burden experienced by beneficiaries.*

Some of the information needed to monitor access can be derived from claims files, but additional access indicators will be needed for a thorough assessment. The commission thus recommends the judicious use of survey data to examine beneficiaries' satisfaction with their care, their self-perceived health status, other measures of access, and the degree of financial burden from out-of-pocket expenses. The commission supports the HCFA's efforts to develop an ongoing survey to gather detailed information on beneficiaries' use of service, out-of-pocket expenditures, and other items. It recommends that full support be provided for implementing the proposed Current Beneficiary Survey.

RECOMMENDATION: *Information gathered on access to care should be integrated into the decision on the annual update.*

Evidence of limited access to a service or category of service could be one consideration for a revision in the payments for those services. Or evidence of limitations in a geographic area could lead to a revision in the geographic multiplier. Finally, evidence on access by the Medicare population as a whole could be relevant to the update in the conversion factor.

Update Process. A fee schedule is not a static policy. It must be revised to reflect changes in physician practice, beneficiary access, and the utilization of services. To update the fee schedule, it will be necessary to revise the conversion factor and revise the relative payments. The conversion factor is likely to be based on a blend of factual data and budget or other policy considerations. Updating the relative payments will be a matter of handling the technical issues involved in adjusting relative values for individual procedures and valuing new procedures, refining the coding system, and modifying geographic multipliers.

The commission has studied the experience in updating fee schedules in Canada, France, and West Germany and has concluded that no single approach used elsewhere can be applied in the United States. It has also considered four methods that might be used for this purpose: a formula approach, a rule-making process, an independent commission, and direct negotiation. It concluded that a process combining elements of each is most compatible with the American political and administrative traditions.

RECOMMENDATION: *The process used to develop the fee schedule proposal— whereby the Physician Payment Review Commission seeks the input of organizations representing physicians, beneficiaries, and other affected parties and develops recommendations to present to Congress—should be used for updating the fee schedule as well.*

That process has been successful in accomplishing the technical and policy development tasks required to date, and has provided organizations representing physicians, beneficiaries, and others affected by the policy a substantial opportunity to participate in the decision making.

Under this process, Congress would set policy regarding updates in the conversion factor, changes in relative values, and adjustments to the fee schedule. The commission would continue to provide the Congress with the necessary data, analysis, and policy advice each year for its update decisions. Groups representing physicians, beneficiaries, and others would participate in both technical refinements and major policy decisions, and the commission would provide the principal forum for their input. The HCFA would continue to be the principal implementing agency, carrying out congressionally defined policies through its administrative and rule-making processes. Both the commission and the HCFA would monitor the implementation of the fee schedule and conduct the technical analyses needed for policy decisions.

Expenditure Targets

The rapid growth of spending on physicians' services in Medicare has diverted substantial public resources from other federal priorities. It has also diverted beneficiary resources that pay for premiums and coinsurance from other needs. If these trends continue, the sacrifices will become much larger than ever before. The commission has therefore proposed that annual increases in the conversion factor under the Medicare fee schedule be based on a comparison of increases in spending per enrollee and a target rate of increase.

RECOMMENDATION: *The conversion factor should be updated annually through an expenditure target formula, so that the rate of increase of Medicare expenditures per enrollee determines in part the size of the conversion factor update.*

In contrast to budget policy in recent years, which has concentrated on reducing price, expenditure targets would provide an opportunity for physicians to help the program achieve its cost containment objectives through actions to slow the increase in the utilization of services. A collective incentive would be given to the medical community to reduce services of little or no benefit to patients. Although it would not provide direct incentives to individual practitioners, such a policy would encourage the leadership of medicine to promote activities that would help inform physicians of the medical benefits and risks of procedures and encourage them to play a more active and constructive role in peer review activities. Expenditure targets would send physicians a message about the need to slow the rate of increase in program and beneficiary outlays and provide them with constructive ways to respond.

The target would reflect increases in a reformulated Medicare economic index (MEI),[13] the growth and aging of the enrollee population, and a policy decision on the degree to which expenditure growth should exceed these factors. This decision would represent a trade-off between beneficiary needs, technological advances, and affordability to beneficiaries and taxpayers.

If actual expenditures during a year equaled targeted expenditures, then the conversion factor update for the following year would be equal to the increase in the MEI. The update would be increased or decreased to reflect differences between actual and targeted expenditure increases. As an example, assume that the MEI will increase by 4 percent, enrollment and aging will increase expenditures by 2 percent, and the volume of services is expected to increase by 7 percent per (age-adjusted) enrollee. This would lead to a 13 percent increase in expenditures from the base year. Now assume that a target of 11 percent per year for two years—2 percentage points less than the projection—is chosen. Thus growth of billed services per enrollee would have to slow to 5 percent for physicians to receive an update equal to the MEI for the following year.

If actual expenditures rise 13 percent, then the conversion factor update for the following year will be 2 percent (the 4 percent increase in the MEI less the 2 percent by which the target was exceeded). If actual expenditures rise only 9 percent, then the conversion factor update will be 6 percent (the MEI increase of 4 percent plus the 2 percent by which expenditures fell short of the target). In either case, the target for the second year would be 111 percent of the first-year target level of expenditures (or 123 percent of expenditures in the base year).

Alternatively, the target could be set further below the projected rate of increase in expenditures—for example, 8 percent. This would hold growth in Medicare physician outlays much closer to increases in the gross national product, but it would increase the probability that smaller conversion factor updates would play a larger role in bridging the gap between the projected and targeted rates of growth of expenditures.

RECOMMENDATION: *Initially, the expenditure target should apply to all physicians' services[14] in the nation. As the policy evolves, it is expected to incorporate a broader range of services and subtargets for regions and/or categories of physicians' services.*

359

Over time, the scope of expenditure targets could be broadened to include other Part B services ordered by physicians and the rate of hospital admissions.[15] Physicians would thus have additional ways to slow expenditure growth. Subtargets could be established for states, carrier areas, or metropolitan areas. These areas conform to the Medicare infrastructure of carriers, intermediaries, and PROs and the medical profession's infrastructure of state and county medical societies and chapters of specialty societies. With regional targets, physicians might think that they could work through their local organizations to meet state or metropolitan targets, while national targets would encompass too many aspects of care beyond their control. In addition, targets could be developed for categories of medical services. Although the commission recommends a relatively simple program to start with, it has already studied several of these options extensively and will continue to do so.

Expenditure targets would not directly alter the financial incentives for individual physicians and their patients. Rather, they would affect the physician community as a whole, which might respond through education of practitioners and support of the existing infrastructure of medical review. For example, the AMA and national specialty societies could develop and disseminate practice guidelines. They could provide technical assistance for carriers and PROs in the development of criteria for review and could support sanctions against physicians who persisted in providing inappropriate and poor-quality care. So that enough time will be set aside to develop the necessary infrastructure to control costs, the commission suggests a cautious approach to setting target increases for the first few years.

Antitrust and tort law may have to be changed to ensure that the physician community develops as effective a response as possible. Although carriers and PROs have immunity from antitrust violations when pursuing their assigned tasks, medical associations and hospital medical staffs may be limited in the activities directed at physicians whose quality of care does not meet recognized standards or who perform unnecessary services. The commission plans to examine the impact of antitrust barriers on medical organizations in order to discern whether limited immunity would be advisable.

Fear of malpractice suits may inhibit change by encouraging physicians to continue prescribing services that have only marginal benefit. Roughly 6 percent of the cost of physician services now goes to pay malpractice premiums, and that does not include the cost of defensive medicine. If the nation wants physicians to heed the urgings of the payers and their peers to practice more efficiently, it needs to concern itself with the magnitude of the malpractice risks that physicians face. The commission plans to examine the medical malpractice issue and to make recommendations concerning possible federal legislation.

Effectiveness Research and Practice Guidelines

Clinical and health services research is clearly needed to improve our knowledge of the effectiveness and appropriateness of medical practices and procedures. Such research would enable us to determine the medical outcomes and costs of clinical alternatives. It would include clinical trials, epidemiological studies using data generated by clinical practice, analysis of the cost effectiveness of alternative ways to organize care, and assessment of the techniques used in managed care to influence physicians' clinical decisions.

Practice guidelines would synthesize the best we know from research and the judgments of practicing physicians into a form that can be readily used. These guidelines should be incorporated into physicians' practices and made available to patients. They should also provide the basis for coverage, payment, and medical review criteria developed by hospital medical staffs, PROs, intermediaries, and carriers.

RECOMMENDATION: *The federal government should support effectiveness research and practice guidelines through increased funding, coordination, and evaluation.*

Several hundred million dollars per year should be provided for clinical research and technology assessment. Tens of millions are needed per year to develop, disseminate, implement, evaluate, and revise practice guidelines and review criteria. These sums are small when compared with the funds spent on research to develop new medical technologies; they are a tiny fraction of the $500 billion spent annually on health care. The medical profession would be expected to continue its support for this important research through contributions of funds and of physician time and expertise.

For effectiveness research, Congress could continue to use existing federal agencies to conduct intramural and sponsor extramural research, or it could direct that a new entity be created in the Department of Health and Human Services for this purpose.

RECOMMENDATION: *For practice guidelines, federal funds should be used to support and build on initiatives by the medical profession and others in the private sector.*

361

Federal funding would be accompanied by federal oversight to safeguard the integrity of the guideline development process—both the quality of the methods used and the validity of the resulting guidelines. The government could also help coordinate the now-fragmented activities in the private sector by facilitating efforts to share information, identify issues, and set priorities. The federal government should evaluate the processes by which guidelines are disseminated to practicing physicians and their effects on clinical practice.

The federal government also administers Medicare. The HCFA should emphasize that medical review must be based on sound criteria by helping PROs and carriers make sure they choose criteria that are consistent with practice guidelines. It should provide the carriers and PROs with funding in support of the dissemination. It should also evaluate the effects of practice guidelines on the outcomes of utilization and quality review activities in Medicare.

Utilization and Quality Review

Programs concerned with Medicare utilization and quality review should ensure that beneficiaries receive necessary and appropriate medical care in a cost-effective manner, and that such care meets recognized standards of quality. Medicare review programs, like those of other payers, were originally designed to focus on individual insurance claims, not to provide for the effective management of the complete range of medical services beneficiaries receive.

If utilization and quality review are to help improve the quality and efficiency of care and control the growth of Medicare expenditures, the Medicare program will have to create a comprehensive medical review system that looks across individual services to complete episodes of care and systematically integrates information drawn from claims data and medical records, analyses of practice variations, and profiles of physician practice. It will take time and additional resources for the carriers and PROs to take on these responsibilities. They will also require more administrative flexibility and the cooperation of the medical community.

RECOMMENDATION: *The commission supports the HCFA's current efforts to move toward a more comprehensive approach to medical review and calls for further actions to strengthen the review process. It has a number of specific recommendations for structuring this transition.*

First, the HCFA should take steps to encourage carriers and PROs to assist in designing the criteria used in utilization and quality review, in developing physician profiling activities, and in investigating physicians suspected of providing inappropriate or substandard care or inappropriate billing.

Second, the HCFA, carriers, and PROs must work together to define the future roles of PROs in the review of care provided by physicians in office settings. One question that needs attention is how the findings from PRO reviews of care in office settings and PRO activities focused on entire episodes of illness should be coordinated with carrier and intermediary medical review responsibilities.

Third, PROs and carriers should consult with the appropriate medical organizations when developing review criteria. The commission believes that the proposed rule published January 30, 1989, would be an important step toward meeting this objective.

Fourth, the HCFA should designate a single entity to support research, demonstrations, evaluations, and technical assistance in quality and utilization review for PROs, carriers, and intermediaries. This office should also serve as a source of information about state-of-the-art review methods and as a conduit for information about new practice guidelines that can be integrated into review criteria.

Strengthening the Infrastructure for Payment Reform

Before a fee schedule and expenditure targets can be set up, the Medicare data system will have to be changed, so that it will be possible both to administer the policies and monitor their effects. The commission applauds the HCFA's efforts to improve the data system, such as the unique physician identifier, by incorporating diagnosis codes on physician claims forms and developing a common working file that includes both Part A and B data. The commission recommends two further changes in the data agency's system to help it implement these payment reforms. It also calls for increased funding for program administration.

Improvements to Data System.

RECOMMENDATION: *Providers should file Medicare claims for all services—both assigned and unassigned—with no charge to beneficiaries. Claims should be submitted within ninety days after the delivery of service.*

This would ensure that the beneficiaries received the benefits to which they are entitled and would facilitate efficient claims processing and accurate and timely program data. Carriers should contact a

363

sample of beneficiaries to determine the accuracy of claims submitted by physicians.

RECOMMENDATION: *The HCFA should establish comprehensive requirements for carrier electronic claims capabilities and should provide technical assistance for carriers.*

Increased use of electronic claims (EMC) could significantly reduce carrier processing costs and improve the accuracy of program data. During the next year, the HCFA should develop an operational plan for more rapid conversion from paper claims to EMC. Congress should make movement to EMC a clear priority for HCFA by writing a timetable for electronic submission of all Part B claims.

RECOMMENDATION: *Electronic claims should be exempted from requirements for minimum processing times.*

One of the main incentives for physicians to use EMC is prompter payment, but current minimum times for processing remove much of that advantage.

Funding. The ability of the carriers to implement a fee schedule, increase EMC usage, and expand their medical review activities depends on adequate and predictable funding. Unfortunately, such funding cannot be taken for granted. Although funding for medical review activities of carriers was increased for the current fiscal year, the president's budget for 1990 would cut funding by 19 percent.

RECOMMENDATION: *The commission urges Congress to provide adequate and predictable funding for program administration.*

Since the HCFA is trying to hold back outlay increases in the range of $4 billion per year, attempts to shave spending for administration (in particular, medical review) are poorly conceived. If we are to attempt major reforms in this program, we must ensure that the administrative resources are there to carry them out.

Criteria for Judging the Recommendations

A Commentary by Joseph P. Newhouse

Paul Ginsburg has presented the rationale for the Physician Payment Review Commission's (PPRC) recommendations. What are reasonable criteria for judging a set of recommendations such as these? How do we determine whether implementing these recommendations would yield a better fee structure than the one we now have?

Incremental and Average Costs

We would be in the best position to appraise the recommendations if we had a criterion for an ideal fee. Mark Pauly gave one such criterion: the fee should be set where the demand curve of an informed consumer cuts the physician's marginal cost curve.[1] Although Pauly admitted that moral hazard would remain for insured consumers, he focused on possible distortions from supplier-induced demand and pointed out that such distortions would vanish if fees were set at marginal cost. In that case, the physician would have no incentive to induce additional services. Indeed, one can interpret calls to rationalize fees, or to reduce fees of "overpriced" procedures, as calls to bring fees closer to marginal cost.

How does Pauly's ideal fee mesh with the proposals of the commission? Unfortunately, neither the demand curve of the informed consumer nor the marginal cost curve of the physician is observed. Hence, it is difficult, perhaps impossible, to use this criterion to appraise empirically any actual fee schedule. Indeed, if there was a consensus on this criterion and if it was simple to implement, there almost certainly would not be a Physician Payment Review Commission asked to render judgment; the HCFA probably would long since have aligned fees with the resulting schedule. Because a straightforward empirical appraisal is not possible, one can use Pauly's criterion to evaluate the commission's proposals only

365

theoretically. This is unfortunate, but, in the absence of criteria for ideal fees that can be implemented empirically, theoretical appraisals are the best one can do.

The commission's starting point is the resource-based relative value scale (RBRVS) developed by William Hsiao. The RBRVS measures (relative) average cost, however, not (absolute) marginal cost, as proposed by Pauly. Moreover, average cost is assumed to be proportional to the total work of the physician. Several issues arise as a result.

One has to do with the correctness of the factor that converts the relative values into an absolute dollar figure. Converting in a budget-neutral fashion is pragmatic, but has little economic claim to optimality. Before making too much of this, however, one should consider the difficulty, perhaps impossibility, of determining an economically optimal conversion factor. For example, in addition to the health policy consequences of alternative conversion factors, one would need to know the deadweight losses from the taxes used to finance the program.

Another serious problem is the allocation of practice cost. Some "practice cost" is true marginal cost and should be allocated to a procedure; for example, both the nursing time used and the risk of malpractice associated with that procedure can in principle be allocated. Such allocations may well not be proportional to physician work (primarily physician time), as the RBRVS assumes. If nursing time, for example, does not vary proportionately with physician work or time (it may well vary inversely), the RBRVS as now constructed will not correctly measure marginal cost.

But even if nursing time and other relevant inputs did vary proportionately with physician time, marginal cost may not be constant. Pauly's notional marginal cost curve is rising; hence, one explicitly confronts the issue of variation with scale. If one sets prices equal to marginal cost, and marginal cost is not constant, where on the marginal cost curve does one wish to be?

Furthermore, nonconstancy may arise for reasons other than scale. For example, the costs of a given procedure may vary over time because of technological change. One rationale for developing the RBRVS was that costs for new procedures, such as coronary artery bypass surgery, did not fall over time as physicians presumably moved down a learning curve. This was used to infer that physician pricing was not competitive. This example also suggests that the costs the fee schedule is trying to match will change over time. The more that costs vary over time, of course, the more difficult the empirical problem will become and the more the need for updating.

366

Marginal costs may also vary over time or space because of variation in patient mix. If patients are older or more difficult, physicians may have a higher supply price. In principle, variation in the type of patient can be addressed by an expansion of codes, but in practice such differences in supply price will be difficult to measure.

Thus, a portion of the practice cost should be allocated to procedures, but not all practice cost should be allocated. For example, the cost of utilities to heat or cool the office is a joint cost that cannot be identified with specific procedures.

Nonetheless, both Hsiao and the PPRC seek to allocate all practice cost. As mentioned above, Hsiao does so through a proportional method; PPRC prefers an additive allocation. But from a theoretical point of view, both allocations are arbitrary, and neither would necessarily be closer to a theoretically optimal price.

Although neither Hsiao nor PPRC handles joint costs correctly from a theoretical point of view, such costs raise a fundamental conceptual problem for Pauly's criterion, because they suggest that prices set at incremental costs may fail to cover average costs. Hence, pricing at marginal or incremental cost may well not be feasible.

In the usual multiproduct firm case in which marginal or incremental costs are less than average costs, one applies the so-called Ramsey rule to find optimal second-best prices; the rule says to mark up marginal costs on each product in proportion to the reciprocal of the demand elasticity of that product, subject to the constraint that average cost be recovered. The Ramsey rule cannot be straightforwardly applied to physician fee schedules, however.

First, the Ramsey rule assumes that the consumer pays the supplier's price; it places higher markups on products with small demand elasticities in order to minimize the departure of quantities bought from the economically efficient quantity. But because of the prevalence of Medigap insurance as well as Medicaid, the price Medicare pays for the procedure will not much influence quantities demanded. Indeed, the issue here is exactly the opposite: How will the quantity supplied be influenced by the price Medicare pays?

Second, the Ramsey rule does not contemplate supplier-induced demand and presumes that the consumer is the best judge of how much should be bought. But a principal rationale for Pauly's reliance on the informed consumer's demand curve and marginal cost pricing is to eliminate incentives to induce demand. Following Pauly's argument, if feasible prices have to be above incremental cost, we again open up the possibility of inappropriate supplier-induced demand. (Inappropriate means care that would be valued by an informed consumer at less than its private opportunity cost. If externalities exist of the kind that the nonelderly are willing to pay something for the elderly's care, then the valuation should reflect the nonelderly's preferences as well. One might say that because the financing of Medicare comes in part from the nonelderly, their preferences are relevant, but that is a separable issue that I will not discuss further.)

Once we allow for supplier-induced demand, one would like to know how the mix of appropriate and inappropriate services changes for various procedures as their fee varies above marginal cost. And if one can only get more appropriate services by accepting more inappropriate services, one needs to know the rate of substitution between appropriate and inappropriate services. This would seem to be the analog in this world to the traditional rule's emphasis on minimizing deadweight losses on the demand side. In other words, the issue here is the optimal departure from marginal cost pricing. I certainly do not know what the optimal departures are, but nothing in the RBRVS methodology suggests that it will arrive at optimal departures or take into account how much appropriate and inappropriate demand will be induced.

In short, many reasons make it difficult to argue a priori from economic theory that an RBRVS-like fee scale, such as the PPRC proposes, will be optimal, or even better than the current situation. Thus, the ultimate test of how good such a fee scale is will have to be an empirical one. Put another way, evaluation will be important.

Specialty Differentials

Although the Hsiao and PPRC methods for allocating practice cost both seem arbitrary from a theoretical point of view, the PPRC method causes less change in interspecialty differentials. Whether this is good, of course, depends upon one's view of current interspecialty differentials. One might say that existing differentials have been distorted by the presence of insurance toward procedure- or inpatient-dominated specialties. In this view, both methods are an improvement, and one cannot say a priori which is preferred. In the RBRVS methodology, however, there is no allowance for nonpecuniary or equalizing specialty differentials. Even setting aside technical problems with linking procedures across specialties (such as the assumption that the errors across linking procedures have a zero expected value, that is, are not correlated), there remains the assumption that the procedures or patients unique to each specialty are on average equally attractive. This may well not be the case.

For example, a common interpretation of why radiologists, anesthesiologists, and pathologists have relatively high incomes is that their work is dominated by procedures that have historically been well insured, but another possibility is that specialists in such fields need to be compensated for the relative lack of patient contact. Pediatrics and psychiatry present a quite different example. A common interpretation is that those specialties are relatively poorly paid because historically there has been little insurance, but another possibility may be that (in contrast to, say, geriatrics) most patients get better, and physicians find that congenial.

Those who wish to assume that nonpecuniary specialty differentials are zero at the margin should consider the fear of some in departments of internal medicine that the combination of AIDS and older, more severely ill patients in the hospital is behind a fall in the attractiveness of their residency programs. This latter example points up that specialty differentials may also change over time.

In sum, the assumption that there are no nonpecuniary differentials across specialties—that the marginal physician will always gravitate to the more highly paid specialty—is suspect. Setting specialty differentials on this assumption may well distort the distribution of physicians across specialties.

Geographic Differentials

One of the PPRC's recommendations that is sure to be controversial is that the physician's take-home portion of the fee should not be adjusted for cost-of-living differences; apart from practice cost differences, the PPRC recommends the same nominal fee in Dubuque as in New York City. This view follows a long literature that has emphasized the variation in nominal total fees, usually concluding that the variation was too high and was in part responsible for a dearth of physicians in rural areas.

Only recently has it been pointed out that real fees and real earnings do not differ that much between metropolitan and nonmetropolitan areas (and may in fact be lower in large metropolitan areas). Ironically, the Physician Payment Review Commission itself has made this argument.[2] Some have also challenged the view that there is a dearth of physicians in nonmetropolitan areas. There is little evidence of access problems for most of the nonmetropolitan population; waits to appointment do not much differ between metropolitan and nonmetropolitan areas, and visit rates do not seem abnormally low in nonmetropolitan areas. Indeed, the picture is consistent with the marginal physician's being close to neutral about location (there is some evidence of a mild preference at the margin for cities of 1,000,000 or more).

369

If the marginal physician is nearly location-neutral, the commission's recommendations would redistribute physicians toward nonmetropolitan areas. If physicians in rural areas are not much more heavily loaded with patients than their counterparts in metropolitan areas, the presumption would be that those in metropolitan areas are not willing to pay to place more physicians in rural areas (that is, there is no externality toward residents of rural areas on this account). If not, the PPRC's recommendation could well bring about an economically inefficient spatial distribution of physicians.

The stated desire of the RBRVS is to emulate the properties of a competitive market. One might argue that cost of living differentials are equalizing; that is, physicians in attractive locations would have lower real incomes in equilibrium and thus that the PPRC recommendation is consistent with competitive behavior (but why then adjust for practice costs, a large portion of which is the wages of ancillary personnel?).

One way to test the proposition that observed differentials are equalizing is to ask what policies multiplant firms have about geographic differentials; although I have not investigated the issue, I would guess that compensation policies do take some account of the local cost of living, at least where the differences are marked. (Such policies may come in forms other than a simple salary differential, for example, differential housing assistance.) If this is right, the PPRC proposal would not emulate a competitive market.

Guidelines

The PPRC calls for a large research effort into the effectiveness and appropriateness of care, with an eye to developing practice guidelines. I heartily endorse this call, but make the point (not novel to me) that such guidelines may not save money. One can illustrate this point through a simple example using two stylized facts from the Health Services Utilization Study: (a) that areas with high procedure rates have rates that are four times those of low-rate areas and (b) that a third of the procedures in both high- and low-rate regions may be inappropriate.[3]

Suppose there are only two areas, and that in one area a given procedure is done four times as frequently as in the other. Table 13–C1 shows the number of procedures now done in both areas and the number that would be done in a hypothetical world in which no inappropriate procedures were done and all appropriate procedures were done, the intent of the guidelines. I make the assumption that because the areas are large, the rate of appropriate procedures is

TABLE 13–C1
POSSIBLE INCREASES IN PROCEDURES FROM GUIDELINES

	Appropriate Procedures	Inappropriate Procedures
Current situation		
High rate area	8	4
Low rate area	2	1
Hypothetical optimal situation		
High rate area	8	0
Low rate area	8	0

SOURCE: Author.

similar in the two areas and equals the rate in the high area. (If some appropriate procedures are not now done in the high rate area, the point is even stronger.)

As can readily be seen, if the guidelines bring about the hypothetical optimal situation, the total number of procedures will increase by one. By assumption, of course, the hypothetical situation is an improvement (assuming taxpayers are willing to pay for all appropriate procedures), but program costs may well increase.

One can add a number of caveats. To know what would happen to program costs one needs to know the cost of an inappropriate procedure relative to an appropriate one. For example, the length of stay in the hospital and the likelihood of complications may not be similar for appropriate and inappropriate procedures. Further, guidelines may be more effective at reducing inappropriate procedures than at increasing appropriate ones. If so, the chances are better that guidelines would reduce program costs. Most important, the studies of appropriateness imply directly that there is substantial inappropriate use; they only yield an inference that there may be substantial underutilization. In particular, some of what I have inferred to be underutilization may be attributable to differences in health status across areas. Nonetheless, the possibility remains that guidelines may not save money.

Data and Administrative Improvements

In recent years the HCFA has moved to upgrade the quality of Part B data, for example, by giving physicians unique identifiers and linking Part A and Part B data. The importance of these improvements for analysis can scarcely be overemphasized. The commission suggests

371

further improvements, including filing all claims. I agree with these recommendations and add two of my own:

1. For the study of how patients with a particular medical problem or diagnosis are treated, especially if the problem is one that is sometimes treated on an outpatient and sometimes on an inpatient basis, a linked A–B file that is larger than the current 5 percent sample should be created. Indeed, there should be a 100 percent sample; because the data are from administrative records, the additional cost of the larger sample should be modest.

2. Although it is not practical to do so in the short run, the HCFA needs to collect data on outpatient services delivered by capitated organizations. This will obviously become more important if the share of the Medicare market held by capitated organizations increases.

Evaluating the Behavioral Response

It is clear that we do not know how the existing stock of physicians will respond to the proposed changes in fee schedules. Some argue that if fees are reduced, quantities will increase,[4] while others are skeptical. Over the longer run, there will presumably be differential entry and exit by specialty that will make the response look more like an upward sloping supply curve. If we do not even know a priori whether the quantities of services consumed will increase or decrease in the short run, however, we cannot be very confident that the proposed changes in Medicare fees will represent an improvement in welfare. Thus, it is important that any changes be introduced in a way that permits as reliable an estimate as possible of their effects.

The draft of the commission's report prepared for the conference suggested a transition to a new fee schedule, but appeared (by silence) to imply that this would be accomplished in a nationally uniform fashion. The strongest design for evaluation would be to introduce the schedule in only part of the country initially. However, if that is precluded by political constraints, it would still be worthwhile to build in some seemingly modest nonuniformities in implementation. For example, the stipulation that hospitals would go onto the Prospective Payment System (PPS) at the beginning of their fiscal years enabled Ginsburg and Carter to compare hospitals that were on the PPS in one quarter with hospitals that were not on the PPS in that quarter.[5] This yielded a highly credible estimate of how much case mix change in the first year of PPS was true change and how much was upcoding. Because of the importance of estimating the effects of any fee schedule changes, it is well worth contemplating how analogous delays in applying any new fee schedule to some physicians might be accomplished.

Alternatives for Setting and Adjusting Fee Schedules III

A Discussion

COMMENT: If you allow a 10 percent return to all training, this implies as much as a 30 percent difference in the value of time across specialties. And those factors, if applied to specific specialties in the Juba-Colby presentation, would change the impact on the specialties a great deal. The percentage changes across the specialties become much closer to zero. In other words, if you incorporate these 10 percent rates of return to training, the specialties are not affected relatively as much as the PPRC's proposed RVS would affect them.

I want to ask about the double-counting problem, because there seems to be a fundamental problem in the PPRC's deciding not to adjust for training. Labor economics has viewed human capital in general as raising the productivity of labor time. And what we are really trying to get at is, what is the product of this physician's time? We can't measure the product. We can't measure the quality. We are trying to control that by using this same CPT, but even in that, there may be a difference in the actual product that is produced by the different specialties.

So it seems that even controlling for work and complexity, you can't be sure that the productivity of that physician time isn't really different for people with different training, and in fact twenty-five years of labor economics would suggest that it is.

So there is a fundamental identification problem in comparing across specialties, even for the same procedure, because we don't know exactly what the product is, and in fact there are differences in training that would suggest that the product might well be different.

PAUL B. GINSBURG: It really depends on how you're going to try to measure the inputs. In the Hsiao study, they asked the physician, how much time does this take, and then, how much skill relative to a

---

Part I of this discussion is on page 255, and part II on page 310.

reference procedure does it take? We are going to pay the physician more when the procedure takes more skill.

Now what we don't know is how much of that skill is coming from the additional specialty training. So you could have a model that says, well, we just want to pay for time, but then we are going to value the time according to a human capital model by the additional specialty training, or we are going to take the other approach. Instead of doing it that way, we'll pay for time and skill. So that is why I said that it would be double-counting to adjust for training. I can't say this with confidence. We'll never know. But it really is a possibility that these are just two different methods, and if we combine them, we pay double for the skill that is acquired through the training.

QUESTION: If marginal costs and average costs do differ, what should Medicare pay? Should Medicare be a prudent purchaser and just pay marginal cost? You know, forget malpractice, forget specialty training. Or should it be fair, and pay average cost?

MR. GINSBURG: It is tempting for Medicare, as the payer with the most market power, to demand the marginal cost price. On the other hand, Medicare would be politically constrained from doing so. Probably, it should come out somewhere between the marginal and average cost.

Interestingly, an example of the marginal-versus-average cost problem has been placed in the commission's lap for some decision after this report. In the catastrophic bill, a new Medicare benefit was created for mammography screening, and the bill actually put in a price that Medicare was going to pay. It was going to pay $50.

That price was apparently determined by some information on what average costs were at specialized facilities that do mammography screening, where the equipment is used pretty much full time. There, average and marginal costs would be nearly equal. A member of one of the committees objected strenuously to that, because she wanted women to be able to have this procedure done at their doctor's office, and not to have to go to these efficient facilities. She didn't get her way, but she did get a request for the commission to report to Congress on that issue. I believe the thinking of the commission is that we don't want to set the price up at the average or even marginal costs of the inefficient provider. Given that patients have access to going to a provider that can go down the marginal cost curve, we might set it at that price.

COMMENT: If you think about this as a mixture of payers, and what price they should pay, each of those payment sources—including the patient paying—involves some distortion. That is, we are in a second-best world. Medicare is tax-financed, in some degree premium-financed; there are distortions from the tax-financed part. There are distortions from the insurance subsidy and there are risks from cost sharing.

It seems that it is reasonable to think that each payer paying above marginal cost would be better than loading it all onto some single payer, since welfare losses increase disproportionately to the distortion. This suggests that Medicare should pay above the marginal cost.

COMMENT: Joe Newhouse suggested that one way of judging whether the PPRC recommendations are appropriate is to look at the goal. The goal, he said, was to reduce distortions in fee schedules.

There are other criteria that you might also want to use, for example, simplifying the payment system. Another criterion would be setting a price, so that the beneficiary and the provider will know before the service is rendered what it is going to cost.

It may well be that if you just give me a price, any price even if it isn't quite as good as the current price, if it simplifies and establishes the price, perhaps many would prefer that.

MR. GINSBURG: If you have a fee schedule, whether it is resource-based or charge-based, physicians can quote a conversion factor. If physicians were willing or were ordered to maintain their relative values in the fee schedule for their prices, so that they could say I'm at 1.1 times the fee schedule, this would simplify purchasers' and patients' work in shopping for price enormously, and that could be quite significant.

QUESTION: What happens to the notion of resource and cost when you choose the conversion factor? Presumably you want to pay the resource cost of each service. No more. Then when you choose the conversion factor and you base it on some budget-neutral or other criteria, is it true that a budget-neutral conversion factor really sets it equal to resource cost, or is it an arbitrary choice?

MR. GINSBURG: Well, all of the focus has been on the relative resource costs. Getting the absolute resource cost is probably more difficult, and certainly politics will play a much bigger role in that than in the relative resource costs.

QUESTION: But how do you know if you are paying too much or not enough? Is it irrelevant after that?

MR. GINSBURG: There are some indicators as to whether we're paying too much or not. We know what the aggregate amount of balance billing is today, and we can make a judgment as to whether, given the system we have with that amount of balance billing, we are paying too much or too little.

There is some feedback information, and that will be thrown into a political process in determining how much to pay. If Medicare paid a lot less, balance bills would go up, and congressmen are concerned about that.

Maybe they are fooling themselves, but beginning in 1984, they kept saying we want to pay less to physicians and we don't want that shifted to the beneficiaries. As a result they concocted many restrictions on balanced billing.

WILLIAM C. HSIAO: The way that we have handled the practice costs through a multiplicative model, and the way that PPRC is using an additive model—the differences are not that great.

The differences in the simulation results came about because the PPRC assumes that physicians will always recapture their current practice cost. Meanwhile, in our simulation, we assume that if a fee's going to go down, the practice cost will go down proportionately. And so it really is due to simulation assumptions rather than the multiplicative versus the additive model.

DAVID C. COLBY: We took the automobiles and the fringe benefits and moved them from practice costs into physician net income. So Bill Hsaio's assumption may be a bit extreme—that is, to say that practice costs are so malleable, they're so much in a sense implicit income built in that they would automatically conform to changes in payments.

MR. HSIAO: I'm not defending it. I'm just saying the difference is from that assumption. It depends on a policy decision—whether you are going to continue to reimburse the physician's practice costs in full or are going to make some changes. We are going from one extreme position, and the commission went to the other extreme. Ultimately, it is probably going to be coming out somewhere in the middle.

MR. COLBY: That's right. We could have produced the same results we've showed there with the multiplicative model. So the difference is not in the functional form. It is in the assumptions about practice costs.

PART THREE

Lessons Learned from Research, Theory, and Experience

On Regulating Prices for Physicians

A Commentary by Roger G. Noll

As many others have concluded, using an administrative process to construct a competitive equilibrium in the structure of physician prices appears to be intellectually impossible for a host of measurement reasons. Hence, the important challenge is to identify the least damaging way to engage in extraordinarily complex price regulation of doctor services. That is, if there is some political imperative, whereby people are holding guns to the heads of officials of the Health Care Financing Administration (HCFA) so that they must engage in price regulation, what ought they to do in order to minimize the damage? I will not address this question, but two others that are related to it: What are the kinds of problems that are likely to emerge when regulation is imposed? What is the nature of the political imperative behind the proposal to regulate? In order to do as little damage as possible, one wants to avoid the major problems, while responding to the political imperative.

Regulation is likely to create three important problems: (1) all ways of allocating joint and common costs will be fundamentally arbitrary; (2) since we have very little knowledge about how to measure quality, we will not be able to quantify the quality implications of any rule that we might undertake; and (3) in examining the components of physician's incomes, we will not have an adequate model to separate opportunity costs from various sorts of rents. These three problems make it almost impossible to regulate doctors' services efficiently. The only way to ensure that serious damage will be avoided is to design a system that will not have much effect. This raises the question of whether a policy that does little is consistent with the political imperative behind its creation, and therefore why people are even interested in it. Why is there a political or bureaucratic demand to play this game in the first place? That is the single most perplexing issue, because only three groups could possibly have anything to gain from this form of regulation.

One group consists of the bureaucrats in the HCFA, who stand to gain because of the enormous increase in information processing that regulation will entail. About 10,000 prices will have to be set just to begin regulating doctors' fees, but eventually the number will be much larger. When the Interstate Commerce Commission was busily engaged in regulating the relatively homogeneous transportation services, it had four billion different prices. But, medical care is less homogeneous than transportation, so the ICC number is probably a lower bound on the number of prices HCFA will have to regulate. Can you imagine the number of people who are going to be employed in the HCFA when they are regulating 10 billion medical service prices?

Of course, the HCFA cannot implement these prices without help. The second group of potential beneficiaries are people who are in the business of providing consulting services for the HCFA and other interested parties. Perhaps the regulation of doctor pricing is coming about because secretly, about a year and a half ago, people like Jan Mitchell and Bill Hsiao met to form a new professional association, the Motherhood of Medical Economists. This group managed to convince some political officials that it was in the national interest to increase the demand for their services by asking them to estimate impossible things. The potential demand for these people, once we embark on the regulation of 10 billion prices, is almost enough to induce me to become a medical economist.

What about the American Medical Association (AMA)? A particularly interesting aspect of the proposal is the combination of cost-based regulation with more or less equality of quality-adjusted labor inputs. That sounds like a union contract. Indeed, because the HCFA's rules for physician payments apply only for services paid by the HCFA, they are really a unilaterally imposed contract rather than a set of regulations. Perhaps the AMA sees itself as the natural countervailing authority for negotiating this contract and senses the possibility of gain from negotiating with the government for a national, quality-adjusted, hourly income for doctors. With budget neutrality, the AMA can pick out a few specialists who receive enormous fees and just beat the hell out of them, then redistribute the benefits through budget neutrality to all of the other members of the AMA.

The preceding scenario creates the opportunity for about 75 or 80 percent of the AMA to have a pay increase, at the expense of 20 to 25 percent. The only problem with all of this is that there might be the slightest bit of efficiency reason for existing wage differentials. If so, those efficiencies must be sacrificed, which in the long run means that the net income of AMA members is going to go down. That is to say, the efficiency loss will be visited in part upon the AMA. The rest of the loss will be experienced by patients in the form of lower quality of care.

Nevertheless, in the short run there could be a substantial net gain for most doctors. Its source is the existing stock of service-specific or specialty-specific investments in human and physical capital. A change in policy could expropriate some of those investments. The courts have not yet handed down a *Smyth v. Ames* decision for medical care. About 100 years ago in *Smith v. Ames*, the Supreme Court ruled that regulation cannot be used for the uncompensated expropriation of capital, but this decision has not been applied to the negotiation of union contracts. Unions can negotiate wage rates that expropriate some of the human capital of some of their workers. (A recent example is the "salary cap" rule in professional basketball, which affects primarily the best players.) The usual effect of these kinds of contracts is that the people whose capital has been expropriated eventually disappear from the industry or defect from the union. But in the short run, at least, other members can expropriate their capital. Because it takes so long to enter the doctor market, there could be a sustainable income redistribution within the AMA for many years.

In addition, some doctors may believe that they would be better off in a bilateral negotiation with the government over their average hourly wage than they would be in the marketplace. The AMA might have the view that if it can set itself up as a union negotiating the incomes of doctors with the government, maybe it would do better for doctors as a whole than simply keep up with the cost of living, which is what doctors have done for the past ten years. And it is perfectly plausible that the formation of an effective cartel for doctors through collective bargaining might improve doctors' incomes. On the other hand, one might caution doctors about recent trends in federal pay, as illustrated in early 1989 by the ill-fated attempt to raise the salaries of judges, members of Congress, and senior executives.

In any case, the adoption of fee regulation would mark a significant change in the way society operates. It would do more completely what has only been done highly imperfectly in the past, which is to convert a professional association into a real union, thereby effectively cartelizing something that has been only imperfectly cartelized for the past 100 years.

Consider now why political actors might be interested in attempting to regulate the prices of doctors' services. The budget-neutral feature brings the AMA into the fold. The deeper question is, What does it do for politicians?

From the standpoint of an elected official, there is much more to the political life, particularly as policy affects Medicare beneficiaries, than simply pleasing doctors and medical economists. Indeed, one of the interesting features of American policy over the past thirty or forty years is the growing political influence of the geriatric set. Moreover, their influence is only going to become stronger in the future because their relative proportion of the population and their relative wealth are both increasing.

Thirty years ago, the elderly were the most likely group to be poor. That is no longer the case. The one group for whom society has significantly reduced poverty—through a generous set of programs—is the elderly. This very accomplishment has increased the demand for more such programs because of their ability to pay the cost of even better political organization.

Consequently, the politics of dealing with the elderly must also be an important component of regulating doctors. And here we come to the core issue of this debate. We have six candidates for the real political reason behind the move to curb the rapidly growing rate of expenditures on Medicare.

1. Of course, some may not see rising medical expenditures as a problem at all, or at best, only a problem in the eyes of people who are paying the bill. For both the political actors and the recipients of care, increasing expenditures on medical care for the elderly may not betoken any kind of economic problem. If so, the regulation of doctors' services is not intended to have much effect on the costs of Medicare, and a weak, ineffective program is optimal both economically and politically.

Alternatively, politicians may be responding to real political problems that have some connection to cost control. If that is the case, budget neutrality is a short-run phenomenon, and the AMA is in for a shock. The real point of controlling the fees of physicians would then be to reduce the long-run rate of growth in Medicare expenditures by somehow controlling doctors' incomes. Rationales two through six all deal with politically significant potential causes of rising costs.

2. Suppose that the purpose of the proposed changes is to eliminate monopoly rents of physicians. Because their actual income is a relatively small fraction of Medicare expenditures, and because some fraction of that must be deserved, the amount of money involved in monopoly rents must be a relatively small part of Medicare costs. Hence, controlling Medicare expenditures by limiting

doctors' incomes cannot possibly be the motive behind these proposals.

3. Some services are thought to be provided more inefficiently than they otherwise could. That was a reason, incidentally, for introducing diagnosis-related groups (DRGs). Before DRGs, the mechanism for paying hospitals provided no means of disciplining inefficient hospitals. The theory was that prospective reimbursement could induce more efficiency in hospital care. For hospitals, this was a perfectly plausible and reasonable economic argument. It seems less reasonable in the case of doctors' services. The "customary and reasonable fee" reimbursement is something that already provides good incentives for doctors. It is in the doctor's interest to minimize cost if the reimbursement schedule is fixed, no matter what form treatment takes. Hence, we already have an incentive structure for production efficiency for doctors services.

4. Perhaps the government seeks to reorganize the medical care delivery system. The preceding argument does not imply that there may not be other forms of care provision that are more efficient than mom and pop doctors. One example may be corporate medicine, not just group practice, but hierarchical organizations for employing doctors to provide services. Whether there are more efficient organizational forms, however, has nothing to do with how we set fees, which is determined by other practices and policies in medicine. Hence, this cannot be the reason for changing the method of calculating the fees.

5. Perhaps the real agenda is to reduce the consumption of medical services, in recognition of the growing perception that medical care does not have much effect on the health of the elderly. This strikes me as the real winner from the perspective of the overall welfare of society. Consider the issue of allocating medical resources between the elderly and the children of the poor. It would obviously make a great deal of cost-effective sense to switch resources from the former to the latter. This, too, is implausible as a political reason. To pursue this objective, political actors would have to be willing to effect a dramatic reduction in the availability of medical care for the elderly. Thus, the government might use supply constraints as the de facto mechanism for reducing expenditures through Medicare. Controlling doctors might well work to achieve this end because doctors are the key to getting into the hospital and to obtaining other kinds of services. If as a result of price regulation half as many doctors treat Medicare patients, and so half as many patients are admitted to hospitals and half as much capital facilities are acquired to treat these patients, then we are talking real dollars. We can effect a big savings.

But such a change would reverse the current political trend of providing more and more support for the elderly as they grow more numerous and more wealthy. That is implausible.

6. Perhaps the proposed controls on physicians' fees are like most of the other deficit-reduction actions of the past few years, a form of short-sighted delusion. Specific kinds of medical care services are provided for the elderly, so that certain kinds of investments are made exclusively to serve the Medicare population which cannot be used to any significant extent elsewhere. Hence, one might be able to extract a lot of money in the short run. In the long run, of course, the services will just not be provided, or will be of drastically lower quality. Because this harms the elderly, the long-run consequence is politically implausible. Hence, the program must be temporary. If this is the case, the program seeks to extract quasi-rents from investments in the short run. Such an explanation seems plausible because it parallels the other budget reduction policies of the past ten years. It sounds exactly like something one does for one or two years to get past the next election or the next Gramm-Rudman target without actually solving the problem of the long-term budget deficit. Note that it is also consistent with the argument given to explain AMA support.

The short-term delusion, then, is the most plausible explanation for the attention that is being paid to the otherwise ludicrous idea of regulating physicians' fees. But this also implies that the system is not intended really to work, or even to last very long. Were it to be effective and durable, it would reduce care for the elderly and harm all doctors, neither of which seems very plausible. Hence, even political leaders must believe that the program will be temporary. If so, the potential economic windfall for medical economists and policy analysts is small, and I can safely remain in the economics of sports without a serious loss of permanent income.

The Passengers at the Station

A Commentary by James F. Rodgers

To paraphrase Jack Hadley, Medicare's physician payment reform locomotive is in the station full of passengers holding tickets to the cost-based fee schedule destination. The passengers know why the current location is unsatisfactory, but they have been more motivated by the thought of leaving than they have been by the offerings of the destination. The chapters in this volume provide a glimpse of that destination.

In examining the implications of Medicare's use of a cost-based fee schedule, it is useful to consider a fee schedule by itself, apart from cost, as a possible basis for determining relative values. A fee schedule or, to be more precise, an indemnity payment schedule that would mimic existing average charges across services and geographic areas in lieu of the current system would cause at least some changes within the marketplace.

The current payment system has become largely a system of physician-specific payment schedules; switching to a more aggregated approach would induce some change in payment rates. First, the existing variation in payment rates for the same services in the same geographic areas across physicians would be removed. It has been argued that such variation is not justifiable for reasons of cost, quality, or market disequilibrium differences. Second, whatever "inherently inflationary" aspects that remain in the current "customary, prevailing, and reasonable" (CPR) methodology for determining Medicare's payment rate for individual services would be removed by a more aggregated schedule.[1] The use of a payment schedule to remove these two bugaboos of the CPR methodology would simplify the payment system, should have little impact on beneficiary outlays, and might introduce a modest incentive for price searching by beneficiaries. Thus, a payment schedule (without balance billing limits) seems to be at worst harmless and probably of some benefit.

A cost-based or modified "resource-based relative value scale"

387

(RBRVS) could be more disruptive in its implementation. Theory and research are said to provide little or no support for the notions that such a massive change would be welfare-enhancing or would move reimbursement rates or fees closer to the relative rates that would prevail in a competitive market. Of course, we cannot say the reverse, either. To the extent that such a change is driven by a desire to change the relative incomes of different specialty groups, David Dranove and Mark Satterthwaite have pointed out that, under a variety of conditions, a modified RBRVS approach is unlikely to have any effect in the long run.

We have heard some other advice on proposed Medicare physician payment reform. Reimbursement rates, if changed, should be changed slowly so as not to be disruptive; in other words, first do no harm. Balance billing should be retained as a safety valve and as an administrative signaling device to indicate how payment rates may need to be modified for either access or beneficiary protection objectives. As John Holahan and Steve Zuckerman indicate, beneficiary protection can be obtained largely via certain inducements without strict price regulation (mandatory assignment of claims). Unfortunately, many of the ideas from this conference are not reflected in the current recommendations to Congress in the report of the Physician Payment Review Commission (PPRC). In particular, that report recommends price regulation in the form of strict permanent limits on balance billing.

A more aggregated type of payment schedule provides a starting point for reforming Medicare physician payment. Some would argue, however, that it would be a rather modest step toward reform and that a more significant change can be effected only by altering the dynamics of the payment system—that is, the incentives. Would there be fundamental change in the structure of beneficiary cost sharing? Would the schedule be updated in a manner that addresses some of the other program objectives, such as efficiency? I have heard very little discussion of those issues.

Why? I sense that we economists are being too constrained in our advice by what we feel is feasible in the current political environment. The parameters of payment reform as reflected in the PPRC report focus on federal outlays with little change in beneficiary outlays or coverage allowed. Without such constraints, economists would be focusing more attention on several measures that would be likely to improve efficiency. Also, it might be possible to implement such changes in a manner that would not redistribute much wealth or that would preserve "beneficiary protection."

Those measures would first include taxing Medigap insurance.

The burden imposed on the program cost of Medicare by this cost-sharing reduction mechanism is well documented, as indicated by Tom McGuire. Second, cost sharing could be restructured in a manner that would be more productive, as suggested by Jesse Hixson. Rather than raising revenue for the program with premiums, deductibles, and co-insurance—which have a dampened or zero effect at the margin—the program could be changed so that the entire amount of revenue from beneficiaries would serve the productive purpose of encouraging consumer search. This means, of course, that cost sharing would have to be in the form of balance billing. Third, armed with these two changes, the information contained in balance bills could be used to update Medicare payment rates according to some explicit access goals of the program.

There are two important aspects of the current PPRC proposal about which little has been said: geographic adjustment of payment rates and expenditure targets. There is no more, and perhaps no less, justification for a cost-based adjustment than there is for a cost-based RVS. Both, as currently envisioned, would use self-reported survey data in their construction. If geographic cost variation changes much over time, the data on which adjustments are made will be obsolete by the time they are used. Following initial implementation, adjustments due to changes in costs would have to be made very bluntly (or very expensively) because such mechanisms rely on a great deal of data. The current work being done on geographic practice cost indexes is based on 1980 data.

On expenditure targets, we have heard that, as currently proposed, they are unlikely to be effective in changing physician behavior because there are no individual incentives. There is only the threat to physicians as a group. Joe Antos has explained that further downward adjustment in reimbursement rates as a penalty for exceeding targets is very similar to the informal exercise that Congress has been implementing for years. Physicians as a group realize that high, rising, or unexpected federal outlays on physician services under Medicare (for whatever reason they may have occurred) lead to substantial pressure to reduce payment rates of the program. This pressure has brought about an actual reduction in payment rates (from those that would have been made with a normal Medicare Economic Index adjustment) for some or all services every year in recent memory. Yet such physician behavior as reductions in fees or services has not been observed. Thus, it is unlikely that explicit expenditure targets will be any more effective.

Let's take a closer look at expenditure targets (ETs). Suspend disbelief for a moment and suppose that the group incentive works

389

to achieve what its designers presumably have in mind. What occurs? A group of physicians develops a list of payment rules that amount to inside limits or coverage decisions. The idea is that doctor groups would decide what services Medicare should not cover. It is hoped that doctors would know what is least valuable to patients and would choose rules that reduce or eliminate those services.

This line of reasoning suggests several questions about ETs. Would they lead to the birth of doctor organizations that would establish volume-reducing rules? And even if you believe the answer is "yes," would the decisions made by such organizations be good ones in any societal sense? And, would the volume-reducing rules reduce expenditures? Effective expenditure targets would reduce federal outlays by reducing coverage or services. They are the equivalent of a supply-constrained market, as Ted Frech has indicated.

Returning to the PPRC locomotive of Medicare Part B reform, the passengers have been waiting quite some time to depart, but I certainly hope that they have some time to exchange their tickets before departure. They are likely to be less satisfied at the end of their trip than before they decided to leave.

The Views of an Internist

A Commentary by Robert A. Berenson

My views about the Hsiao concept and the PPRC recommendations are somewhat different from others expressed in this volume. I am an internist and think of myself as besieged and underpaid—and that certainly colors everything else that I will say. I also wrote an article with Jack Hadley a few years ago that anticipated a few of the criticisms of the Hsiao resource-based relative value scales (RBRVS). My concerns seem to be quibbles alongside others, but let me go through a few of them.

One problem is that the RBRVS is not nearly as objective and scientific as advertised. A number of policy decisions described in this volume really determine what the outcome of the RVS consensus process is going to be. These decisions represent actual compromises.

We are dealing with a political process. Over the past few years, Dr. Hsiao has achieved a consensus within the medical profession, although the AMA is beginning to show some splintering. In general, however, the political process behind the RBRVS was a successful one.

The RBRVS measures how professionals value their own service. Interestingly, some of the changes from prevailing charges to relative values are very small. If he had defined different groups of experts— not physicians drawn from a given specialty, but perhaps medical directors of large group practices or health maintenance organizations (HMOs)—Dr. Hsiao might have come up with significantly different relative values. That does not invalidate his effort. It is a terrific starting point; there is just not as much science to it as advertised. It is the result of a political process, and with the kinds of changes that PPRC is recommending, it will be a viable compromise with which to begin reforming the way Medicare pays fees for services.

There should be notions of effectiveness in how we set up relative value scales and fee schedules. Professionals like to think that what they do is worthwhile. But we have evidence that in some cases what physicians do isn't terribly useful to patients. Simply because physicians spend a lot of time and value the time highly, should Medicare reward them for performing activities that do not help the patient?

A resource-based relative value scale provides a starting point. Then the burden of proof to alter it will be pretty high. But we should start altering it—that is one of the points in Jack Hadley's paper.

Let me give you a concrete example concerning something as simple as a routine history and physical. The *Annals of Internal Medicine* recently published a review article on the routine physical examination; the basic conclusion was that there's no real proof that it does any good for the patient. Certain specific components of the physical exam do seem to lead to differences in outcomes, but most of it represents a long-term rite that continues without foundation.

One of the conclusions emanating from the simulations we've seen here is that Medicare is going to pay more for a routine history and physical because it is a time-intensive evaluation and management service. As a member of the Health Care Financing Administration (HCFA) or as a congressman, I would not recommend cutting the reimbursement for the history and physical right now. That is the kind of discussion that should take place, however, and we need to accumulate more data before we can begin to change incentives and thus influence physician behavior. Even if physicians continue to perform the history and physical for cultural and social reasons— which is why I will continue to do it—Medicare as a prudent payer should not allocate as much of its budget to that activity, whether or not the price change reduces the volume of histories and physicals provided. In summary, it is reasonable to start with a resource-based RVS, but it should not be the end result of the reform effort.

As for mandatory assignment, I have taken it since I started practicing eight years ago. I have also had the dubious honor of having to represent Michael Dukakis's candidacy to physicians, explaining why mandatory assignment would be good for them. I am personally persuaded by the argument that as a safety valve and as an administrative correction factor, the option of balance billing should be maintained for now.

Note, however, that the PPRC proposal essentially calls for two fee schedules, and not what the contributors to this volume mean by balance billing. The PPRC recommends establishing a 15 or 20 percent limit over the new fee schedule for physician charges to the patient. In some areas and in some specialties, most charges would exceed that limit. Those physicians whose charges are restrained by the 15–20 percent limit in effect have a choice of fee schedules, neither of which bears much relation to their own charges. I am concerned that this PPRC proposal restricts balance billing too much.

At the same time, because of the pervasive influence of health insurance, the pricing mechanism does not really help consumers select quality in the medical marketplace, as some have argued. In a market with an excess of doctors, who are able and willing to see a greater volume of patients, the increased volume of patients generated though patient recommendations and physician referrals becomes a way of rewarding quality. Such recognition need not come through higher prices for individual services.

What do physicians do when they judge they are not earning enough? If we extrapolate from the data presented by William Marder, we find that an internist makes $36 an hour. If true, that seems low. The Urban Institute pays me more than that for consulting, and it is a nonprofit organization.

David Dranove and Mark Satterthwaite suggest that there is a compensating differential, such that physicians will continue to work for that low income. I agree, but only after an income threshold is met. What if the threshold is not being reached? The idea that the most able students and young doctors will select other, higher-paying specialties is disturbing, particularly because internal medicine has always drawn the "best and the brightest." There are entry barriers that prevent established physicians from formally moving into higher-paying specialties—the next generation might do that.

In fact, what is going on now is a real-world test of the absence of licensure or certification barriers, whereby internists and other primary care physicians are redefining themselves as specialists. With little formal training, we are now becoming dermatologists, noninvasive cardiologists, endoscopists, radiologists, gynecologists, for purposes of getting procedural reimbursement. There are obviously some limits on this activity, but many physicians are acquiring specialist skills and other technologies to alter their practices. This phenomenon is not widely recognized.

Some doctors are responding to diminished earnings by becoming entrepreneurs; that is the subject of the Stark legislation limiting the financial interests of physicians in organizations that they can then refer patients to. We can argue whether that is good or bad. The point is, this is another thing that happens when physicians do not earn what they want.

Demand creation occurs. I sit in meetings with my practice partners in which we ask at least once a month, "How are we going to create new demand this month?" Really.

Also note that for Medicare beneficiaries the time costs associated with revisits are low. Anecdotal conversations with people managing HMOs suggest that there has been an explosion of office visits from people being brought back—because there is no reason not to. There are no out-of-pocket expenses for the patient and no strictures from their employers. Time costs do not necessarily exert a brake on demand creation.

I endorse Mark Pauly's concept that physician discomfort is a limiting factor for demand creation—that is, physicians do not wish to deviate from what they regard as the best practice. But when you have incentives that say more is better, the best practice becomes a more-is-better practice. The differing constraints in the health care systems in England and in the United States, for example, produce different operational definitions of the best practice.

Costs, Competition, and Controls under Medicare

A Commentary by Robin Allen

The proponents of resource-based relative value scales (RBRVS) tell us that this mechanism is a more equitable method of reimbursement than other schemes and that it gives physicians more incentive to provide cognitive services and less incentive to provide surgical services. Many economists have cautioned, however, that RBRVS is no panacea and, that it does not address fundamental issues concerning, for example, the volume of care. I would like to add another word of caution: Under physician price controls, fewer innovative cost-saving and quality-improving techniques may be adopted or even developed.

Note that when the trucking and airline industries were regulated, rates were set for passage between one city and another. Once these industries were deregulated, the ensuing price competition caused prices to be significantly lower than they otherwise would have been. Furthermore, deregulation gave trucking and airline firms the freedom to decide not only *what* price to charge, but *what service to* price.

Before deregulation of the trucking industry, for example, one rate was assigned to any given haul. Since deregulation, trucking firms have been allowed to charge lower rates to customers who are more flexible about when their orders arrive, and higher rates to firms that need fast deliveries at a specific time. This combination of speed and reliability has enabled American firms to cut their inventory costs and to adopt modern inventory techniques such as the "just-in-time" method used by the Japanese.

Before the deregulation of the airline industry, trunk carriers were allowed to provide service only between larger cities, and local

The opinions expressed are the author's and not necessarily those of the Department of Justice.

service carriers were allowed to serve only designated regional areas. A passenger who traveled from a city served by a trunk carrier to one served by a regional carrier (or vice versa) could find the trip long and inconvenient because schedules might not be coordinated and might require long layovers. There could also be long walks between terminals and a greater risk of losing baggage during the transfer. Since deregulation, airlines have adopted the more efficient hub-and-spoke system, which facilitates connections in most of the cities that cannot support nonstop service. In fact, a 1986 Brookings study concluded that the time saved from these networks in 1983 alone was most likely worth more to airline passengers than the savings from lower fares.[1]

Another improvement in the airline industry is comparable to the new array of price-reliability combinations available in the deregulated trucking industry: Fare/flight frequency/load factor combinations now vary according to whether the cities served are primarily tourist or "time-sensitive" centers. On the one hand, many tourists are happy to give up frequent departure times in order to travel inexpensively. Such flights tend to have higher load factors. On the other hand, time-sensitive travelers (mostly business travelers) are willing to pay more for frequent departures. These flights tend to have lower load factors.

The message is clear: regulators decide not only *what* price to set but *what to* price. In both cases, if there is no market mechanism to guide these decisions, the welfare loss may be severe. In particular, when regulators choose *what to* price incorrectly, firms have little incentive to set up the more efficient arrangements that they would settle on if they had the freedom to choose what to price.

Ironically, in the past year or so there has been much talk about effectiveness research becoming a key factor in future efforts to contain costs and to improve the quality of care. Last fall, Bill Roper announced that effectiveness research was his "number one priority."[2] The Physician Payment Review Commission has also come out in favor of effectiveness research as a way to address volume and quality issues. Physician price controls (or for that matter, any system other than one that reimburses at the health insurance level), however, provides little incentive to contain costs voluntarily through measures such as medical practice standards. Price controls also tend to reduce the private demand for such research.

Suppose, for example, that some HMOs developed a new system of protocols for a certain diagnosis that made it possible to use fewer physician services and fewer hospital resources for the average person with that diagnosis at no reduction in the patient's health. Would a Medicare RBRVS cause physicians to adopt this set of protocols for serving Medicare patients? It is quite unlikely. First, there is no financial incentive for physicians to adopt this protocol. Hospitals may also be reluctant to do so if it reduces the number of procedures performed (although there is some incentive if the resources used for a given DRG are reduced). Furthermore, because physicians and hospitals are not linked, either contractually or corporately, there are no organizations, as there are in alternative delivery systems, to facilitate the cooperation needed to implement this set of protocols.

Of course, some may argue that even though physicians may not voluntarily adopt such medical practice standards, the Health Care Financing Administration (HCFA) could force them to do so through utilization review. I am not in favor of this approach for two reasons. First, this would be a step backward in HCFA's general efforts to streamline the amount of bureaucracy in the Medicare program. Second, for a given amount of savings achievable through utilization review, these decisions are probably best made through a private health plan. Such organizations have greater flexibility (and arguably, greater incentive) to respond to physician and patient dissatisfaction with the review process. Organizational flexibility is particularly important because physicians and patients are heterogeneous.

Clearly, the alternative delivery plans and managed care systems—and, more generally, the payers—have the strongest incentive to adopt efficient medical practices. They also have the strongest incentive to innovate or to help fund research on efficient medical practices. It is not surprising, for example, that the HCFA, the Health Insurance Association of America, and the Blue Cross/Blue Shield Association have been among the strongest supporters of medical effectiveness research.

To summarize, the greatest potential for saving on HCFA costs and improving the quality of services for Medicare beneficiaries seems to be in the area of establishing medical practice guidelines. The HCFA has pledged support and funding for this area of research. Ironically, it is also investigating another method of payment that does little to promote the voluntary pursuit of efficient medical practices or the private funding of research in this area. Admittedly, Medicare can try to enforce efficient medical practices through utilization review, but this can only be accomplished at significant bureaucratic cost and in a less effective and less sensitive manner than is possible through private health plans, which are able to incorporate physician and consumer views into the review process more effectively.

To a certain degree, unrestricted balance billing might address some of the efficiency problems introduced when the government decides not only *what* price to set but *what to* price. Suppose, for example, that the most efficient way to deal with a certain medical problem is for the physician to spend an hour counseling the patient. Also, suppose that Medicare only pays enough to allow the physician to counsel the patient for fifteen minutes. Clearly, the physician and patient are both better off if the patient pays more and the visit lasts longer. Balance billing does not solve all efficiency problems, however, particularly in situations where the Medicare price is too high.

RBRVS may or may not be an improvement over the current Part B reimbursement. If the system is eventually adopted by HCFA, I hope it is only an interim solution and that HCFA's long-term goal will be to pay for Medicare beneficiaries' private health plans of their own choice.

A "Safe Harbor" Plan

A Commentary by Glenn M. Hackbarth

As a lawyer-bureaucrat in the private sector, I must confess to being a little perplexed by the economics of the proposed payment procedures. I do accept as axiomatic that primary care physicians are paid too little and that the procedure-oriented specialties are paid too much—at least, relative to one another. And you might improve long-run efficiency if you could send "better" price signals to physicians. Nevertheless, I have been, and continue to be, a critic of the effort to develop a resource-based relative value scale (RBRVS) for the Medicare program.

It is a serious misallocation of our resources—political, analytical, and administrative—to spend so much effort trying to derive the "right" price for each of thousands of different procedures and services provided by physicians. The primary issue facing the Medicare program, indeed, the country, is not how to perfect fee-for-service payment, but how to impose limits on it, and how to encourage the use of other forms of health care financing and delivery.

The original appeal to physicians of fee-for-service was, at least in substantial part, that it maximized their clinical freedom, freeing them to act as the agents of their patients. That, at least, was the theory. Sheltering physicians against unwarranted interference is a legitimate goal.

One of my sources for this interpretation of the history of insurance is an interesting historical document, the 1932 report of a blue-ribbon commission, the Committee on the Cost of Medical Care. Back then, more or less the same issues were being debated. The majority of this blue-ribbon panel recommended that health care services be financed and delivered through organizations that would today be called health maintenance organizations (HMOs).

A stinging dissent, however, was filed by physician representatives who argued that the prospect of physicians being employed by lay-controlled organizations was unacceptable. They feared the end result would be intrusion on the clinical freedom of physicians, with adverse consequences for the patient. In historical fact, the committee's minority report was much more influential than the majority report on the development of health care financing and delivery in the United States.

So we set off on a fifty-year experiment with the view of the minority—that, yes, we could have widespread access to health care; we could have high-quality health care; we could have efficient health care under a system that coupled indemnity insurance, fee-for-service payment, with decentralized, if not fragmented, delivery of services. The results of that experiment are clear: astronomical costs and deteriorating access to care, which is attributable at least in part to the escalating cost of care. As far as quality is concerned, it can be said that we have health care of unsurpassed technical virtuosity, but whether that is synonymous with high quality is open to considerable debate. Rather than trying to perfect this system of indemnity insurance, fee-for-service payment and free choice of provider at the point of service, the Congress, the Health Care Financing Administration (HCFA), and everybody interested in health care financing should be devoting all their efforts to moving the health care delivery system away from fee-for-service payment and delivery.

Our dependence on this form of payment has had a number of adverse effects, but the one most often discussed by economists is that fee-for-service payment provides poor incentives for efficiency. A much more fundamental problem is that it has fragmented the delivery of health care services, both from the standpoint of financial and medical accountability. We have a health care system that consumes more than 11 percent of the gross national product, yet is organized, to a considerable degree, as a cottage industry. People and organizations provide slivers of service, without assuming responsibility for a full range of services.

In order to minimize the adverse financial consequences of this form of financing and delivery, fee-for-service insurers, including Medicare, have adopted a host of administrative controls—some directed at fees, some at trying to control utilization through prior certification of nonemergency admissions, concurrent review, retrospective review, and so on.

At one point I was somewhat hopeful that we could improve the efficiency and effectiveness of the system through these efforts, but my experience in the government has caused me to despair. We will not significantly improve the quality and efficiency of our health care system through these tacked-on administrative controls.

One of the worst results of this approach is the demoralizing effect that it is bound to have on the *best* of the physicians. More and more physicians are just beside themselves at the prospect of repeatedly having to call nurses for approval to do things that they know are appropriate. Regrettably, a lot of physicians do need that supervision, but the problem with these administrative controls is that they apply evenly to all physicians. So a crisis of morale has developed among good and bad physicians, alike.

Our primary goal ought to be to change the paradigm, to try to get away from this dependence on fee-for-service, free choice of provider, indemnity insurance. Instead of spending all of our resources trying to perfect it, we should be taking the recommendations of the Physician Payment Review Commission (PPRC) on expenditure targets and shaping them into a strategy that, in the long run, might lead us away from this inappropriate emphasis on fee-for-service practice.

If I were the HCFA administrator, what I would be saying to the Congress is, "That's the part of the report that you ought to pay attention to." We need to impose some constraints on the fee-for-service sector, and then allow physicians the opportunity to find "safe harbors," where they would police themselves, where they would have an incentive and an opportunity to develop their own rules for practicing more effective, more efficient medical care.

The "safe harbors" would be defined in two ways. First, they would be organizations (like HMOs) that assumed the medical responsibility for providing the full range of services to an enrolled group of Medicare patients. Second, they would assume the full financial risk for such services by agreeing to provide them in exchange for a fixed capitation payment. Physicians who elected to participate in Medicare through those organizations would be exempt from the increasingly arbitrary controls placed on the fee-for-service sector.

In effect, Medicare would be giving physicians a choice. They could continue to practice in the fee-for-service portion of Medicare, which would look increasingly like a giant, government-sponsored independent practice association HMO. Physicians electing to do so would be subject to potentially arbitrary cuts in their fees based on the performance of all their fee-for-service colleagues in a given area. Alternatively, the physician could choose his or her own business partners by electing to participate in a qualified "safe harbor" plan. Then, the physician would not be responsible for what happens in the unconstrained fee-for-service sector, but only for the actions of physicians of his or her own choosing.

What Have We Learned from Research, Theory, and Experience?

A Discussion

ROBERT HELMS: There is another way to look at the attention Congress has focused on physician expenditures under Medicare. The way savings are calculated under the Gramm-Rudman-Hollings Act is to compare new projected spending to projected growth under current law. Therefore, to find large savings, it is helpful to target programs with high rates of growth, as well as those with high current levels of spending. Since Medicare has been growing at an annual rate of about 20 percent, this feature of the Gramm-Rudman-Hollings Act attracts additional attention to Medicare's physician spending, perhaps more attention than might seem reasonable.

THOMAS G. McGUIRE: Politically, there is some willingness to use supply constraints to restrict what the elderly get. The diagnosis-related groups (DRGs) did that. The balanced-budget analysis is a little misleading. The DRGs were also balance-budgeted in the first year. And that's not really the point. Once the Health Care Financing Administration (HCFA) gets all of the update factors, they don't need to be balance-budgeted as time goes on.

ROGER G. NOLL: Perhaps we disagree about the effectiveness of the DRGs in terms of controlling Medicare expenditures.

MR. McGUIRE: But here's the question. You asked how I would change prices the least painful way possible and still meet these goals. Do you have any ideas about this?

MR. NOLL: The only nonpainful way to do it is short-term expropriation of the human and physical capital investments of those particular physicians who not only practice primarily for Medicare populations,

402

but are gatekeepers for physical investments and other human capital investments that are engaged mainly in providing services for Medicare patients. They are going to have the smallest elasticities of substitution for other services with the imposition of a big price reduction.

If you could target that group of people, there would be a short-term, one-shot expenditure reduction until the effect began curtailing supply. Then there would be the political issue of whether the first observations of nonprice rationing to the Medicare population would cause a political backlash.

This whole program would most likely have no effect at all on Medicare expenditures simply because of the mechanics of implementing it. If there were an effect, it would be a relatively short-run one of a few years until the supply response was visible.

There could be some supply response without passing the threshold of political saliency, but if a significant Medicare population was eventually being denied a service that it wanted—through nonprice rationing, as opposed to the economic mechanism—they would indeed renew the political demand to reestablish some sort of a policy to restore the *status quo ante*. This has two possible outcomes: One is nothing, and the other is a short-term budgetary saving that would be reversed in the future.

WILLIAM C. HSIAO: I am in total support of Glenn Hackbarth's argument that the à la carte method of delivering medical care and of getting payments is not the optimum system and that he is offering a better alternative.

For about sixteen years or more, we have had experience in promoting health maintenance organizations (HMOs). Why hasn't that form of delivery, and the market organization, moved farther along than it has? In other words, are we holding out a "noble vision" that is impractical, for whatever reason?

Now you are in favor of a prepaid plan. Are you willing to put up $100,000 to commission a series of papers, examining that strategy in a critical sense—to really look at the extent to which the market forces and competitive forces can work in a capitated system, and to consider issues such as adverse selection, or the level of competition, or product differentiation? This has not been critically examined, at least not in the context of Medicare.

GLENN M. HACKBARTH: Those are legitimate questions. Reorganizing the delivery and integrating financing and delivery are a necessary condition, though not a sufficient condition, for success. There are

403

two reasons why those in the HMO world have not done what a lot of us would have hoped to see accomplished.

One reason is that HMOs continue to do business in a predominantly fee-for-service market, which has a significant effect on the ability of an HMO to rationally organize and purchase services. The amounts that HMOs must pay physicians are dictated by market prices. They're not unilaterally set by HMOs.

In the state of Massachusetts, the amount we pay for hospital services and our ability to move people out of hospitals are heavily regulated, and in many ways adversely so. It is impossible to find skilled nursing facility beds in Massachusetts, so that we can move Medicare beneficiaries out of the hospital more quickly. That is the perverse result of regulation.

The other reason that HMOs have not attained everything that I would have liked is that it is not just a matter of having the right organizational form or the right economic incentives. An organization needs to know how to manage care. Physicians need information that they can use in choosing among competing therapies.

Such information has been in short supply in the health care world. Indeed, that was one of the reasons why Bill Roper and I called for a significant increase in public funding for effectiveness research. That sort of research provides a public good—information— which the market is obviously undersupplying.

PETER ZWEIFEL: Robin Allen's point on innovation merits closer attention. Quite a few European countries have had fifty years of experience with fee schedules that are not openly cost-based, but tend to be resource-based, and that is exactly what is happening. You should distinguish between product innovation and process innovation. Although it is already hard enough to get the new products on the list, it is possible because there is some competition among those social and health insurers that you wouldn't have with Medicare.

Process innovation—getting the same type of good produced at lower cost, more efficiently—is more difficult. European medical practice, especially in the ambulatory care sector, seems to be lagging behind in this.

A problem is coming up for the United States in this regard. If you wanted to have Medicare as one block and to use those resource-based fee schedules, process innovation would be retarded. The hospitals that have DRG fixed-price schemes now went into process innovation pretty quickly in order to stay in the market. And that is exactly the drive being taken out now in the ambulatory care sector.

MR. NOLL: Isn't the serious issue—especially for Medicare patients—whether, on balance, technological innovation is beneficial or harmful? A lot of it has been costly and used for extending very low-quality life, and its value has not been entirely obvious.

Assuming Jan Mitchell's characterization is right, we have a system now where, in order to innovate, people charge very high prices initially, and then the Medicare system attenuates the speed at which the price falls. A market would attenuate the price faster, but it would still start off high. New products always start off more expensively than they eventually end up.

The third possibility is the mechanism that is proposed. It supposedly eliminates the temporary high price for the innovator, and that would in fact reduce innovation. This might be an advantage if one could confine the absence of the incentive to innovate to those things where the marginal value of the service seems extremely low, and retain the current overpricing of innovation in areas where the marginal value is very high, like neonatal care.

That is, the dynamics of price change through time, an interesting potential instrument out there that is not working now. Markets could certainly be tracked better, but it is not necessarily bad to go from overpricing to underpricing, depending on the type of service involved.

MR. ZWEIFEL: What you are arguing for is to go straight to the outcome measurement obtained for health outcomes. You wouldn't have to take the route via resource-based fees.

MR. NOLL: I agree. The RBRVS is the nineteenth-best solution.

GEORGE GREENBERG: Obviously, we are talking about differences in the fee-for-service system. If Congress chooses to go that way, we have to address the issues, but we should look at them more as a continuum, with the current customary, prevailing, and reasonable (CPR) system at one end and resource-based relative value scales (RBRVS) at the other, and many stopping points in between.

Instead of talking about either/or choices, one has to ask what one gains by moving along the continuum. The charge-based fee schedule is based on the physician's own past charges. Then you have to ask, what do you gain by dropping the customary charge? Without it, you are going to pay a number of doctors who charge less than the market more than they would be willing to accept. Inevitably, the question is how would you recapture this, and is the national

405

expenditure target an adequate mechanism for recapturing the additional payments?

The difference between the charge-based RVS and the resource-based RVS is simply how you calculate the relative fees. They are certainly easier to calculate under a system based on charges. The HCFA already has the data, and the system could be implemented within a short period of time. It may not take as many resources as some economic and medical experts suggest. It allows for adjustments. If, however, you really believe that the market is terribly distorted, then it does not provide an adequate pricing mechanism.

But if you go to the resource-based mechanism, you are going to a cost-based system that is moving in a completely different direction from hospital payments, where we are moving away from costs and toward something else.

You have to price 8,000 procedures a year and you have to remeasure resource cost periodically. What bureaucratic mechanism is going to do that? Are you going to have an FDA-type entry mechanism on procedures because Medicare won't pay their price? Does that really tell a physician not to use an innovative procedure until it is priced by Medicare? What are the regulatory implications?

ROBERT A. BERENSON: When I tried to help a *de novo* preferred provider plan (PPO) develop a fee schedule to accomplish a few specific goals, we didn't have an existing physician base. We had to try to recruit some doctors, and did so in part with a new innovative fee schedule.

We wanted the eager participation of primary care physicians, but we also wanted specialists. Those are not the same things. We wanted to meet the actuarial targets that underwriters had set so they could price their product in the marketplace. Also, we wanted to try to influence behavior somewhat.

And we came up with a hybrid technique. It was my belief, going in, that the greatest distortion was not between knee surgery and arm surgery performed by an orthopedist. It was the relationship between procedures and emergency medical services.

Once you recognize that, you can base charges on the concept that there are families of procedures. Since there are nondistortions within families, we can use charges to establish fees. We took actual charges for about 600 or so procedures and visit codes in a geographic area and simply set a percentile. We took the 80th percentile for visits and the 40th percentile for the 600 procedures and thereby established new relative values. It was fairly crude. After that, we plugged them into an existing McGraw-Hill charge-based RVS. You could use the California relative value scale or you could use almost anything else to calculate the other 7,000 fees that we did not have.

And then we did one final thing, which was what Jan Mitchell discussed: We looked at outliers, which were still greatly over- or underpriced. We went after the high-volume ones and made some corrections. And we developed a fee schedule—in about fifty hours.

For our marketplace, this schedule probably accomplishes what we want it to. We have now used it for about six or eight months. For EM services, we pay out 85 percent of charges. For surgical procedural services, we pay out 75 percent of charges.

As the PPRC has pointed out, some procedures that need a special look are the ones where physicians don't do anything. They read a computerized report that a machine generates and charge an outrageous amount. We are paying much less for these test interpretations, probably around the 50th percentile.

So we have accomplished some goals. The primary care physicians are happy, and the surgeons have accepted 25 percent discounts. Also, we are really going after the nonuseful procedures that physicians have always used to pad their income. The system is charge-based but it is not structured according to the existing relationship of charges and it is easier to work with.

I have also had some experience with a partly capitated system. That is, we got a capitation for each patient, but as a group of ten internists we decided to reallocate it among ourselves like a fee for service, but with greatly altered relative values. And we cut the EKG interpretation to what we thought was the marginal cost, which was the level at which physicians would continue to do it, unless the test was unnecessary. There was no profit in it at all. You can do that sort of thing in small groups. That is why I support the notion of decentralizing all of this and going into competitive plans.

MR. HELMS: The interesting question is, when the HCFA had the highly competitive contract negotiations to develop this thing, why didn't you win the contract instead of Bill Hsiao?

MARVIN KOSTERS: So far, the discussion has moved along two tracks. One has to do with the technical merits of different kinds of formulas, often with budget neutrality as part of the suggested goal, and the other has to do with cutting cost in this sector, which is said to be the real problem. Another way of looking at these subjects is to say that we have fortunately been able to identify an overpaid group that we can tax, or take something away from, in order to accomplish the budget objective.

But are people on the panel convinced that changing relative values would be preferable to what seems like a "meat ax" approach of simply slashing rates of growth across the board? Is there a good case for combining the relative price shifts with a budget-cutting plan?

Mr. Hackbarth: Having worked in the HCFA, I would say that we have to choose between the two. As I pointed out earlier, the procedure-oriented folks are paid too much and we need to redistribute, but I am not enough of an expert to criticize Bill Roper's methodology or the PPRC's approach. My perspective is much more pragmatic. I know the scope of the HCFA's abilities and the "attention span" of the relevant people in the Department of Health and Human Services and the Congress.

There are only so many things of this scale that an organization can do. Even if you accept that going in the direction of an RBRVS would be a good thing, it is not free. It takes political, research, and administrative resources, and I'm simply saying that the price is too high. We can't do both. We have to choose because of the limits on managerial attention that the agency faces. Establishing the overall limit is a much higher priority for the Medicare program.

Mr. Noll: You can arrive at a similar conclusion in a slightly different way. Economists have focused on two kinds of fundamental policy changes that would make the delivery of medical care more efficient. One would shift more financial responsibility for medical care to the patient, through things like deductibles, coinsurance, and balance billing. And the other would change the institution to one that provides medical care, preferably closed-panel provision.

The political constraints really cut here. It is not in the cards to do either of these two things: that is, to substantially increase the exposure of individuals to financially burdensome medical care or to have wide and obvious disparities in the availability of medical care by socioeconomic class, or age, or sex, or things like that.

The only solution may be the institutional one favoring HMOs and preferred provider organizations (PPOs), or perhaps there is no solution. If the institutional buggy doesn't fly and a better organizational form of the provision of medical care produces few economic gains and if the political constraints are as I've described them, then we are going to see a large fraction of GNP devoted to medical care, both privately and publicly, for the indefinite future.

This last remark about misplaced emphasis is exactly on target. That is why the conclusion is the same. The only way that the administrative approach of changing fees can get away without politically damaging the status quo is if it has no effect.

In the short run, it could reduce the budget, but if it exposes old people to more financial problems in getting access to medical care, or if it creates a two-tiered medical system in which working-age people and their children get a substantially different kind of medical care than elderly people do, the system will just self-destruct. Except for short-run palliatives on the short-term budget crisis, the only solution is the institutional one, and even that may not work. The argument against the institutional (PPO, HMO) change has always been, "Yes, but we need to get through the next fiscal year; how are we going to deal with the short-term problem?" If we had gone the institutional route in 1970, we would now know whether it could work. The long run turns out to be not that long after a series of ineffective short-run palliatives.

JOSEPH R. ANTOS: Something implicit throughout these discussions is the idea that if the right business organizations come together to negotiate or somehow deal with the payers, everything will be all right. This might be an HMO or a PPO. The entity that has been left out of this, however, is the patient, the person upon whom the medical experiment is performed.

The person with the greatest interest is probably not the person who has a financial stake in this. And that is the essential problem here. Fee schedules don't have any impact on decision making in the health system, and I don't see that any of the other proposals really address that problem.

It is not true that the ignorant beneficiary entrusts himself to the all-knowing fee-for-service physician or to the HMO and then accepts whatever he gets. Over some period of time, that ignorant consumer learns and marches out and finds some other provider. So that piece of the puzzle hasn't really been looked at.

COMMENT: Another point that hasn't been raised is that we must be cautious of the Medicaid experience. In many states we've created a second-level tier of care and in some states a very poor level of care. We did this by lowering fees and prohibiting balance billing.

Part of the reason you have so few people covered under Medicare competition (HMO) programs is all the requirements that exist. Medicare has been relatively careful about who it contracts with, and you haven't gotten scandals. But, there is some danger of scandals. And, frankly, Congress is far more sensitive about problems with the aged than problems with the poor.

FREDERICK R. WARREN-BOULTON: We need some historical perspective here. We've had 2,000 years of experience with cost-based regulation. Recall that when Emperor Diocletian marched his armies into certain areas, lo and behold, the price of food would go way up. People thought there must be a lot of profiteering going on, so he put price controls on.

Controls have been used where technical change is very rapid, where there is a lot of risk and uncertainty, where there are a lot of rents (for example, in the case of natural gas or quasi rents in the case of housing), but the supply curve is considerably more elastic in the long run than in the short run. Also, it has been common where there is either no monopoly power or a large number of competitors, where consumers are politically powerful or where, with the prospect of a large transfer of rents, they can become politically powerful, and where the regulation involves a large expenditure on bureaucracy.

Now, the results in all those situations have been twofold. First, cost-based regulation with restricted or prohibited balance billing, which is what the RBRVS would be like, has been extraordinarily inefficient and expensive; second, it has been almost as costly to remove once it's been in place. The question is, do the people who like this system, and for whom hope springs eternal, expect anything any different in this case than every other situation that we've had?

JOEL IRA FRANCK: It is not going to be different. If you believe that health care is a right, a free good, a public good—whatever phrase you want to use—and therefore that the government, the agent of force, is to supply it, then you have to advocate total price control. You are going to reach a fee schedule, whether it is resource based or whether it is the phases of the moon, or whether it is the AMA leadership—whoever is going to administer it is going to establish complete price control.

What constituency is there for that? Why are we discussing a proposal for cost-based fee regulation? Nobody benefits from that and nobody claims to benefit from that.

If, on the other hand, you believe that health care is an economic good and that with all economic goods it is best expanded and achieved by markets, by voluntary exchange, which will enhance technology and competition and free interaction among people, then the ideal would be to get the government out of health care—because everywhere else that they have attempted control, as we've just pointed out, was a disaster. And it has been no different for the past twenty-five years in medical care.

Instead of picking a particular model, like the HMO as the ideal model, why don't we stop being social engineers? Why don't we say that we don't know what doctors should earn? We don't know what procedures should be done. It is something we can't design. Doctors don't know. Doctors don't know what's good or bad yet in most instances. (At any medical meeting you'll hear discussion about the simplest procedures, debates on whether they are worthwhile.)

Why don't we simply say that the government, on an interim basis before it totally got out of health care, could allow the market to determine what's going on by giving each consumer who they believe should be helped (the elderly and the poor) a voucher and say, "You want to go to Joel Franck and see if he can guarantee all your health care? Fine. You want to go to the Harvard PPO or HMO? Fine." And let the market determine by natural experience, by competition, all the ideal arrangements.

That would have the maximum constituency, politically. It would be politically palatable to go up to Congress and say that. Why isn't anybody saying it? Why are we focusing on a number scheme of price control that will benefit nobody?

Mr. Hackbarth: Roger Noll and some others have tried to figure out a sophisticated explanation of why there are supporters of a resource-based relative value scale. It doesn't really require a lot of sophistication, only a little understanding of how decisions are made in Washington.

The basic appeal is straightforward. It is an appeal to equity. There is a gut feeling that the procedure-oriented folks are paid too much. They get thousands of dollars for doing a forty-five-minute operation, while the primary care physicians are struggling, and it seems that they are providing a valuable service.

Just a few people have to be sold on that simple notion. And that has happened. A few key members of Congress have bought on to that simple premise. And they have kept this going. They have mandated an HCFA study of the issue, provided the funding. They do all the talking in the relevant subcommittee and committee meetings, they shape the views of their colleagues who find this all hopelessly arcane, and it is just a relatively simple phenomenon, an appeal to equity and a few embracing it and willing to act on it, and they have the influence to make it happen.

The ideal way to run Medicare would be to convert it from an entitlement to a fee-for-service payment to a fixed amount. The government will pay X dollars per month to help you buy your health insurance coverage. And let a thousand flowers bloom as far as the delivery organizations, delivery physician relationships is concerned.

411

But you have to cap the fee-for-service portion for Medicare. As long as capitation is only one of the options, costs under the fee-for-service option can grow unrestrained and that affects the dynamics of physician choice. It means physicians find it more appealing to practice fee-for-service Medicare as opposed to the more constrained alternatives. It affects the resource prices that the HMOs, PPOs, and other such groups have to pay.

The problem is what do you do with the fee-for-service portion of Medicare during the transition period? We already offer the capitation option to Medicare beneficiaries. One million have elected it. They enroll in capitated organizations. One reason that the number is so low is that the fee-for-service portion of the program is still too comfortable. It's unconstrained.

We should have Ross Arnett say, "Here's the per capita cost of fee-for-service." Then, we estimate how much it is going to increase, and Medicare beneficiaries who elect to stay in fee-for-service have to start paying the incremental, out-of-pocket costs associated with staying in a very ineffective, inefficient delivery system.

Mr. Noll: Dr. Franck made two political assertions, both of which are false.

The first is that everybody loses in price regulation. That's not true, and it's not what Rick Warren-Boulton said. What happens is that price regulation confers benefits on some people and costs on others. The costs it imposes on others are much larger than the benefits it does confer on those who benefit. Nonetheless, some people benefit.

In the case of the medical care business, it seems that a lot of wealth is at stake in the institutional arrangements being as they are. A lot of people have oriented their lives toward optimizing in the current institutional environment. And they stand to lose if another institutional form dominates.

The transition to something more efficient would be costly, especially to people with investments that depend on the government continuing to do what it already does. So they fall back on something like a contract argument. You set up this weird system, and we've oriented our life to it; now don't screw us in the middle. That's the first thing.

The second part of the story is that institutional change is not a novel idea. It has been around for twenty years. People have been testifying in Congress, writing books, making statements at these conferences, and proposing the voucher mechanism—where you choose between fee-for-service or HMO or any other kind of intermittent institutional form you can think of—for some time.

It is not because people are unaware of it that they have refused to adopt such a mechanism. One thing we know about politics is that if the organizations—the General Motors of medical care that don't exist yet—are pitted against the institutions that do exist, then the guys who are going to benefit are going to be unorganized; they are not even going to know who they are, and they are not going to be as powerful in the political system as the guys who know that their ox can be gored.

That's why what Rick Warren-Boulton says is true. It is extraordinarily difficult to change these systems. Usually, some sort of really important economic dislocation or other form of social dislocation has to occur that is so bad that it gets the attention of people even though there are all these inertia effects to overcome.

MARK V. PAULY: It doesn't make sense to be too rough on fee-for-service medicine. Recently, I chose Blue Cross/Blue Shield 100, the most expensive fee-for-service insurance policy. My employer makes a contribution, but it costs me the extra deduction of a few thousand a year. I think I have a comparative advantage of saying no to doctors and demanding my rights. And there was no cap, no limit on the rate of growth, as far as I know, in the Blue Cross/Blue Shield 100. We ought to cap the government's contribution, the government transfer, and then allow beneficiaries to supplement that if they want to buy into an unconstrained open-ended situation.

MR. BERENSON: People have misunderstood what RVS is supposed to be doing. We have price regulation in Medicare. We've had it at least since 1972. The RBRVS is not supposed to do what everyone on the panel wants to talk about, which is make fundamental institutional changes in health care. There should have been more tinkering, more leadership from HCFA, so it didn't have to become a congressional level issue.

Another point: You can get away with expenditure caps a little easier if there is some way of placating some of the equity concerns. You then can be more arbitrary about imposing expenditure targets.

H. E. FRECH III: Where does the support for this Rube Goldberg machine, the RBRVS, come from? At one level it is mysterious. Roger Noll has a more or less straightforward public choice story, where one group is ripping off another group in the short run, taking quasi rents and saving some budgetary money for a year or two, maybe

413

three. Glenn Hackbarth added a philosophical or aesthetic point, which is this concern with equity, a feeling that certain doctors are getting too much relative to other doctors, and that's aesthetically unappealing.

But there's still another attraction of the RBRVS, and it is also a noneconomic, aesthetic, or philosophical one. The RBRVS is tremendously arbitrary. There are judgment calls from the very beginning, from writing the vignettes of care to linking unrelated specialties. But to those on the outside—which means to the congressmen and their staffs—it is a scientific black box, like a computer. To them it seems scientific and objective and mechanical. It seems devoid of human judgment or values.

And that is what they want. There has always been a tremendous demand in economic matters for getting the economics out of it, to make it somehow technocratic, mechanical, automatic. No moral judgments, no empirical judgments, no value judgments. Let me give a couple of examples.

First is the internal rate of return rule for investment decisions. It seems to avoid the necessity of observing the market and making empirical judgments about the right interest rate. This apparent technocratic nature is the appeal of that rule. And the internal rate of return rule cannot be beaten down. I get students who have had a couple of courses in accounting and I have to beat the internal rate of return idea out of them before I start telling them how to make investment decisions correctly.

The other example is growth theory. Remember the way old-fashioned growth theory was done fifteen years ago? There were no value judgments. The golden rule growth path depended only on technology growth, and population growth. There was no problem choosing among different generations because automatically if you got to that golden rule path, consumption was higher for every generation. It seemed to take all the judgment out of economic growth problems.

Well, you can't take the economics out of economics. There has to be empirical judgment, continuing management, and thought. Somehow, the real enthusiasts for the resource-based relative value scale are trying to do without these matters of scientific and moral judgment. An important part of the support for the RBRVS comes from its appearance of scientific objectiveness.

COMMENT: This fee schedule might be useful in instilling competition in the fee-for-service sector. Right now, part of the reason why it is difficult to search for prices is that doctors don't know what reimbursement they are getting a lot of times, and the price each doctor is getting under Medicare is a little bit different. So if consumers wanted to find out how much it is going to cost, they would have to spend a great deal of time doing so.

If you went to an RBRVS, however adjusted—geographically corrected, whatever—and instead of going to mandatory assignment you went to mandatory nonassignment and you had unlimited balance billing (where the patient was responsible for the entire difference between what the physician charged and what Medicare was going to pay), then it would be very easy for the patient to say to the doctor, can you do it for the Medicare price? The patient does not even have to know what the Medicare price is. He just says, "Can you do it for the Medicare price?"

And if the answer is no, then it will be very clear what the patient's liability would be. It is the difference. It will be 100 percent on the patient. Then the fee-for-service sector might have to compete. For example, if Dr. Franck's surgery cost $1,000 more than the next neurosurgeon down the street, he would have to have a good reason for it. The patient would be able to call and say, "Will you do my surgery for the Medicare price? If not, Smith down the road will do it for that price."

MR. HACKBARTH: The problem is what do you have to invest to get to that point? And do you think that the benefits of competition at this level are going to be sufficient to justify the investment? The investment of political, administrative, and research resources needed to develop that system is substantial, given the way the agency operates and all the other things it has to do. And I don't think that the benefits of that form of competition are great.

They are not zero, but just not large enough to justify giving precedence to this particular investment of scarce resources. And it seems to be that we ought to go in other directions.

COMMENT: One of the things that muddles our thinking is the way we use the term "fee schedule." To people who aren't normally working in this physician services market, it sounds like price regulation.

Sometimes the term "fee schedule" is used, when we are really talking about an indemnity payment schedule as is used in the private insurance industry. If balance billing is unrestricted, as it is for those with private insurance, then deciding on a fee schedule, even a bad one, is very different from price control. We often get confused and

415

use that single term to refer to two different things, often in the same sentence.

MR. HELMS: It seems that this panel has voiced some interesting and serious criticisms of the resource-based relative value scale. A question in many minds is why Congress would really want this. Others predict that it is coming despite all of the reservations of policy experts.

Notes

CHAPTER 1: OVERVIEW OF POLICY ISSUES, *H. E. Frech III*

1. See Lee Benham's chapter for more discussion of entry limitation in physician services.

2. For more on the idiosyncratic relationship between consumers and their physicians, see the chapter by David Dranove and Mark Satterthwaite.

3. See H. E. Frech III and Paul B. Ginsburg, *Public Health Insurance in Private Medical Markets: Some Problems of National Health Insurance* (Washington, D.C.: American Enterprise Institute, 1978), or the more technical "Imposed Health Insurance in Monopolistic Markets: A Theoretical Analysis," *Economic Inquiry,* vol. 13, no. 1 (March 1975), pp. 55–70; or Joseph P. Newhouse and Vincent Taylor, "How Shall We Pay for Hospital Care?" the *Public Interest,* vol. 23 (Spring 1971), pp. 78–92; Joseph P. Newhouse and Vincent Taylor, "The Subsidy Problem in Hospital Insurance: A Proposal," *Journal of Business,* vol. 43, no. 4 (October 1970), pp. 452–56; or Mark V. Pauly, "Indemnity Insurance for Health Care Efficiency," *Economic and Business Bulletin,* vol. 4, no. 4 (Fall 1971), pp. 53–59, for more on the advantages of indemnity insurance.

4. H. E. Frech III, "Preferred Provider Organizations and Health Care Competition," in *Health Care in America: The Political Economy of Hospitals and Health Insurance,* ed. H. E. Frech III (San Francisco: Pacific Research Institute for Public Policy, 1988), pp. 353–70.

5. See the chapters by David Dranove and Mark Satterthwaite, Jack Hadley, John Holahan and Stephen Zuckerman, and Mark Pauly.

6. See the chapter by William Marder and Richard Willke and the commentary of Joseph Newhouse for more on the higher psychic costs of specialties with little patient contact like pathology and surgery.

7. Restrictions under the Maximum Allowed Actual Charges (MAAC) program are minor for most existing physicians, although some of the higher-priced ones find their balance bills reduced. They are fairly strict for new physicians, since they are limited to the fiftieth percentile of charges. But the MAAC restrictions are mild compared to what the PPRC is proposing.

8. The recommendation of the PPRC is summarized in Paul Ginsburg's paper in this volume. The full length version is in *Annual Report to Congress: 1988* (Washington, D.C.: Physician Payment Review Commission), April 1988 (hereafter *PPRC, 1989*).

9. See Joseph Antos's paper in this volume for more on this and other policy issues.

10. Gail Lee Cafferata, *Private Health Insurance Coverage of the Medicare Population,* NCHRS National Medical Care Expenditures Study, Data Preview 18, DHHS Publication No. (PHS) 84-3362 (September 1984), p. 15.

11. *PPRC, 1989,* p. 21.

12. Thomas Rice and Nelda McCall, "Factors Influencing Physician Assignment Decisions under Medicare," *Inquiry,* vol. 20, no. 1 (Spring 1983), pp. 52–54.

13. Janet B. Mitchell and Jerry Cromwell, "The Impact of an All-or-Nothing Assignment Requirement under Medicare," *Health Care Financing Review,* vol. 4, no. 4 (Summer 1983), p. 68.

14. Margo L. Rosenbach, Sylvia Hurdle, and Jerry Cromwell, *An Analysis of Medicare's Physician Participation Agreement Program.* Final Report, Submitted to National Opinion Research Center re HCFA Contract No. 500-83-0025. Needham, Massachusetts: Health Economics Research, Inc. (October 29, 1985), chap. 4, p. 13.

15. *PPRC, 1989,* p. 18.

16. H. E. Frech III and Paul B. Ginsburg, "Competition among Health Insurers, Revisited," *Journal of Health Politics, Policy and Law,* vol. 13, no. 2 (Summer 1988), pp. 279–91.

17. William C. Hsiao and William Stason, "Toward Developing a Relative Value Scale for Medical and Surgical Services," *Health Care Financing Review,* vol. 1, no. 2 (Fall 1979), pp. 23–38.

18. Jack Hadley and Robert A. Berenson, "Seeking the Just Price: Constructing Relative Value Scales and Fee Schedules," *Annals of Internal Medicine,* vol. 106, no. 3 (March 1987), pp. 461–66.

19. David Juba, "The Effects of Health Insurance on Absolute and Relative Prices of Physicians' Services," in "Final Report on Alternative Methods of Developing a Relative Value Scale of Physicians' Services," Report No. 3075-07, ed. Jack Hadley (Washington, D.C.: Urban Institute, April 1985).

20. Joseph Newhouse maintains that the 3 percent rate of combined dropping out or flunking out of medical school does not indicate that poor performers get through because medical schools are very selective. But I would expect more than 3 percent, however well selected, would drop out for lack of interest, before even counting the poor performers.

21. Recently, the catastrophic program was dropped. Some form of it will probably be presented again soon, however.

22. His specific reference was to H. E. Frech III and Paul B. Ginsburg, *Public Health Insurance,* 1978. But he could have mentioned our earlier, more technical piece, "Imposed Health Insurance," *Economic Inquiry* (1975), pp. 55–70. Other references on the importance of balance billing are Newhouse and Taylor, "How Shall We Pay for Hospital Care?" *Economic Inquiry* (1971), pp. 78–92; Newhouse and Taylor, "The Subsidy Problem in Hospital Insurance," *Economic Inquiry* (1970), pp. 452–56; or Pauly, "Indemnity Insurance," *Economic Inquiry* (1971), pp. 53–59.

23. Edward F. X. Hughes, Victor Fuchs, J. E. Jacoby, and E. W. Lewit, "Surgical Workloads in a Community Practice," *Surgery,* vol. 71, no. 3 (March 1972), pp. 315–27.

24. Roger Noll, Joseph Antos, Clark Havighurst, and Glenn Hackbarth were especially vehement on this matter.

25. Mark V. Pauly, "Overinsurance and Public Provision of Insurance: The Roles of Moral Hazard and Adverse Selection," *Quarterly Journal of Economics*, vol. 88, no. 1, (February 1974), pp. 44–62; and Mark V. Pauly, "Overinsurance: The Conceptual Issues," in Mark V. Pauly, ed., *National Health Insurance: What Now, What Later, What Never*, pp. 201–19 (Washington, D.C.: American Enterprise Institute, 1980).

26. The most intellectually serious case for the cost-based approach can be found in a few pages of chapter 3 of the *Annual Report to Congress: 1988*. Washington, D.C.: Physician Payment Review Commission, April 1988. But the topic demands several articles or books devoted entirely to it.

27. See especially the chapters and commentary by William Marder and Richard Willke, Jody Sindelar, Mark Satterthwaite and David Dranove, Jack Hadley, Frank Sloan, Joseph Newhouse, and Roger Noll.

28. See the chapter by William Marder and Richard Willke and the commentary by Jody Sindelar for the details on amortizing training costs over physicians' lifetimes.

29. For more on this see Jack Hadley's chapter and Joseph Newhouse's and Roger Noll's commentaries.

30. There was wide assent to the idea that balance billing provides an important safety valve and would be even more important if the RBRVS were to be instigated. See especially the Holahan and Zuckerman chapter.

31. Paul B. Ginsburg, Lauren B. LeRoy, and Glenn T. Hammons, "Medicare Physician Payment Reforms," *Health Affairs*, vol. 9, no. 1 (Spring 1990), pp. 179–88.

32. It is a matter of semantics whether we call insurance with limits to balance billing price control or simply a particular type of procurement of services. After all, the physician can simply refuse to treat the patient. But the same statements could be made about a price-control law.

33. Physician Payment Review Commission, *Annual Report to Congress: 1989* (Washington, D.C.: Physician Payment Review Commission, April 1989), p. 141.

CHAPTER 2: POLICY CONTEXT OF PHYSICIAN PAYMENT, *Joseph R. Antos*

1. This sense of frustration is evident in Representative Pete Stark's open letter to the president. See Fortney H. Stark, "Open Letters to a New President," *Health Management Quarterly* (First Quarter 1989), pp. 15–17.

2. See articles by Professor William Hsiao and his colleagues and the accompanying commentary in the September 29, 1988 issue of the *New England Journal of Medicine* and the October 28, 1988 issue of the *Journal of the American Medical Association*. The full study is described in William Hsiao, Peter Braun, Edmund Becker, et al., *A National Study of Resource-Based Relative Value Scales for Physician Services: Final Report to the Health Care Financing Administration* (Boston: Harvard University School of Public Health, 1988), publication 17-C-98795/1-03.

3. See Mark Chassin, Jacqueline Kosecoff, Rolla Park, et al., "Does Inap-

propriate Use Explain Geographic Variations in the Use of Health Care Services?" *Journal of the American Medical Association,* vol. 258, no. 18 (November 13, 1987), pp. 2533–37.

4. About 20 percent of physician bills are unassigned claims, on which the patient is balance-billed. Private supplemental insurance frequently covers part of this balance billing. Such insurance usually limits allowable charges eligible for reimbursement, but the limits may exceed Medicare's allowed charge.

5. Growth of the Medicare population refers to increases in the number of beneficiaries. The number of individuals reaching age sixty-five every year has been growing and is expected to continue growing for several more decades. Because of greater longevity, the Medicare population is also aging. Both the greater number of beneficiaries and the greater average age of those beneficiaries contribute to growing costs of the Medicare program.

6. See U.S. Department of Health and Human Services, *Paying Physicians: Choices for Medicare* (Baltimore, Md.: Health Care Financing Administration, 1987).

7. See William Hsiao, Peter Braun, Nancy Kelly, and Edmund Becker, "Results, Potential Effects, and Implementation Issues of the Resource-Based Relative Value Scale," *Journal of the American Medical Association,* vol. 260, no. 16 (October 28, 1988), pp. 2429–38.

8. This analysis is based on an additive RBRVS model with separate payment amounts for practice cost and for physician work (modified by relative-opportunity cost). The geographic practice-cost adjustment is applied to both payment amounts in the RVS model. Technical details are contained in U.S. Department of Health and Human Services, *Medicare Physician Payment* (Baltimore, Md.: Health Care Financing Administration, 1989). New impact estimates available since this paper was written are contained in Jesse Levy et al., "Impact of the Medicare Fee Schedule on Payments to Physicians," *Journal of the American Medical Association,* vol. 264, no. 6 (August 8, 1990), pp. 717–22.

CHAPTER 3: PHYSICIANS' FEES, INCOMES, SPECIALTIES,
Dranove and Satterthwaite

1. W. Hsiao et al., "Results and Policy Implications of the Resource-Based Relative-Value Study," *New England Journal of Medicine,* September 29, 1988, pp. 881–88.

2. W. Hsiao et al., "Estimating Physicians' Work for a Resource-Based Relative-Value Scale," *New England Journal of Medicine,* September 29, 1988, pp. 835–41.

3. See the calculations of Hsiao et al., "Results and Policy Implications," on the impact of an RBRVS on compensation rates and the distribution of Medicare payments to specialties. See P. Burnstein and J. Cromwell, "Relative Incomes and Rates of Return for U.S. Physicians," *Journal of Health Economics,* vol. 4 (1985), pp. 63–78, for evidence that incomes corrected for length of training, etc., vary substantially across specialties.

4. A more complete exposition of fee setting under monopolistic competition may be found in M. A. Satterthwaite, "Competition and Equilibrium as a Driving Force in the Health Services Sector," in R. P. Inman, ed., *Managing the Service Economy: Prospects and Problems* (New York: Cambridge University Press, 1985), pp. 239–67. Extension of the model to include physicians' decisions about the qualitative attributes of their practice may be found in D. Dranove and M. Satterthwaite, "Monopolistic Competition When Price and Quality Are Not Perfectly Observable," December 1988, unpublished.

5. See J. Newhouse et al., "Some Interim Results from a Controlled Trial of Cost Sharing in Health Insurance," *New England Journal of Medicine*, December 17, 1981, pp. 1501–7; W. Manning et al., "Health Insurance and the Demand for Medical Care: Evidence from a Randomized Experiment," Rand Report R-3476-HHS (Santa Monica, Calif.: Rand, February 1988).

6. R. Lee and J. Hadley, "Physicians' Fees and Public Medical Care Programs," *Health Services Research*, vol. 16 (1981), pp. 185–203; T. McCarthy, "The Competitive Nature of the Primary-Care Physician Services Market," *Journal of Health Economics*, vol. 4 (1985), pp. 93–117.

7. Throughout this analysis physicians are assumed to be income maximizers. This is a crude approximation; physicians do have a variety of goals that may lead them not to exploit fully their monopoly power. Thus, if an RBRVS that lowers their fees for Medicare is imposed, surgeons may "cost shift" by increasing fees to non-Medicare patients and, to an extent too difficult to determine, induce demand by adopting a less rigorous standard for deciding when surgery is indicated. See D. Dranove, "Pricing by Non-Profit Institutions: The Case of Hospital Cost-Shifting," *Journal of Health Economics*, vol. 7 (1988), pp. 47–57, concerning cost shifting, and both Dranove, "Pricing by Non-Profit Institutions," and J. Cromwell and J. Mitchell, "Physician-Induced Demand for Surgery," *Journal of Health Economics*, vol. 5 (1986), pp. 293–314, concerning demand inducement.

8. M. Satterthwaite, "Consumer Information, Equilibrium, Industry Price, and the Number of Sellers," *Bell Journal of Economics*, vol. 10 (1979), pp. 483–502; Dranove and Satterthwaite, "Monopolistic Competition."

9. Satterthwaite, "Consumer Information," see pp. 494–98. M. Pauly and M. Satterthwaite, "The Pricing of Primary Care Physicians' Services: A Test of the Role of Consumer Information," *Bell Journal of Economics*, vol. 12 (1981), pp. 488–506, provide empirical evidence for the importance of search and information costs.

10. Dranove and Satterthwaite, "Monopolistic Competition"; equation (3.18).

11. Ibid.

12. Satterthwaite, "Consumer Information"; see pp. 491–94.

13. Pauly and Satterthwaite, "Pricing of Primary Care Physicians' Services"; Satterthwaite, "Competition and Equilibrium."

14. This decision is affected by the details of Medicare payment rules. Since Jack Hadley, in chapter 5, discusses these details, we focus only on those aspects that directly influence the physician's decision.

15. The behavior of a firm that faces a kinked demand curve is analyzed in many intermediate microeconomic and industrial organization textbooks. See F. M. Scherer, *Industrial Market Structure and Economic Performance* (Chicago: Rand-McNally, 1980), pp. 164–68.

16. Hsiao et al., "Results and Policy Implications."

17. W. Marder, "Theory of Job Shopping and Physician Location Choice," (1989, unpublished).

18. Satterthwaite, "Competition and Equilibrium."

19. Cromwell and Mitchell, "Physician-Induced Demand for Surgery"; see table 2, regression 4. The argument here is confined to Cromwell and Mitchell's interpretation of their regression 4. Their paper contributes to an understanding of demand inducement.

20. Ibid., p. 305.

21. Ibid. Cromwell and Mitchell also state that their result "is true even after purging surgeon availability of the feedback effect of higher fees on surgeon location." They used two-stage least squares to estimate the price regression, with surgeons per thousand treated as an endogenous variable. Using two-stage least squares, however, does not establish the direction of causation. In particular their price equation can be derived from a monopolistically competitive model of the industry just as easily as they derived it from a perfectly competitive model.

22. Cromwell and Mitchell's elasticity estimate can be interpreted as evidence of great market power on the part of surgeons. To make the calculation easy, assume that in each community the demand for surgery is fixed and perfectly inelastic. If each surgeon's individual elasticity of demand is -1.1 and the cost is constant, then a 10 percent increase in surgeon's fees must be associated with a 9 percent increase in the number of surgeons in the community. Otherwise surgeons' incomes would not be constant across communities.

23. Interestingly Marder, "Theory of Job Shopping," presents evidence that the returns to ability may vary across geographic markets. Thus one might see persistent income differentials across geographic markets due to the same selection-by-ability effect that in the next section is identified with specialty choice.

24. M. Noether, "The Effect of Government Policy Changes on the Supply of Physicians: Expansion of a Competitive Fringe," *Journal of Law and Economics*, vol. 29 (October 1986), pp. 231–62.

25. The process of applying for a residency may help medical students to evaluate themselves. Those specialties that contain concentrations of high-ability physicians and thus have high average incomes may have long queues of students wishing to gain entry. The residency program may select among the applicants on the basis of ability because low-ability physicians will be painfully inadequate if they are admitted. Medical students' success in gaining admission to residency programs may therefore signal to the students their ability.

26. Dranove and Satterthwaite, "Monopolistic Competition," develop a

model in which better observability of ability (or quality) results in more elastic demand with respect to ability.

27. G. Akerlof, "The Market for 'Lemons': Quality Uncertainty and the Market Mechanism," *Quarterly Journal of Economics*, vol. 84 (1970), pp. 488–500.

CHAPTER 4: LICENSURE AND COMPETITION, *Lee Benham*

1. Before rejecting the argument that licensure has general consequences for foreign policy, one should consider the implications of licensure for the training of foreign physicians, who are a principal elite group in most third world countries. Aspiring students from other countries have virtually no chance of admission to U.S. medical schools. In unlicensed fields foreign students are well represented at American universities. John A. D. Cooper, "Health Resources: The United States and the Third World," *Health Affairs*, Summer 1984, p. 150.

2. Lincoln Moses and Frederick Mosteller, "Institutional Differences in Postoperative Death Rates," *Journal of the American Medical Association*, vol. 203, no. 7 (February 12, 1968), p. 151.

3. Staff of the Stanford Center for Health Care Research, "Comparison of Hospitals with Regard to Outcomes of Surgery," *Health Services Research*, vol. 11, no. 2 (Summer 1976), pp. 112–27.

4. Harold Luft, John Bunker, and Alan Enthoven, "Should Operations Be Regionalized?" *New England Journal of Medicine*, vol. 301, no. 25 (December 20, 1979), p. 1364.

5. Harold Luft, "The Relations between Surgical Volume and Mortality: An Exploration of Causal Factors and Alternative Models," *Medical Care*, vol. 18, no. 9 (September 1980), pp. 940–59.

6. "Peer Review," *Professional Regulation News*, April–May 1983, p. 8.

7. "Regulatory Update," *Professional Regulation News*, February 1983, p. 1.

8. "AMA Presidents Blame Courts & FTC," *Professional Regulation News*, April–May 1983, pp. 9–10.

9. Some sensitivity by the Association of American Medical Colleges is evident in its comments on this issue.

Although student evaluation is rigorous, the rate of attrition in U.S. medical schools is low—less than 3 percent. Students with detected deficiencies in knowledge or skills are provided counseling and assistance. Usually, students who are having difficulties are offered the opportunity to repeat course work. However, all faculties reserve the right to drop students whose academic or personal characteristics are found to be incompatible with the professional responsibilities of a physician in this society.

Association of American Medical Colleges, *Medical School Admissions Requirements, 1989–90*, 39th ed. (Washington, D.C.: AAMC, 1988), p. 4.

10. Ibid., pp. 10–11.

11. Ibid., p. 9.

12. An illustration of some peculiarities of the system, college graduates with a major in biology have had lower starting salaries than even humanities graduates ("Labor Letter," *Wall Street Journal*, July 31, 1984, p. 1). Because of the attraction of medicine as a career, many more students study biology than would otherwise do so. Some are unsuccessful at gaining admission to medical schools; others decide late against a medical career. Both patterns lead to more trained biologists than would be the case without the attraction of a medical career. Consequently the cost of research is lowered, and innovation is encouraged. This is not the usual rationale for the current system.

13. "Florida Medical Discipline," *Professional Regulation News*, February 1984, p. 4.

14. "Good Doctors Know Who the Bad Ones Are," *Professional Regulation News*, April–May 1983, pp. 5–6.

15. Ibid., pp. 8–9.

16. Ibid., p. 9.

17. "Regulatory Update," *Professional Regulation News*, February 1983, p. 1.

18. "Legislative News," *Professional Regulation News*, August 1982, p. 1.

19. Gary D. Hailey, Jonathan R. Bromberg, and Joseph P. Mulholland, *A Comparative Analysis of Cosmetic Contact Lens Fitting by Ophthalmologists, Optometrists, and Opticians* (Washington, D.C.: Bureau of Consumer Protection, Bureau of Economics, Federal Trade Commission, December 1983). This is frequently described as Eyeglasses II.

20. Ibid., p. 14. See also Benham and Benham, "Regulating through the Professions: A Perspective of Information Control," *Journal of Law and Economics*, October 1975.

21. See Benham and Benham, ibid.; also FTC, *State Restrictions on Vision Care Providers: The Effects on Consumers* (Washington, D.C.: Bureau of Consumer Protection, FTC, 1980).

22. See Hailey, Bromberg, and Mulholland, *Comparative Analysis of Cosmetic Contact Lens Fitting*, pp. 9–19.

23. At 10 percent levels of significance. See ibid., pp. D9–D18. In two of the twelve statistical tests of specific measures, noncommercial optometrists showed significantly lower quality at the 10 percent level of significance. In eight of the twelve tests, the estimated quality was higher for commerical optometrists (chi-square value of parameter estimate = 2.8, 3.6, .02, 2.1, 1.9, 1.0, 0.0, .3); in the remaining four cases the estimated quality was higher for noncommercial optometrists (chi-square = 0.0, 0.1, 0.0, 0.1).

24. *Professional Regulation News*, February 1984, p. 3.

25. *Professional Regulation News*, January 1984, pp. 4–5.

26. Valerie Cheh, *The Effect of Commercial Competition on Health Care Quality: Evidence from the Contact Lens Market* (St. Louis: Washington University, Department of Economics, 1990).

PROTECTING THE MEDICAL PROFESSION, *A Commentary by Peter Zweifel*

1. OECD, *Measuring Health Care 1960–1983. Expenditure, Cost, and Performance* (Paris: OECD, 1985).

2. For the case of Germany, see P. R. Kleindorfer and J. M. von der Schulenburg, "Intergenerational Equity and Fund Balances for Statutory Health Insurance," in J. M. von der Schulenburg, ed., *Essays in Social Security Economics* (New York: Springer, 1986), pp. 108–29.

3. R. A. Kessel, "Price Discrimination in Medicine," *Journal of Law and Economics*, vol. 1, no. 5 (1958), pp. 20–53.

4. W. G. Manning et al., "Health Insurance and the Demand for Medical Care: Evidence from a Randomized Experiment," *American Economic Review*, vol. 77 (1987), pp. 251–77; G. J. Wedig, "Health Status and the Demand for Health: Results on Price Elasticities," *Journal of Health Economics*, vol. 7, no. 2 (1988), pp. 151–64.

5. J. P. Acton, "Nonmonetary Factors in the Demand for Medical Service: Some Empirical Evidence," *Journal of Political Economy*, vol. 83, no. 3 (1975), pp. 595–614; OECD, *Measuring Health Care*.

6. OECD, *Measuring Health Care*.

CHAPTER 5: FOUNDATIONS OF THE RBRVS, *Jack Hadley*

1. W. Hsiao et al., "Resource-based Relative Values," *Journal of the American Medical Association*, October 28, 1988, pp. 2347–60; emphasis added.

2. Ibid.

3. Physician Payment Review Commission, *Annual Report to Congress* (Washington, D.C.: PPRC, 1988).

4. M. Pauly, "Reflections on Using Physician Agents to Minimize the Cost of Health," *Journal of Health Economics*, March 1985, pp. 79–82.

5. M. Pauly and M. Satterthwaite, "The Pricing of Primary Care Physicians' Services: A Test of the Role of Consumer Information," *Bell Journal of Economics*, vol. 12 (1981), pp. 488–506.

6. D. Juba, "The Effects of Health Insurance on Absolute and Relative Prices of Physicians' Services," in Jack Hadley et al., *Final Report on Alternative Methods of Developing a Relative Value Scale of Physicians' Services*, report 3075-07 (Washington, D.C.: Urban Institute, April 1985).

7. R. Lee, "Insurance and Medical List Prices" (Chapel Hill, N.C.: University of North Carolina, 1988; unpublished); R. Lee and J. Hadley, "Physicians' Fees and Public Medical Care Programs," *Health Services Research*, Summer 1981, pp. 185–203; D. Yett et al., "Fee Screen Reimbursement and Physician Fee Inflation," *Journal of Human Resources*, Spring 1985, pp. 278–91.

8. F. Sloan and R. Feldman, "Monopolistic Elements in the Market for Physicians' Services," in W. Greenberg, ed., *Competition in the Health Care Sector: Past, Present, and Future* (Germantown, Md.: Aspen Systems, 1978), pp. 45–102.

9. T. McCarthy, "The Competitive Nature of the Primary-care Physician Services Market," *Journal of Health Economics*, June 1985, pp. 93–118; M. Stano, "An Analysis of the Evidence on Competition in the Physician Services Market," *Journal of Health Economics*, September 1985, pp. 197–212.

10. J. Newhouse and F. Sloan, "Physician Pricing: Monopolistic or Competitive: Reply," *Southern Economic Journal* (April 1972), pp. 577–80.

11. American Medical Association, *Profile of Medical Practice 1981* (Chicago: AMA, 1981).

12. Ibid.

13. Pauly and Satterthwaite, "Pricing of Primary Care Physicians' Services."

14. Mark Pauly raised this possibility at a conference held several years ago. The phenomenon of hospital pricing to cross-subsidize care from privately insured to uninsured patients is similar, although care to the uninsured presumably has different motivations. J. Hadley and J. Feder, "Hospital Cost Shifting and Care of the Uninsured," *Health Affairs*, vol. 4 (Fall 1985), pp. 67–80; and J. Hay, "The Impact of Public Health Care Financing Policies on Private-Sector Hospital Costs," *Journal of Health Politics, Policy and Law*, vol. 4 (Winter 1983), pp. 945–52.

15. P. Danzon, W. Manning, and M. Marquis, "Factors Affecting Laboratory Test Use and Prices," *Health Care Financing Review*, Summer 1985, pp. 23–32.

16. P. McMenamin, "Medicare Part B Carrier Approved Charges: 1988 Summary," April 7, 1989, unpublished.

17. T. Cowing and A. Holtmann, "Multiproduct Short-Run Hospital Cost Functions," *Southern Economic Journal* (January 1983), pp. 637–53; T. Cowing, A. Holtmann, and S. Powers, "Hospital Cost Analysis: A Survey and Evaluation of Recent Studies," in *Advances in Health Economics and Health Services Research* (Greenwich, Conn.: JAI Press, 1983), pp. 257–303; T. Grannemann, R. Brown, and M. Pauly, "Estimating Hospital Costs: A Multiple-Output Analysis," *Journal of Health Economics* (June 1986), pp. 107–27; J. Hadley and K. Swartz, "The Impacts of Hospital Costs between 1980 and 1984 on Hospital Rate Regulation, Competition, and Changes in Health Insurance Coverage," *Inquiry*, Spring 1989, pp. 35–47.

18. Hsiao et al., "Results, Potential Effects, and Implementation Issues," p. 2431.

19. E. Becker et al., "Relative Cost Differences among Physicians' Specialty Practices," *Journal of the American Medical Association*, October 28, 1988, pp. 2397–2408; W. Hsiao et al., "Results, Potential Effects, and Implementation Issues of the Resource-based Relative Value Scale," *Journal of the American Medical Association*, October 28, 1988, pp. 2429–38.

20. J. Hadley and K. Swartz, "Impacts of Hospital Costs."

21. W. Kelley et al., "Extrapolation of Measures of Work for Surveyed Services to Other Services," *Journal of the American Medical Association*, October 28, 1988, pp. 2379–89.

22. P. Braun et al., "Cross-Specialty Linkage of Resource-based Relative Value Scales," *Journal of the American Medical Association*, October 28, 1988, pp. 2390–96.

23. This section borrows extensively from J. Hadley and R. Berenson, "Seeking the Just Price: Constructing Relative Value Scales and Fee Schedules," *Annals of Internal Medicine*, March 1987, pp. 461–66.

24. American Society of Internal Medicine, "Reimbursement for Physi-

cians' Cognitive and Procedural Services: A White Paper" (Washington, D.C.: American Society of Internal Medicine, January 1981).

25. J. Hadley et al., "Alternative Methods of Developing a Relative Value Scale of Physicians' Services," Working Paper 3075–4, chapter 2 (Washington, D.C.: Urban Institute, February 1983).

26. J. Hadley, "How Should Medicare Pay Physicians," *Milbank Memorial Fund Quarterly*, Spring 1984, pp. 279–99.

BEYOND PAYMENT REFORMS, *A Commentary by Charles E. Phelps*

1. The same result would also occur if the supply of some complementary factor, for example, availability of operating rooms, were restricted. Chapter 3, by Dranove and Satterthwaite, provides some excellent analyses of some situations where differential returns to surgical specialties could arise from reasons other than entry restrictions. In particular they analyze conditions where differential skill led to systematic sorting of better doctors into the higher-paying specialties. Their models are both useful and appropriate.

2. Chapter 13, by Marder and Willke, provides new evidence on rates of return using current data. They show comparable returns as have previous studies, except they show much higher returns for radiologists, pathologists, and anesthesiologists than previous studies have shown, and indeed higher than for any other specialty analyzed.

3. They also completely ignored differences in the ratios of physician to nonphysician inputs across procedures, assuming specifically that such ratios were constant. Hadley's concern with this omission in chapter 5 is valid.

4. W. E. Roper, W. Winkenwerder, G. M. Hackbarth, and H. Krakauer, "Effectiveness in Health Care: An Initiative to Evaluate and Improve Medical Practice," *New England Journal of Medicine*, vol. 319, no. 18 (1988), pp. 1197–1202.

5. A modestly complete bibliography of this literature contains more than 100 references. Representative works include J. E. Wennberg, "Small Area Analysis and the Medical Care Outcome Problem," in L. Sechrest, E. Perrin, and J. Bunker, eds., *Research Methodology: Strengthening Causal Interpretation of Non-Experimental Data*, U.S. Department of Health and Human Services Report PHS90-3454 (Rockville, Md., 1990), 177–213; N. P. Roos, "Hysterectomy: Variations in Rates across Small Areas and across Physicians' Practices," *American Journal of Public Health*, vol. 74 (1984), pp. 327–35; M. R. Chassin et al., "Variations in Use of Medical and Surgical Services by the Medicare Population," *New England Journal of Medicine*, vol. 314, no. 5 (1986), pp. 285–90; K. McPherson, J. E. Wennberg, O. B. Hovind, and P. Clifford, "Small-area Variations in the Use of Common Surgical Procedures: An International Comparison of New England, England, and Norway," *New England Journal of Medicine*, vol. 307, no. 21 (1982), pp. 1310–14.

6. W. G. Manning et al., "Health Insurance and the Demand for Medical Care: Evidence from a Randomized Experiment," *American Economic Review*, vol. 77, no. 3 (1987), pp. 251–77.

7. J. E. Wennberg, J. L. Freeman, and W. J. Culp, "Are Hospital Services Rationed in New Haven or Over-utilised in Boston?" *Lancet 1*, May 23, 1987, pp. 1185–88.

THE ART OF PAYING PHYSICIANS, *A Commentary by Clark C. Havighurst*

1. Lawrence Goldberg and Warren Greenberg, "The Effects of Physician-controlled Health Insurance: U.S. v. Oregon State Medical Society," *Journal of Health Politics, Policy and Law* (Spring 1977), pp. 48–78.
2. Charles Weller, " 'Free Choice' as a Restraint of Trade in American Health Care Delivery and Insurance," *Iowa Law Review* (July 1984), pp. 1351–92.
3. Clark Havighurst and Philip Kissam, "The Antitrust Implications of Relative Value Studies in Medicine," *Journal of Health Politics, Policy and Law* (Winter 1979), pp. 48–86.

CHAPTER 6: BALANCE BILLING AND PAYMENT REFORM, *Zuckerman and Holahan*

1. W. C. Hsiao, P. Braun, D. Dunn, and E. R. Becker, "Resource-based Relative Values," *Journal of the American Medical Association*, vol. 260 (October 28, 1988a), pp. 2347–60.
2. Janet B. Mitchell and Jerry Cromwell, "Physician Behavior under the Medicare Assignment Option," *Journal of Health Economics*, vol. 1, no. 3 (December 1982), pp. 245–64; Lynn Paringer, "Medicare Assignment Rates of Physicians: Their Responses to Changes in Reimbursement Policy," *Health Care Financing Review*, vol. 1, no. 3 (Winter 1980), pp. 75–89.
3. Janet B. Mitchell, Margo L. Rosenbach, and Jerry Cromwell, "To Sign or Not to Sign: Physician Participation in Medicare, 1984" *Health Care Financing Review*, vol. 10, no. 1 (Fall 1988), p. 17.
4. See Jack Hadley and Roberta Lee, "Supplying Physicians' Services to Public Medical Care Programs," Urban Institute Working Paper no. 1145-17 (Washington, D.C., November 1978); David Juba, Margaret Sulvetta, and William Scanlon, "Physician Behavior under an All or None Assignment Policy," Urban Institute Working Paper no. 1306-02-10 (Washington, D.C., May 1985); Mitchell and Cromwell, "Physician Behavior"; Paringer, "Medicare Assignment Rates of Physicians"; Frank Sloan, J. Cromwell, and J. Mitchell, "Physician Participation in State Medicaid Programs," *Journal of Human Resources*, vol. 13 (1978), p. 211.
5. Other assumptions can be made about the physician's objective. Two prominent alternatives assume the physician is a utility maximizer. In one instance, utility is a function of income, leisure, and demand creation. See Robert G. Evans, "Supplier-induced Demand: Some Empirical Evidence and Implications," in M. Perlman, ed., *The Economics of Health and Medical Care* (London: Macmillan, 1974), pp. 162–73. These models suggest that physicians tend toward a "target income" because of the disutility associated with

demand creation. A second alternative treats the medical practice as a price-taking firm that maximizes utility instead of profits because of the essential role of the physician's own input in the production process. See Harvey E. Lapan and Douglas M. Brown, "Utility Maximization, Individual Production, and Market Equilibrium," *Southern Economic Journal*, vol. 55, no. 2 (October 1988), pp. 374–431. This second model can yield a negatively sloped product supply curve if the physician exhibits a backward-bending labor supply curve that exceeds the practice's ability to substitute other inputs for physician time. We chose the profit-maximizing framework as the basis for this study because it is consistent with the literature on assignment behavior and because it highlights clearly the primary issues associated with prohibiting balance billing.

6. Hadley and Lee, "Supplying Physicians' Services"; Sloan et al., "Physician Participation in State Medicaid Programs."

7. If the relationship between D_p and D_e is close to that represented by the curves drawn, then mandatory assignment would lead to higher private fees. We are aware that this result is not generalizable and is due largely to the degree of inelasticity of D_p relative to D_e in figure 1. If D_e were sufficiently inelastic relative to D_p, private quantity would fall after mandatory assignment, as would the private price (P_1).

8. Under current policy, nonparticipating physicians face a shift in D_e equal to about $0.05*R$. The adverse financial consequences of choosing nonparticipating status will be less than those of "opting out" because the case-by-case assignment option is still available.

9. Juba et al., "Physician Behavior under an All or None Assignment Policy."

10. Philip J. Held and John Holahan, "Containing Medicare Costs in an Era of Growing Physician Supply," *Health Care Financing Review*, vol. 7, no. 1 (Fall 1978).

11. Sloan et al., "Physician Participation in State Medicaid Programs."

12. Janet B. Mitchell and R. Schurman, "Access to Private Obstetrics/Gynecology Services under Medicaid," *Medical Care*, vol. 22 (1984), p. 1026.

13. Janet B. Mitchell, "Medicaid Participation by Medical and Surgical Specialists," *Medical Care*, vol. 21 (1983), p. 929.

14. Jack Hadley, "Physician Participation in Medicaid: Evidence from California," *Health Services Research*, vol. 14 (Winter 1979), p. 266.

15. John Holahan, Margaret Sulvetta, and William Scanlon, "Medicaid Fee Controls and Physician Behavior: Preliminary Evidence for California," Urban Institute Working Paper no. 1250-03 (Washington, D.C., March 1981).

16. Held and Holahan, "Containing Medicare Costs in an Era of Growing Physician Supply."

17. Janet Perloff, Philip R. Kletke, and Kathryn M. Neckerman, "Recent Trends in Pediatrician Participation in Medicaid," *Medical Care*, vol. 24 (1986), pp. 749–60.

18. Janet Perloff, Philip R. Kletke, and Kathryn M. Neckerman, "Physicians' Decisions to Limit Medicaid Participation: Determinants and Policy

Implications," *Journal of Health Politics, Policy and Law*, vol. 12, no. 12 (Summer 1987), p. 221.

19. Michael Schwartz, Suzanne G. Martin, Deborah D. Cooper, Greta M. Ljung, Bernadette J. Whalen, and Joseph Blackburn, "The Effect of a Thirty Percent Reduction in Physician Fees on Medicaid Surgery Rates in Massachusetts," *American Journal of Public Health*, vol. 71, no. 4 (April 1981).

20. Held and Holahan, "Containing Medicare Costs."

21. Hadley, "Physician Participation in Medicaid."

22. Mitchell, "Medicaid Participation by Medical and Surgical Specialists."

23. Perloff et al., "Recent Trends in Pediatrician Participation," and "Physicians' Decisions to Limit Medicaid Participation."

24. Holahan et al., "Medicaid Fee Controls and Physician Behavior."

25. Held and Holahan, "Containing Medicare Costs."

26. Schwartz et al., "The Effect of a Thirty Percent Reduction."

27. Mitchell and Cromwell, "Physician Behavior under the Medicare Assignment Option."

28. Paringer, "Medicare Assignment Rates of Physicians."

29. James F. Rodgers and Robert A. Musacchio, "Physician Acceptance of Medicare Patients on Assignment," *Journal of Health Economics*, vol. 2, no. 1 (March 1983), pp. 55–73.

30. Thomas Rice and Nelda McCall, "Factors Influencing Physician Assignment Decisions under Medicare," *Inquiry*, vol. 20 (Spring 1983), pp. 45–56.

31. Thomas H. Rice, "Determinants of Physician Assignment Rates by Type of Service," *Health Care Financing Review*, vol. 5, no. 4 (Summer 1984), pp. 33–42.

32. Mitchell et al., "Physician Participation in Medicare."

33. Mitchell and Cromwell, "Physician Behavior under the Medicare Option."

34. Evans, "Supplier-induced Demand"; Mark Pauly, "Issues Related to the Volume and Intensity of Physician Services," University of Pennsylvania Working Paper no. 99-C-99169/5-01 (Philadelphia, 1988).

35. Juba et al., "Physician Behavior under an All or None Assignment Policy"; Lapan and Brown, "Utility Maximization, Individual Production, and Market Equilibrium."

36. Thomas H. Rice, "The Impact of Changing Medicare Reimbursement Rates on Physician-induced Demand," *Medical Care*, vol. 21 (August 1983), p. 803.

37. John Holahan, Avi Dor, and Stephen Zuckerman, "Medicare Physician Expenditures: Sorting Out the Reasons for Growth," Urban Institute Working Paper 3650-06 (Washington, D.C., January 1989).

38. John Holahan and Stephen Zuckerman, "Mandatory Assignment: An Unnecessary Risk for Medicare," *Health Affairs* (Spring 1989), p. 65.

39. Such a policy exists in France, where patients with low incomes, any of twenty-five designated illnesses, hospital stays of longer than thirty days, and long costly treatments resulting in payments of more than 90 French francs per month are exempt from coinsurance payments. See M. Duriez, C.

Glarmet, and S. Sandier, "Physician Compensation in France" (1984, photo-copied).

MAINTAINING MARKET DISCIPLINE, *A Commentary by Jesse S. Hixson*

1. H. E. Frech III and Paul B. Ginsburg, *Public Insurance in Private Medical Markets: Some Problems of National Health Insurance* (Washington, D.C.: American Enterprise Institute, 1978).
2. Patrick S. Cotter, "Physician Service Coverage under Medicare: History, Performance, and Evaluation," discussion paper presented at Leonard Davis Institute and American Medical Association Research Conference on the Medicare Part B Projection Residual, Philadelphia, November 29, 1988.

CHAPTER 7: MEDICARE'S DEMAND-SIDE POLICIES, *Thomas G. McGuire*

1. General Accounting Office (GAO), "Medigap Insurance: Law Has Increased Protection against Substandard and Overpriced Policies," GAO/HRD-87-8 (Washington, D.C.: October 1986), p. 11.
2. Amy K. Taylor, Pamela Farley Short, and Constance M. Horgan, "Medigap Insurance: Friend or Foe in Reducing Medicare Deficits," in H. E. Frech III, ed., *Health Care in America: The Political Economy of Hospitals and Health Insurance* (San Francisco: Pacific Research Institute for Public Policy, 1988).
3. Regulatory concern about Medigap has focused on consumer protection issues. Federal regulation of the terms of Medigap policies stemmed from concern for protecting consumers against unfair pricing and marketing policies, and misleading coverage features. See Gail Lee Cafferata, "Private Health Insurance of the Medicare Population and the Baucus Legislation," *Medical Care*, vol. 23, no. 9 (1985), pp. 1086–96. Section 507 of the Social Security Amendments of 1980, known as the Baucus legislation, sets federal standards for state certification of private insurance sold to Medicare beneficiaries after July 1982. A main feature of the federal minimum standards is the required coverage of Part A and Part B copayments. The Baucus legislation also sets targets for the loss ratio. Policies must return a minimum of 690 percent of premiums in benefits for individual policies and 75 percent for group policies. In a recent survey of 142 policies, GAO (1986) found most to meet minimum standards and where standards were not met, the discrepancy was minor. Many policies exceeded standards. Loss ratio targets were met or exceeded by large carriers, BC/BS, and large commerical carriers. For the 376 policies of commercial carriers studied, the average loss ratio was only 60 percent, which indicates that many fell below the target.
4. GAO, "Medigap Insurance."
5. Thomas Rice, "An Economic Assessment of Health Care Coverage for the Elderly," *Milbank Quarterly*, vol. 65, no. 4 (1987), pp. 488–520.
6. Health Care Financing Administration, Office of Research and Dem-

onstrations, *Impact of the Medicare Hospital Prospective Payment System*, 1985 Annual Report, publication no. 03251 (Washington, D.C., August 1987).

7. John Holahan, Avi Dor, and Stephen Zuckerman, "Medicare Physician Expenditures: Sorting Out the Reasons for Growth," Urban Institute Working Paper no. 3650-06 (Washington, D.C., January 1989).

8. Alma McMillan, James Lubitz, and Delores Russell, "Medicare Enrollment in Health Maintenance Organizations," *Health Care Financing Review*, vol. 8, no. 3 (Spring 1987), pp. 87–93.

9. John K. Iglehart, "Medicare's New Benefits: 'Catastrophic' Health Insurance," *New England Journal of Medicine*, vol. 320, no. 5 (February 2, 1989), pp. 329–35.

10. Mark Pauly, "Overinsurance: The Conceptual Issues," in M. Pauly, ed., *National Health Insurance* (Washington, D.C.: American Enterprise Institute, 1980), p. 208.

11. Sandra Christensen, Stephen H. Long, and Jack Rodgers, "Acute Health Care Costs for the Aged Medicare Population: Overview and Policy Options," *Milbank Quarterly*, vol. 65, no. 3 (1987), p. 409.

12. Congressional Budget Office, *Containing Medical Care Costs through Market Forces* (Washington, D.C.: Government Printing Office, May 1982).

13. Paul Ginsburg, "Public Insurance Programs: Medicare and Medicaid," in Frech, ed., *Health Care in America*, p. 212.

14. H. E. Frech, "Introduction," in Frech, ed., *Health Care in America*; Taylor et al., "Medigap Insurance: Friend or Foe."

15. Ibid.

16. William S. Cartwright, Teh-wei Hu, and Lien-fu Huang, "The Impact of Varying Medigap Insurance Coverage on the Use of Medical Services by the Elderly" (Berkeley: University of California School of Public Health, n.d.).

17. Thomas Rice and Nelda McCall, "The Extent of Ownership and Characteristics of Medicare Supplemental Policies," *Inquiry*, vol. 22 (Summer 1985), pp. 188–200.

18. GAO, "Medigap Insurance."

19. Christensen et al., "Acute Health Care Costs for the Aged Medicare Population."

20. Taylor et al., "Medigap Insurance: Friend or Foe."

21. Teh-wei Hu, Lien-fu Huang, and William S. Cartwright, "Supplemental Health Insurance Enrollment, Premium Payment, and the Effects of Insurance on Health Care Expenditures among the Elderly," paper presented at the Allied Social Sciences Association Annual Meeting, December 28–30, 1987, Chicago, Ill.

22. Holahan et al., "Medicare Physician Expenditures."

23. Richard M. Scheffler, "An Analysis of 'Medigap' Enrollment: Assessment of Current Status and Policy Initiative," in Pauly and Kissick, eds., *Lessons from the First Twenty Years of Medicare* (Philadelphia: University of Pennsylvania Press, 1988).

24. See, for example, the summary of the results from the Rand study in W. G. Manning, J. P. Newhouse, N. Duan, E. B. Keeler, A. Leibowitz, and

M. S. Marquis, "Health Insurance and the Demand for Medical Care," *American Economic Review*, vol. 77, no. 3 (June 1987), pp. 251–77.

25. Average expenditures were estimated to be $3,351 in 1987 for all beneficiaries. This includes those with Medicaid or Medigap insurance. See Christensen et al., "Acute Health Care Costs for the Aged Medicare Population."

26. Ibid.

27. Ibid.

28. See Manning et al., "Health Insurance and the Demand for Medical Care." It should be noted that the elderly were excluded from the Rand study, and that all insurance plans in the study included a stop loss. Thus, for all families with very large expenditures, care was free at the margin.

29. A risk-aversion parameter of .0005 was recently used in a simulation model of the elderly's demand for Medigap coverage; see Lien-fu Huang, William S. Cartwright, and Teh-wei Hu, "Demand for Medigap Insurance by the Elderly: A Micro-Simulation Analysis," *Applied Economics*, 1989. This value was also chosen by M. S. Feldstein and B. Friedman, "Tax Subsidies, the Rational Demand for Insurance, and the Health Care Crisis," *Journal of Public Economics*, vol. 25, no. 3 (Fall 1988), pp. 364–73; and E. G. Keeler, D. T. Morrow, and J. P. Newhouse, "The Demand for Supplementary Health Insurance, or Do Deductibles Matter?" *Journal of Political Economy*, vol. 85, no. 4 (1977).

30. Iglehart. "Medicare's New Benefits."

31. To be complete in the social welfare calculation, we should value the extra services consumed after the purchase of Medigap, the area corresponding to DEF in figure 1. We ignore this in what follows, essentially assuming that the medical welfare of beneficiaries is unchanged with or without Medigap.

32. Iglehart, "Medicare's New Benefits."

33. Sara S. Bachman, Thomas G. McGuire, and David Pomeranz, "Preferred Provider Organizations: Options for Medicare Policy," Final Report, March 8, 1988. Work performed under cooperative agreement no. 99-C-98526/1-04 with the Health Care Financing Administration. A shortened version of this report is in *Inquiry*, Spring 1989.

34. Marjorie C. Feinson, Stephen Hansell, and David Mechanic, "Factors Associated with Medicare Beneficiaries' Interest in HMOs," *Inquiry*, vol. 25, no. 3 (Fall 1988), pp. 364–73.

35. M. Susan Marquis and Charles E. Phelps, "Price Elasticity and Adverse Selection in the Demand for Supplementary Health Insurance," *Economic Inquiry*, vol. 25, no. 2 (1987), pp. 299–313.

36. See Charles E. Phelps, *Demand for Health Insurance: A Theoretical and Empirical Investigation*, Rand Report R-1054-OEO (Santa Monica, Calif., July 1973); Gerald S. Goldstein and Mark V. Pauly, "Group Health Insurance as a Local Public Good," in Richard N. Rosett, ed., *The Role of Health Insurance in the Health Services Sector* (New York: National Bureau of Economic Research, 1976), pp. 73–110; Amy K. Taylor and Gail R. Wilensky, "Tax Expenditures

and the Demand for Private Health Insurance," in Jack Meyer, ed., *Market Oriented Reforms in Federal Health Policy* (Washington, D.C.: American Enterprise Institute, 1983), pp. 163–84; Martin Holmer, "Tax Policy and the Demand for Health Insurance," *Journal of Health Economics* (December 1984), pp. 203–41; Pamela Farley and Gail Wilensky, "Household Wealth, and Health Insurance as Protection against Medical Risks," in Martin David and Timothy Smelding, eds., *Horizontal Equity, Uncertainty, and Economic Well-Being* (Chicago: University of Chicago Press, 1986).

37. Randall P. Ellis, "The Effect of Prior-Year Health Expenditures on Health Coverage Plan Choice," in Scheffler and Rossiter, eds., *Advances in Health Economics and Health Services Research*, vol. 1 (Greenwich, Conn.: JAI Press, 1985), pp. 149–70.

38. Alan S. Friedlob and James P. Hadley, "Marketing Medicare in a Competitive Environment," Health Care Financing Administration, Office of Research and Demonstrations Evaluative Studies Staff (Washington, D.C., April 1985).

39. Steven A. Garfinkel, William E. Schlenger, Kenneth R. McLeroy, et al., "Choice of Payment Plan in the Medicare Capitation Demonstration," *Medical Care*, vol. 24, no. 7 (July 1986), pp. 628–40. Also see Hu et al., "Supplemental Health Insurance Enrollment," where they use 1977 data to study the determinants of buying Medigap. Limits of the data prevented them from studying a price effect. One finding that runs counter to adverse selection was that Medicare beneficiaries who are in poor health and are poor are less likely to purchase Medigap coverage.

40. Rice, "An Economic Assessment of Health Care Coverage for the Elderly."

CHAPTER 8: ADJUSTED-CHARGE RELATIVE VALUE SCALE, *Mitchell et al.*

1. See O. R. Bowen, *Pacemaker Surgery and Medicare Physician Payment: Report to Congress* (Washington, D.C.: Department of Health and Human Services, 1987); Jerry Cromwell, Janet B. Mitchell, and William B. Stason, "Learning by Doing in CABG Surgery," *Medical Care*, vol. 28 (January 1990), pp. 6–18.

2. William C. Hsiao et al., "Estimating Physicians' Work for a Resource-based Relative Value Scale," *New England Journal of Medicine*, vol. 319, no. 13 (September 29, 1988), pp. 835–41.

3. Each service was identified by its CPT-4 code number and by the written description that accompanies the code in the CPT-4 manual.

4. Margo L. Rosenbach, *Surgeons' Billing Practices for Selected Surgical Procedures*, final report submitted to Assistant Secretary for Planning and Evaluation under HHS contract no. 100-86-0023 (Needham, Mass.: Health Economics Research, February 1988).

5. Janet B. Mitchell and Stephen M. Davidson, "Geographic Variation in Medicare Surgical Fees," *Health Affairs*, vol. 8, Winter 1989, pp. 113–24.

6. Mean time and complexity were calculated only for physicians who

reported that they performed the procedure at least once a month because we were concerned that those who performed the procedure less frequently would not be able to provide accurate estimates. In general, however, reported times and complexity scores were similar, regardless of frequency of performance.

7. William C. Hsiao and William Stason, "Toward Developing a Relative Value Scale for Medical and Surgical Services," *Health Care Financing Review*, vol. 1 (Fall 1979), pp. 23–28.

8. A. C. Chiang, *Fundamental Methods of Mathematical Economics*, 2d ed. (New York: McGraw-Hill, 1974).

9. Another way of creating a weighted average complexity rating based on both procedure and pre/post time was rejected because the long pre/post surgical times generated a downward bias in the average complexity rating. This had the effect of systematically overpredicting surgical fees for short procedures with long pre/post times. We did not have an independent estimate of the complexity of pre/post time itself. If pre/post time is separated from procedure time, however, the multivariate regression has the flexibility of assigning a lower marginal value to the former when physicians or patients view pre/post time as being less complex.

10. The model was also estimated separately for medical and surgical specialists to test the assumption that they were reporting X rays and other procedures along a different complexity scale; see Jerry Cromwell, Janet B. Mitchell, Margo L. Rosenbach, William B. Stason, and Sylvia Hurdle, "Using Physician Effort to Identify Mispriced Procedures," *Inquiry*, vol. 26 (Spring 1989), pp. 7–23. Procedure time coefficients were .55 and .59, respectively, for medical and surgical specialists, which is nearly identical to the .55 coefficient shown in table 8–2. The corresponding complexity coefficients were .55 and .54 versus .49 in table 8–2. Because the activities of medical and surgical specialists overlapped, the pooled regression had fifteen fewer procedures and therefore we did not perform a formal F test of the pooled model.

11. N. Duan, W. Manning, C. Morris, and J. Newhouse, *A Comparison of Alternative Models for the Demand for Medical Care*, Report no. R-2754-HHS, Appendix B (Santa Monica, Calif.: Rand Corporation, January 1982).

12. J. Kmenta, *Elements of Econometrics* (New York: Macmillan, 1971), p. 363.

13. For a more complete presentation of services and procedures, see Cromwell et al., "Using Physician Effort to Identify Mispriced Procedures."

14. Other more complex procedures not shown in table 8–1 included craniectomies, secondary hip revisions, total knee replacements, carotid thromboendarterectomies, CABG operations including more than three grafts, scleral buckling, and trabeculectomy.

15. Recall from table 8–3 that the predicted payment for this service is identical to its actual reimbursement. Furthermore, simulations conducted by one of the authors (Janet B. Mitchell) revealed that an RBRVS-based payment for chest X-ray interpretation and report would be very close to

435

current fees (simulated payment was $14.40, versus an average reimbursement of $14.81 in 1988).

16. Overall, nonphysician cost shares are very similar for surgeons (55.2 percent) and for medical specialists (53.9 percent); see Stephen Zuckerman, W. P. Welch, and G. Pope, *The Development of an Interim Geographic Medicare Economic Index*, report submitted to the Health Care Financing Administration under grant no. 18-C-98326/1-01 (Washington, D.C., December 1987), table III-3. Their malpractice cost share, however, is twice as high: 6.6 percent for surgeons versus 3.1 percent for medical specialists. But surgeons' use of nonphysicians is naturally less. Orthopedic surgeons and ophthalmologists exhibit somewhat higher practice cost shares, primarily because of higher malpractice and equipment costs; see Zuckerman et al., *The Development of an Interim Geographic Medicare Economic Index*, table III-2.

17. There are two exceptions: operative laryngoscopy and cystourethroscopy with tumor resection. The RBRVS values these procedures somewhat more highly than the ACRVS does.

18. This linkage was performed by identifying services and procedures of equivalent work effort (which includes time).

19. See, for example, the chapter by Colby and Juba in this volume; Roger A. Reynolds et al., *The Impact of Medicare Payment Schedule Alternatives on Physicians*, Monograph from the American Medical Association (November 1988).

CHAPTER 9: PRICING PHYSICIANS' SERVICES, *Hsiao and Dunn*

1. U.S. Congress, Office of Technology Assessment, *Payment for Physician Services: Strategies for Medicare*, Publication no. OTA-H-294 (Washington, D.C.: Government Printing Office, 1986); American Medical Association, *Medicare Physician Reimbursement: An AMA Perspective* (Chicago: American Medical Association, 1987).

2. Physician Payment Review Commission, *Medicare Physician Payment: An Agenda for Reform*, annual report to Congress (Washington, D.C.: Government Printing Office, 1987), p. 27.

3. B. B. Roe, "The UCR Boondoggle: A Death Knell for Private Practice?" *New England Journal of Medicine*, vol. 305 (1981), pp. 41–45; S. F. Jencks and A. Dobson, "Strategies for Reforming Medicare's Physician Payments: Physician Diagnosis-Related Groups and Other Approaches," *New England Journal of Medicine*, vol. 312 (1983), pp. 1492–99.

4. J. E. Wennberg and A. Gittelsohn, "Variations in Health Care Delivery," *Science*, vol. 182 (1973), pp. 1102–8.

5. R. Kessel, "Price Discrimination in Medicine," *Journal of Law and Economics*, vol. 1 (October 1958), pp. 25–26.

6. *New York Times*, February 10, 1989.

7. J. P. Newhouse et al., *Some Interim Results from a Controlled Trial of Cost Sharing in Health Insurance* (Santa Monica, Calif.: Rand Corporation, 1982).

8. W. C. Hsiao, P. Braun, D. Dunn et al., "Resource-based Relative Values:

An Overview," *Journal of the American Medical Association*, vol. 260 (1988), pp. 2347–53; W. C. Hsiao, D. B. Yntema, P. Braun et al., "Measurement and Analysis of Intraservice Work," *Journal of the American Medical Association*, vol. 260 (1988), pp. 2361–70; D. Dunn, W. C. Hsiao, T. R. Ketcham et al., "A Method for Estimating the Preservice and Postservice Work of Physicians' Services," *Journal of the American Medical Association*, vol. 260 (1988), pp. 2371–78; P. Braun, D. B. Yntema, D. Dunn et al., "Cross-Specialty Linkage of Resource-based Relative Value Scales: Linking Specialties by Services and Procedures of Equal Work," *Journal of the American Medical Association*, vol. 260 (1988), pp. 2390–96; N. Kelly, W. C. Hsiao, P. Braun et al., "Extrapolation of Measures of Work for Surveyed Services to Other Services," *Journal of the American Medical Association*, vol. 260 (1988), pp. 2379–84; E. R. Becker, D. Dunn, and W. C. Hsiao, "Relative Cost Differences among Physicians' Specialty Practice," *Journal of the American Medical Association*, vol. 260 (1988), pp. 2397–2402; W. C. Hsiao, P. Braun, E. R. Becker, et al., *A National Study of Resource-Based Relative Value Scales for Physician Services: Final Report to the Health Care Financing Administration*, publication 18-C-98795/1-03 (Boston: Harvard School of Public Health, September 1988).

9. The advisory committee consisted of Eli Ginzberg, Ph.D.; Walter J. McNerney; Frank A. Sloan, Ph.D.; Samuel O. Thier, M.D.; and James S. Todd, M.D.

10. W. C. Hsiao and W. Stason, "Toward Developing a Relative Value Scale for Medical and Surgical Societies," *Health Care Financing Review*, vol. 1 (1979), pp. 23–28; W. C. Hsiao, P. Braun, P. Goldman et al., *Resource-Based Relative Values of Selected Medical and Surgical Procedures in Massachusetts: Final Report on Research Contract for Rate Setting Commission, Commonwealth of Massachusetts* (Boston: Harvard School of Public Health, 1985).

11. S. S. Stevens, *Psychophysics* (New York: John Wiley and Sons, 1975); T. Sellin and M. Wolfgang, *The Measurement of Delinquency* (New York: John Wiley and Sons, 1964); G. W. Bohrnstedt, "A Quick Method for Determining the Reliability and Validity of Multiple-Item Scales," *American Social Review*, vol. 34 (1969), pp. 542–48; L. J. Cronbach, "Coefficient Alpha and Internal Structure of Tests," *Psychometrika*, vol. 16 (1951), pp. 297–334.

12. C. M. Fanta, A. J. Finkel, C. G. Kirschner et al., *Physicians' Current Procedural Terminology*, 4th ed. (Chicago: American Medical Association, 1986).

13. A conceptually similar approach was proposed by J. Hadley, D. Juba, R. Berenson et al., *Final Report on Alternative Methods of Developing a Relative Value Scale of Physicians' Services* (Washington, D.C.: Urban Institute, 1984).

14. S. Sprachman and M. Rosenbach, *Report to Respondents Participating in the Physician's Practice, Cost, and Income Survey* (Chicago: Univ. of Chicago, National Opinion Research Center, 1989).

15. Center for Health Policy Research, *1988–1989 Directory of Graduate Medical Education Programs* (Chicago: American Medical Association, 1988).

16. Center for Health Policy Research, *The Demographics of Physician Supply: Trends and Projections* (Chicago: American Medical Association, 1987); Center

for Health Policy Research, in cooperation with the Division of Survey and Data Resources and the Governing Council of the AMA Resident Physicians Section, *Survey of Resident Physicians* (Chicago: American Medical Association, 1987); Stevens, *Psychophysics.*

17. American Medical Association, Center for Health Policy Research, *Socioeconomic Characteristics of Medical Practice, 1987* (Chicago, 1987), p. 137.

18. B. J. Winer, *Statistical Principles in Experimental Design,* 2d ed. (New York: McGraw-Hill, 1971), pp. 283–87.

19. Ibid.

20. W. C. Hsiao, P. Braun, D. Yntema et al., "Estimating Physicians' Work for a Resource-Based Relative Value Scale," *New England Journal of Medicine,* vol. 319 (1988), pp. 835–41.

21. F. Mosteller and J. W. Tukey, *Data Analysis and Regression: A Second Course in Statistics* (Reading, Mass.: Addison-Wesley, 1977), pp. 133–63.

A PHYSICIAN AND MARKET PERSPECTIVE, *A Commentary*
by *Joel Ira Franck*

1. William Hsiao et al., "Resource-Based Relative Values: An Overview," *Journal of the American Medical Association,* vol. 260, no. 12 (October 28, 1988), p. 2347.

2. As quoted in Don Lavoie, *Rivalry and Central Planning* (Cambridge: Cambridge University Press, 1985), p. 71.

3. Hsiao et al., "Results, Potential Effects, and Implementation Issues of the Resource-Based Relative Value Scale," *Journal of the American Medical Association,* vol. 260, no. 16 (October 28, 1988), p. 2363.

4. S. S. Stevens, *Psychophysics: Introduction to Its Perceptual, Neural and Social Prospects* (New York: John Wiley and Sons, 1975).

CHAPTER 10: COMPARISONS BY SPECIALTY, *Marder and Willke*

1. Gary S. Becker, *Human Capital: A Theoretical and Empirical Analysis, with Special Reference to Education* (New York: National Bureau of Economic Research, 1964).

2. William D. Marder and Douglas E. Hough, "Medical Residency as Investment in Human Capital," *Journal of Human Resources,* vol. 18 (Winter 1983), pp. 33–49.

3. William C. Hsiao, Peter Braun, Nancy L. Kelly, and Edmund R. Becker, "Results, Potential Effects, and Implementation Issues of the Resource-Based Relative Value Scale," *Journal of the American Medical Association,* vol. 260, no. 16 (October 28, 1988), pp. 2429–38.

4. Ibid., pp. 2437–38.

5. Catherine M. Bidese, *1986 U.S. Medical Licensure Statistics: 1987 Licensure Requirements* (Chicago: American Medical Association, 1988).

6. For medical and surgical subspecialties, we did not consider practicing as a generalist to be the alternative during the subspecialty training years, as

did the RBRVS study, for two reasons. First, we do not know whether the decision to be a subspecialist is made at the beginning of residency training or at the end of the general part of training. If it is the former, the investment undertaken should be considered a single decision, with a single alternative. Second, and of more practical importance here, if the goal is to calculate an *average* rate of return across all years of residency for a given subspecialist, only the base earnings are necessary. If equation (10.2) is expanded to allow both generalist and subspecialist training with the same rate of return, the earnings of the generalist during the subspecialty training years appear as both costs and benefits and exactly cancel out of the calculation.

7. We regress log earnings on a quadratic function of experience with dummies for the other variables mentioned, as well as a dummy for part-year work in the first year of practice. Predicted earnings are constructed using the formula for the expectation of a log-normal distribution. For a recent discussion of the determinants of physicians' earnings, see Robert L. Ohsfeldt and Steven D. Culler, "Differences in Income between Male and Female Physicians," *Journal of Health Economics,* vol. 5 (December 1986), pp. 335–46.

8. Retirement and mortality probabilities are calculated using the results presented in William D. Marder, Phillip R. Kletke, Anne B. Silberger, and Richard J. Willke, *Physician Supply and Utilization by Specialty: Trends and Projections* (Chicago: American Medical Association, 1988), p. 46.

9. For full details of the estimation procedure and results, see William D. Marder and Richard J. Willke, "The Value of Physician Time: Comparisons across Specialties," AMA Center for Health Policy Research Discussion Paper 89-2 (Chicago, 1989). The typical physician is defined as board certified, with a proportion being female and self-employed, the same as in the entire sample of practicing physicians. We also provide alternative estimates of the rate of return under different assumptions about length of residency, board certification, and self-employment status.

10. Cotton M. Lindsay, "Real Returns to Medical Education," *Journal of Human Resources* (Summer 1973), pp. 331–48.

11. Anne B. Silberger, Sara L. Thran, and William D. Marder, "The Changing Environment of Resident Physicians," *Health Affairs,* vol. 7, no. 2 (Supplement 1988), pp. 121–33.

12. Lindsay, "Real Returns to Medical Education," p. 334.

13. Ibid.

14. For full details on estimation, see Marder and Willke, "The Value of Physician Time." We investigated the possibility of nonconstant hourly wages but were unable to obtain significant evidence that they were in fact not constant over the relevant range.

15. See Lindsay, "Real Returns to Medical Education." Lindsay may not have intended hours of work to be adjusted during the training period, so his conclusions may not apply here.

16. See appendix C for details of the incorporation of retirement and mortality adjustments into this formula.

17. This formula is not formally presented by Hsiao et al. in "Results, Potential Effects, and Implementation Issues of the Resource-Based Relative Value Scale." On p. 2437, however, they show a formula that, when given constant income (except for their assumption about real growth) within a specialty during the postinvestment period, generates the present value of specialty income and leads to (10.7) as shown in the text. Using (10.7), with allowance for retirement, we were able to replicate the markup factors and ASTs that they present.

18. Ibid.

19. Sherwin Rosen, "The Theory of Equalizing Differences," in Orley Ashenfelter and Richard Lyard, eds., *Handbook of Labor Economics*, vol. 1 (Amsterdam: North Holland, 1986), p. 642.

20. Barriers to entry in medicine are discussed by Monica Noether, "The Effect of Government Policy Changes on the Supply of Physicians: Expansion of a Competitive Fringe," *Journal of Law and Economics*, vol. 29 (October 1986), pp. 335–46.

21. Milton Friedman and Simon Kuznets, *Income from Independent Professional Practice* (New York: National Bureau of Economic Research, 1945).

22. See Frank Sloan, "Lifetime Earnings and Physicians' Choice of Specialty," *Industrial and Labor Relations Review*, vol. 24 (October 1970), pp. 47–56; Rashi Fein and G. I. Weber, *Financing Medical Education, An Analysis of Alternative Policies and Mechanisms* (New York: Carnegie Commission on Higher Education and the Commonwealth Fund, 1971).

23. Lindsay, "Real Returns to Medical Education."

24. Stephen T. Mennemeyer, "The Effect of Government Policy Changes on the Supply of Physicians: Expansion of a Competitive Fringe," *Journal of Human Resources*, vol. 13 (Winter 1978), pp. 75–90.

25. Philip L. Burstein and Jerry Cromwell, "Relative Incomes and Rates of Return for U.S. Physicians," *Journal of Health Economics*, vol. 4 (March 1985), pp. 63–78.

26. Marder et al., *Physician Supply*.

27. For the details of this survey, see Silberger et al., "The Changing Environment of Resident Physicians."

28. See Marder et al., *Physician Supply*.

CHAPTER 11: FEE SCHEDULES AND UTILIZATION, Mark V. Pauly

1. William Hsiao et al., *A National Study of Resource-based Relative Value Scales for Physician Services: Final Report* (Boston, Mass.: Harvard University School of Public Health, 1988).

2. R. R. Bovbjerg, P. J. Held, and M. V. Pauly, "Privatization and Bidding in the Health Care Sector," *Journal of Policy Analysis and Management*, vol. 6, no. 4 (Summer 1987), pp. 648–66.

3. Hsiao et al., *A National Study of Resource-based Relative Value Scales for Physician Services*.

4. J. M. Eisenberg, L. P. Myers, and M. V. Pauly, "How Will Changes in

Physician Payment by Medicare Influence Laboratory Testing?" *Journal of the American Medical Association*, vol. 258, no. 6 (August 14, 1987), pp. 803–8.

5. See Robert G. Evans, "Supplier-Induced Demand: Some Empirical Evidence and Implications," in M. Perlman, ed., *The Economics of Health and Medical Care* (London: Macmillan, 1974), pp. 162–73; Mark V. Pauly, *Doctors and Their Workshops* (Chicago: University of Chicago Press, 1980).

6. Physician Payment Review Commission, *Annual Report to Congress*, March 1988.

7. I am indebted to John Eisenberg for suggesting this approach.

8. David Dranove, "Demand Inducement and the Physician-Patient Relationship," *Economic Inquiry*, vol. 26 (April 1988), pp. 281–98.

9. Pauly, *Doctors and Their Workshops*.

10. See Pamela Farley, "Theories of the Price and Quantity of Physician Services: A Synthesis and Critique," *Journal of Health Economics*, vol. 5 (December 1986), pp. 315–34; Jose J. Escarce, "Relative Prices for Physicians' Services," Leonard Davis Institute of Health Economics, University of Pennsylvania (December 1988, photocopied).

CHAPTER 12: OUT-OF-POCKET COSTS AND PHYSICIAN PAYMENTS, *Colby and Juba*

1. Robert H. Lee and Jack Hadley, "Physicians' Fees and Public Medical Care Programs," *Health Services Research*, vol. 16 (Summer 1981), pp. 185–203.

2. Donald E. Yett, William Der, Richard L. Ernst, and Joel W. Hay, "Fee-Screen Reimbursement and Physician Fee Inflation," *Journal of Human Resources*, vol. 20 (Spring 1985), pp. 278–91.

3. Physician Payment Review Commission, *Medicare Physician Payment: An Agenda for Reform: Annual Report to Congress* (Washington, D.C., March 1987), pp. 46–50.

4. This chapter was written before the passage of physician payment reform in the Omnibus Budget Reconciliation Act of 1989. Although the legislation is very similar to that proposed by the PPRC and shown in the simulations, there are two differences. Since the legislation limits submitted charges to 115 percent of the fee schedule payment, the reduction in balance bills would be slightly greater than indicated in this chapter. In addition, the legislated reform includes a partial adjustment for geographic variations in the opportunity cost of physician time and effort. This would slightly reduce the changes across geographic areas.

5. Physician Payment Review Commission, *Annual Report to Congress* (Washington, D.C., March 1988), pp. 45–54.

6. American Medical Association, "Report AA of the American Medical Association Board of Trustees: The National Study of Resource-based Relative Value Scales for Physician Services: Evaluation of Final Report of Phase I and Implementation Issues" (Chicago, December 1988, photocopied).

7. William C. Hsiao, Peter Braun, Edmund Becker, Nancyanne Causino, Nathan P. Couch, Margaret DeNicola, Daniel Dunn, Nancy L. Kelly, Thomas

Ketcham, Arthur Sobol, Diane Verrilli, and Douwe B. Yntema, "A National Study of Resource-based Relative Value Scales for Physician Services," Final Report for HCFA Contract no. 17-C98795/1-03 (Cambridge, Mass., September 27, 1988); William C. Hsiao et al., "A National Study of Resource-Based Relative Value Scales for Physician Services," Supplemental Report for HCFA Contract no. 17-C98795/1-03 (Cambridge, Mass., December 8, 1988).

8. Physician Payment Review Commission, *Annual Report to Congress* (Washington, D.C., April 1989), pp. 29–57.

9. For a discussion of the limitations of the Hsiao estimates of relative work values for evaluation and management services, see ibid., chap. 3.

10. The simulation uses practice costs derived from specialty-specific cost ratios that are different from those used in the Hsiao study. The PPRC recommends, however, using practice cost factors that apply to categories of services, not to specialties.

11. The geographic multipliers are based on Stephen Zuckerman, W. P. Welch, and Gregory C. Pope, "The Development of an Interim Geographic Medicare Economic Index," Interim Report for HCFA Grant no. 17-C-98758/1-03 (Washington, D.C.: Urban Institute and Center for Health Economics Research, December 1987).

12. Revenue received by the physicians and expenses of the beneficiaries may differ from the reported amounts because of (1) the failure to collect some debts and (2) the failure to submit some claims.

13. William C. Hsiao, Peter Braun, Nancy L. Kelly, and Edmund R. Becker, "Results, Potential Effects, and Implementation Issues of the Resource-Based Relative Value Scale," *Journal of the American Medical Association*, vol. 260, no. 16 (October 28, 1988), pp. 2429–38.

14. The seventeen selected procedures in table 1 accounted for 23 percent of Medicare program payments for physician services in 1986.

15. The allowed charge is the amount the Medicare program approves as payment for a procedure. The program pays 80 percent of the allowed charge and the beneficiary pays the remaining 20 percent. In addition, the beneficiary is responsible for any unmet deductible payment and for any balance bill if the claim is not assigned.

16. Since the codes for evaluation and management services must be revised, the fee schedule amounts for specific evaluation and management services are illustrative. See PPRC, *Annual Report to Congress* (1989), chap. 3.

17. These results are different from those reported by Hsiao et al. owing to the changes in work values for evaluation and management services, different practice cost estimates, extrapolation methods, and the incorporation of policy changes occurring between 1986 and 1988. In addition, Hsiao assumed that the ratio of practice costs to physician revenue would be the same for each specialty under a fee schedule as it is now. This assumption resulted in a large overstatement of changes in charges. For comparison, see Hsiao et al., "Results, Potential Effects, and Implementation Issues of the Resource-Based Relative Value Scale."

18. The Congressional Budget Office estimated that beneficiaries had $561

442

total Medicare out-of-pocket liabilities in 1987. See U.S. Congress, House, Committee on Ways and Means, *Background Material and Data on Programs within the Jurisdiction of the Committee on Ways and Means* (Washington, D.C.: Government Printing Office, 1988), p. 181. Medicare out-of-pocket expenses include Part A and Part B deductibles, coinsurance, and balance bills. Beneficiaries also have additional non-Medicare health expenses. See Dwight Waldo and Helen C. Lazenby, "Demographic Characteristics and Health Care Use and Expenditures by the Aged in the United States: 1977–1984," *Health Care Financing Review*, vol. 6, no. 1 (1984), pp. 1–29.

19. The impact on balance bills is large because of the distribution of balance bills. Under CPR, 28 percent of the beneficiaries had no balance bills, while 10 percent were liable for 71 percent of total balance bills. The average of submitted to allowed charges on unassigned claims was 1.3; the median was 1.2.

20. Some have argued that some physicians who have lower payments under the fee schedule may balance-bill in order to recapture lost income. If that were to happen, the reductions in balance bills would be smaller than reported in table 12–2.

21. The unit of analysis for the physician simulations is a practice, not an individual physician. The term "physician" in the text actually refers to a practice of one or more individuals with the same Medicare billing identification number.

22. "Medical" and "surgical" refer to specialties meeting three conditions: they were surveyed in Phase I of the Hsiao study; they are among the top twenty-five specialties in terms of total Medicare program expenditures; and they posed no special data problems. Medical specialties meeting the conditions are internal medicine, family practice, and dermatology. Surgical specialties meeting the conditions are ophthalmology, general surgery, orthopedic surgery, urology, thoracic surgery, otolaryngology, and obstetrics/gynecology. Anesthesia, an important hospital-based specialty, was excluded from the simulations.

23. Pure RVS effects are from a simulation (not shown) comparing total specialty payments under a national average charge-based fee schedule and under the MFS, both having the same geographic adjustment.

24. Harry T. Paxton, "How Much Cheer Do Third Parties Bring You?" *Medical Economics* (December 21, 1987), pp. 108–23.

25. Medicare receipts were computed under the assumption that changes in payments do not affect assignment rates and that balance bills are collected. Receipts from all payers are based on specialty-specific ratios of Medicare revenues to gross practice revenues.

26. W. Hsiao, P. Braun, D. Dunn, E. Becker, M. DeNicola, and T. Ketcham, "Results and Policy Implications of the Resource-Based Relative-Value Study," *New England Journal of Medicine*, vol. 319, no. 13 (September 29, 1988), pp. 884–86.

27. Roger A. Reynolds, "The Impact of Medicare Payment Schedule Alternatives on Physicians," (Chicago: American Medical Association, Center for Health Policy Research, November 1988).

28. The Social Security Act defines "physician" as a doctor of medicine or osteopathy. Dentists, optometrists, podiatrists, and chiropractors are included for specific services. The physician file includes podiatrists and chiropractors. The beneficiary file includes dentists, optometrists, podiatrists, and chiropractors. In the simulations, however, these nonphysician providers are paid at the baseline CPR-allowed amount.

29. U.S. Department of Commerce, Bureau of Census, Current Population Survey, March 1986 (machine-readable data file), produced by the Bureau of Census for the Bureau of Labor Statistics (Washington, D.C., 1986).

30. Although the PPRC recommends the adoption of a procedure-specific approach to practice costs, that methodology has not been developed yet. The methodology used in the simulations is an additive specialty approach.

31. Zuckerman et al., "The Development of an Interim Geographic Medicare Economic Index."

THREE SIMULATIONS, *A Commentary by Roger A. Reynolds*

1. William C. Hsiao, Peter Braun, Daniel Dunn, Edmund Becker, Margaret DeNicola, and Thomas Ketchum, "Results and Policy Implications of the Resource-based Relative-Value Study," *New England Journal of Medicine*, vol. 319, no. 13 (September 29, 1988), pp. 881–88.

2. Roger A. Reynolds et al., *The Impact of Medicare Payment Schedule Alternatives on Physicians*, Monograph from the American Medical Association (November 1988).

3. W. P. Welch, S. Zuckerman, and G. C. Pope, "The Geographic Economic Index: Alternative Approaches," Final report to The Health Care Financing Administration (Baltimore: HCFA, June 1989).

CHAPTER 13: PPRC RECOMMENDATIONS, *Paul B. Ginsburg*

1. Although there is a positive correlation between fees for a procedure and practice costs in an area, the correlation seems smaller than one would expect in competitive markets in which resources can migrate relatively freely.

2. Evidence suggests that some of the measured increase in services per enrollee reflects changes in the use of codes by physicians.

3. Estimates of relative physician work should continue to be refined after the fee schedule is implemented. A regular update of relative values should be carried out for new services and procedures and existing services and procedures should be modified on the basis of new information about costs.

4. Specialty differentials need not result from the use of specialty-level practice costs factors. The factor applied to a service could be a weighted average of the factors for each of the specialties that provide the service.

5. This is relevant to certain diagnostic and therapeutic services performed in a physician's office in which a combined payment is made for

professional and technical services. The estimate of physician work from the Hsiao study would be relevant only to the professional component of the fee.

6. Omnibus Budget Reconciliation Act of 1986 (P.L. 99-509), Section 9331 (d)(2).

7. The version currently used by Medicare does not include the factor for patient condition.

8. By focusing on prices faced, differences in amenity levels from one locality to the next would not affect the index. For example, if physicians in one area tend to have large offices in luxury buildings and those in another area have small offices in more modest surroundings, the index, rent per square foot of a standardized grade of space, would not reflect this behavior. Weights are taken from a national survey of physicians' practice costs. The index was developed by the Urban Institute and the Center for Health Economics Research.

9. Fees in Canadian provinces tend to be uniform except for remote areas, where they are higher. Fees are often uniform nationwide in Europe.

10. The index also measures variation in premiums for professional liability insurance, but this will be reflected in the separate practice cost factor described above.

11. Lyle Nelson, Anne Ciemnecki, Nancy Carlton, and Kathryn Langwell, "Assignment and the Participating Physician Program," Background Paper no. 89-1, Physician Payment Review Commission, September, 1989.

12. Four of the thirteen members of the commission filed a minority report in support of mandatory assignment.

13. The MEI measures annual increases in physicians' costs of practice. It includes a component for the opportunity cost of the physician's time and effort, as well as components for the prices of nonphysician inputs.

14. Laboratory services, whether provided in the physician's office or in an outside laboratory, would be included in the targets, along with physician services, but the subsequent conversion-factor adjustment would apply only to physicians' services.

15. Since Medicare already determines payments per admission, expenditure targets could be limited to the rate of admissions.

JUDGING THE RECOMMENDATIONS, A Commentary by Joseph P. Newhouse

1. Mark V. Pauly, Doctors and Their Workshops (Chicago: University of Chicago Press, 1980).

2. See Physician Payment Review Commission, Annual Report to Congress (Washington, D.C., March 31, 1988), chap. 8; Joseph P. Newhouse, Albert P. Williams, William B. Schwartz, and Bruce W. Bennett, "The Geographic Distribution of Physicians: Is the Conventional Wisdom Correct?" (Santa Monica, Calif.: Rand Corporation, October 1982).

3. Mark R. Chassin, Robert H. Brook, R. E. Park, Joan Keesey, Arleen Fink, Jacqueline Kosecoff et al., "Variation in the Use of Medical and Surgical Services by the Medicare Population," New England Journal of Medicine, vol.

314, no. 5 (January 30, 1986), pp. 285–90; Mark R. Chassin, Jacqueline Kosecoff, R. E. Park, Constance M. Winslow, Katherine L. Kahn, Nancy J. Merrick et al., "Does Inappropriate Use Explain Geographic Variation in the Use of Health Care Services? A Study of Three Procedures," *Journal of the American Medical Association*, vol. 258, no. 18 (November 13, 1987), pp. 2533–37.

4. John Holahan and William Scanlon, "Price Controls, Physician Fees, and Physician Incomes from Medicare and Medicaid" (Washington, D.C.: Urban Institute, 1978); Janet B. Mitchell, Gerard Wedig, and Jerry Cromwell, "The Medicare Physician Fee Freeze," *Health Affairs*, vol. 8, no. 1 (Spring 1989), pp. 21–33.

5. Paul B. Ginsburg and Grace M. Carter, "Medicare Case Mix Increase," *Health Care Financing Review*, vol. 7, no. 4 (Summer 1986), pp. 51–65.

PASSENGERS AT THE STATION, *A Commentary by James F. Rodgers*

1. Conventional wisdom that CPR is inherently inflationary has been challenged in a recent paper. See D. W. Lee and D. W. Mandy, "The Effects of Medicare CPR Reimbursement on Physicians' Profits, Service Levels, and Fees," AMA Center for Health Policy Research Discussion Paper (Chicago, Ill., January 1989).

COSTS, COMPETITION, CONTROLS, *A Commentary by Robin Allen*

1. Steven Morrison and Clifford Winston, *The Economic Effects of Airline Deregulation* (Washington, D.C.: Brookings Institution), pp. 24–36.
2. *Modern Health Care* (November 18, 1988), p. 37.

A NOTE ON THE BOOK

This book was edited by Venka V. Macintyre and by Dana Lane of the
publications staff of the American Enterprise Institute.
The figures were drawn by Hördur Karlsson.
The text was set in Palatino, a typeface designed by
the twentieth-century Swiss designer Hermann Zapf.
Coghill Composition Company, of Richmond, Virginia,
set the type, and Edwards Brothers Incorporated,
of Ann Arbor, Michigan, printed and bound the book,
using permanent, acid-free paper.

The AEI PRESS is the publisher for the American Enterprise Institute for Public Policy Research, 1150 17th Street, N.W., Washington, D.C. 20036: *Christopher C. DeMuth*, publisher; *Edward Styles*, director; *Dana Lane*, editor; *Ann Petty*, editor; *Cheryl Weissman*, editor; *Susan Moran*, editorial assistant (rights and permissions). Books published by the AEI PRESS are distributed by arrangement with the University Press of America, 4720 Boston Way, Lanham, Md. 20706.